W9-CQJ-050

DISCARD

THE *Dream*
OF THE
PERFECT CHILD

BIOETHICS AND THE HUMANITIES
Eric M. Meslin and Richard B. Miller, editors

THE *Dream*
OF THE
PERFECT CHILD

Joan Rothschild

Indiana University Press

BLOOMINGTON AND INDIANAPOLIS

This book is a publication of
Indiana University Press
601 North Morton Street
Bloomington, IN 47404-3797 USA

http://iupress.indiana.edu

Telephone orders   800-842-6796
Fax orders   812-855-7931
Orders by e-mail   iuporder@indiana.edu

© 2005 by Joan Rothschild

All rights reserved

*No part of this book may be reproduced or utilized in any form or
by any means, electronic or mechanical, including photocopying and
recording, or by any information storage and retrieval system, without
permission in writing from the publisher. The Association of American
University Presses' Resolution on Permissions constitutes the
only exception to this prohibition.*

*The paper used in this publication meets the minimum
requirements of American National Standard for Information
Sciences—Permanence of Paper for Printed Library Materials,
ANSI Z39.48-1984.*

MANUFACTURED IN THE UNITED STATES OF AMERICA

Library of Congress Cataloging-in-Publication Data
Rothschild, Joan.
The dream of the perfect child / Joan Rothschild.
p. ; cm. — (Bioethics and the humanities)
Includes bibliographical references and index.
ISBN 0-253-34565-0 (cloth : alk. paper) — ISBN 0-253-21760-1 (pbk. : alk. paper)
1. Abnormalities, Human—Prevention. 2. Genetic disorders—Prevention. 3. Prenatal
diagnosis—Moral and ethical aspects. 4. Medical genetics—Moral and ethical aspects. 5. Human
reproductive technology—Social aspects. 6. Reproductive health—Social aspects. 7. Eugenics—
History. 8. Perfection. 9. Bioethics.
[DNLM: 1. Abnormalities—prevention & control. 2. Genetics, Medical—ethics.
3. Infant, Newborn, Diseases—prevention & control. 4. Prenatal Diagnosis.
5. Reproductive Medicine—ethics. QS 675 R8476d 2005] I. Title. II. Series.
RG626.R68 2005
616'.042—dc22
2004024477
1   2   3   4   5   10   09   08   07   06   05

CONTENTS

CONTENTS

PART THREE
COUNTER-DISCOURSES

PREFACE AND ACKNOWLEDGMENTS

When I was asked to give a paper at a colloquium at Lehigh University in the fall of 1986 on the theme "Technology and the Ideology of Progress," I interpreted progress to mean human progress. To me progress for human beings was tied to striving to improve, its ideology to achieve the age-old quest for perfection. But for most of human history that pursuit was more dream than reality. The critical change came in the Enlightenment, when the quest was secularized and science and medicine replaced faith as the route to perfect human beings and society. But it was not until the late twentieth century that science, technology, and medicine would combine to produce a growing capability to engineer birth. As prenatal diagnosis was making it possible to choose the kinds of children that would be born, birth engineering was happening in reproductive medical practice. This became the focus of my colloquium paper.

As this paper, "Engineering Birth: Toward the Perfectibility of *Man*?," grew into a book, I began to ask myself why I, a woman past childbearing age and who had no children by choice, was focusing my research on pregnancy and the process of prenatal testing. Were women, as they sought a defect-free child, in some ways seeking a perfect child? Were they indeed reflecting today that societal quest for the perfect? As a feminist, I was concerned with reproductive issues and how they affected women's choices. Having written about feminist and social aspects of technology, I was also interested in what was happening in reproductive technologies. But the more I thought about it, what became clear to me was another motivation: my own desire to be perfect.

From childhood on, I was held to exacting standards: When I proudly brought home a 99 on a test, I was asked, Why not 100? As a teenager, my appearance had to be perfect down to the utmost detail. As an adult and a professional, I set perhaps unreachable standards not only for myself but also for others. I had internalized the quest to be perfect and then pro-jected it outward to others and to the world. And yet, solipsistic as my feelings were, it seemed that the quest in various ways was shared by others, even if unwittingly. And so my research led me to explore the perfect's underside, the imperfect.

Inquiry into the imperfect became the most critically important part of my research. As I explored social attitudes, past and present, I found that although these attitudes had perhaps become less harsh, they still appeared to stay the same. My own reactions changed, sometimes markedly, as I met with and read about those who are physically or mentally impaired; those whom society labels as unappealing, even ugly; those whose shapes and forms are called imperfections. Meanings began to change for me, as did the perspectives for my own and others' imperfections. As a colleague once reminded me, "We are all imperfect in some way."

And so, first, I must thank the research process itself, how it can lead to self-examination and self-awareness, to intellectual and emotional insights, to viewing even one small part of one's world differently. Writing this book has been a long and revealing experience, taking many turns along the way. And so my profound thanks to the many people and institutions who helped and encouraged my journey.

The initial stages of my research were supported by grants from the National Science Foundation. These included a postdoctoral research fellowship in the History and Philosophy of Science; a summer scholars award in NSF's Studies in Science, Technology (HPST) Program; an award from the NSF Program in Ethics and Values Studies, which was co-supported by the National Center for Human Genome Research of the National Institutes of Health; and an NSF Studies in Science, Technology and Society (SSTS) scholars award, which was also supported by NSF's Ethics and Values Studies Program. The postdoctoral research fellowship, awarded when I was on leave from teaching at the University of Massachusetts Lowell, was undertaken at the Philosophy and Technology Studies Center at Polytechnic University in Brooklyn. Carl Mitcham, the center's director at the time, provided a stimulating home and collegial atmosphere for my research. Thank you.

At Indiana University Press, my initial thanks to Don Ihde, general editor of the Indiana Series in the Philosophy of Technology, for recommending my proposed book to Janet Rabinowitch, then a senior editor. My warmest thanks to Janet, now director of the Press, for never giving up on me for all the many years it took to complete the manuscript, and for enthusiastically welcoming it when finally submitted. Bob Sloan, editorial director of the Press: how can I thank you enough for taking over as my editor, for your counsel and advice, and for guiding the manuscript through the many critical decisions from the editing phases, to cover design, to marketing and promotion. Your skillful coordination of all of these facets has been invaluable. Jane Lyle, as managing editor, you were key to the process. Your job to move a book from manuscript to finished product—never a completely smooth process—was further compounded with difficulties as balky printers and copiers went awry. I admire the way you coped so efficiently and calmly through it all. Finally, the promotion and marketing staffs require special recognition for your work as you focused skillfully on the qualities and potential of the book for a wide audience.

The readers of the manuscript, or portions of it, contacted by the Press must remain anonymous. I thank them for their critical appraisals and constructive suggestions. The revised final manuscript benefited enormously from two additional readers whose appraisal I asked for in their areas of expertise. Thank you, Carole Browner and Diane Paul. Your corrections, comments, and suggestions were invaluable. Thanks to Barbara Katz Rothman for your comments on my work over the years and more recently—and for uncovering an elusive citation for me, and providing a laugh on doing it!

For a book so long in preparation, inevitably those who have played instrumental roles at various stages tend to become obscured. I can only highlight a few. My thanks to Steven Goldman and Stephen Cutcliffe for inviting me to the Lehigh colloquium, for publishing my paper, and for seeing its potential for a book. To the "feminist community"—its members too numerous to name—thank you for your supports; for your excellent, incisive scholarship, which I have relied on in so many ways; and for the friendship and encouragement of so many of you who are both friends and colleagues. The Society for the History of Technology (SHOT) and its Women in Technological History (WITH) interest group have been a mainstay for me during my long association, now reaching twenty-five years. Nowhere in my professional life have I met with a more delightful and stimulating group of colleagues, a more welcoming atmosphere (as I arrived as a non-historian with my feminist critique of technological history), a better forum for my work, or more continuing opportunities to combine social and intellectual exchange, than I have experienced at SHOT and WITH. Thank you. To the many individuals from a wide variety of institutions in the U.S. and many parts of the world who over the years have invited me to speak, my sincere thanks. These conferences and forums provided important feedback as my research continued.

When this project began, there was no internet widely available for research, no e-mail. I relied on traditional sources: libraries, news and journal reports, telephone and letter exchanges, and much photocopying. I am particularly grateful for the access granted to me as a Cornell alumna to the Weill Cornell Medical Library in New York, even though my degree was a B.A. many years ago in Arts and Sciences (major in English literature!). In the recent and final stages of research, I came to rely on the Internet as an invaluable resource to keep current with work in fields critical to the book, a resource supplanted by e-mail correspondence with these sources and with helpful friends and colleagues.

Inevitably, in a book that draws on events in the fast-changing worlds of genetics and reproductive technologies, materials based on them can become outdated almost before the information appears in print or on the screen. The researcher can only hope to anticipate and hold the door open for discoveries or breakthroughs, for changes in procedures, for new statistics that could affect and question statements or conclusions that appear in the pages of my book. I was not able to consult material published after the book went to press in the fall of 2004.

In the end, of course, this book is not perfect; it cannot hope to be without fault or error. I can only absolve all my sources, institutional and human, for any errors that do occur, for any misrepresentations of fact or opinion. The work herein is my own, and I take full responsibility. It has been a long process to bring this book into print. But at some point one must call a halt to revising, and let the finished product speak for itself. I have tried to do my best to provide the reader with thoughtful and provocative ideas, and to do so in interesting ways. I hope some of what I have learned will be imparted to the reader.

Joan Rothschild
New York City

THE *Dream*
OF THE
PERFECT CHILD

INTRODUCTION

Beautifully Perfect:
The Technological Dream

Perfectly beautiful . . . Isn't that what we wish for every baby born? Isn't that what we expect? And yet the miracle of a healthy baby does not happen every time. . . .

We will continue to strengthen our commitment to a healthier future. Those goals reinforce my personal dream . . . of the day when every baby is born perfectly beautiful and beautifully perfect.[1]

So read the opening message to *Perfectly Beautiful,* a special advertising supplement to the Sunday *New York Times Magazine* in March 1993, sponsored by the March of Dimes Birth Defects Foundation.

The following year a *Times* display ad was headlined

A Campaign for Healthier Babies!

advising potential advertisers in the 1994 supplement that "Your ad in *Perfectly Beautiful* will provide direct assistance to the campaign for healthier babies."[2]

Prepared by the March of Dimes, these advertising sections were paid for by the beauty industry.[3] On the covers were the babies, of varying hues, cuddly and irresistible. Inside, flawlessly beautiful adult models graced full-page, full-color ads for cosmetics and perfumes: Chanel, Revlon, Lancôme, Christian Dior, Gianni Versace among them.[4] In the text, parents, health care professionals, and financial supporters were described as "working together" with the March of Dimes Birth Defects Foundation "toward a common dream": a dream of "children born free of sickness and disability, with the best possible chance for a healthy, productive life."

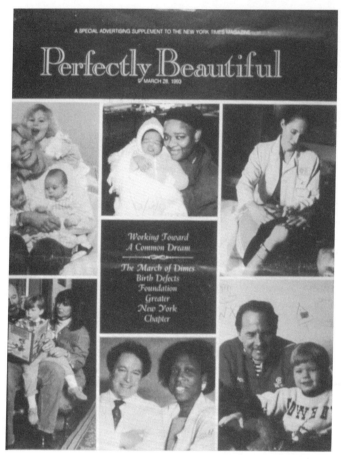

1. "Perfectly Beautiful," cover, March of Dimes advertising supplement to the *New York Times Magazine*, March 28, 1993. Courtesy Greater New York Chapter, March of Dimes Birth Defects Foundation.

A beautiful dream, one we all can share. But in the pages of *Perfectly Beautiful, healthy* and *perfect* are seamlessly conflated. The dream of healthy babies is transposed into "beautifully perfect" babies, who are as flawless and wrinkle-free as are the culture's icons of youth and beauty.[5] Medical science and technology, acting to prevent birth defects, will make it so. Wielding seductive power, the representation of beauty imagery and the promise of technology add up to more than a dream. They become the discourse of the perfect child. Embedded in reproductive medical practice, the discourse is double-edged. Masked by the dream of the perfectly beautiful and beautifully perfect child is the discourse of the imperfect child. This is the unwanted child, the child with birth defects, who cannot be allowed to happen. For the dream is not propelled by hopes alone. It is born equally of deep fears that the child will not be perfect, that it will bear some incurable and disfiguring disease or deformity. As childbearing is postponed and parents plan to have fewer children, each child has come to be a "priceless" investment. Beginning in the 1970s, parents fearful of bearing a less than healthy baby could gain some reassurance that their fetus might be free from some inheritable or congenital disease or "defect."[6] When these March of Dimes supplements appeared in the mid-'90s, prenatal diagnosis methods and genetic research had advanced to include a widening range of such defects, with the ability to screen or test earlier and earlier in the pregnancy. In the language of the supplements, the "miracle" of medical science and technology would spare parents the "tragedy" of birth defects. Not pictured in their pages, the imperfect infant was nevertheless acutely present: it was an ugly evil to be avoided at all costs. Today, the numbers of diagnosable conditions have grown almost exponentially, discoverable as far back as the pre-embryo and the germ cells themselves. The defining characteristics of the imperfect infant have both multiplied and sharpened, while the possibilities for attaining the perfect child grow and the discourse of the perfect child gains cultural strength.[7]

In the more than three decades since the first practices of testing fetuses for possible defects began and gained momentum, the discourse of the perfect child has almost silently become embedded in the dominant culture. Its locus is in practice. The discourse comes into being in the clinical setting, as prenatal diagnosis has become an increasingly routine part of reproductive medical practice. Genetics, molecular biology, and medical technologies have made such practice scientifically and technologically possible. Obstetrics, led by the gatekeepers of reproductive medicine, made the practice medically feasible and promotable. Parents' hopes and fears have fed demands for such prenatal screening and testing. Science and technology, medical professionals, and parents meet in the doctor's office. This privatized setting is the site for individual decisions: whether to test or not, whether to keep a pregnancy or terminate it, and

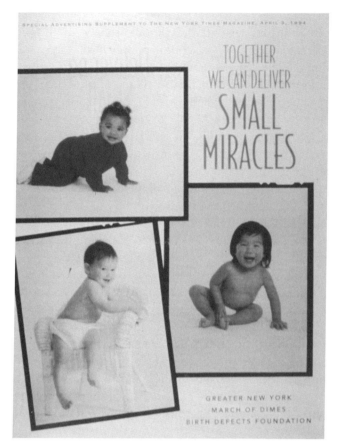

2. "Together We Can Deliver Small Miracles," cover, March of
Dimes advertising supplement to the *New York Times Magazine,*
April 3, 1994. Courtesy March of Dimes Birth Defects
Foundation.

for which diagnosed "defect." Each decision becomes another judgment as
to which conditions, and which children, are acceptable or not. As they
aggregate over time, individual decisions add up to a selection process,
marking the imperfect, those who may be dispensed with, while certifying
those worthy to be born. This process constitutes the discourse of the
perfect child.

Despite their privatized and individualized nature, prenatal diagnosis
decisions do not occur in a vacuum, but rather within a broader, if often
unacknowledged, context. Labeling and selecting out the imperfect and
delineating the contours of the perfect take place in a climate of long-held

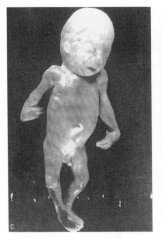 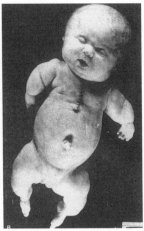

3. Postmortem photographs of fetuses with skeletal
anomalies: left, fetus with trisomy 18; right, 31-week fetus
with osteogenesis imperfecta. From John P. McGahan, MD,
and Manuel Porto, MD, eds., *Diagnostic Obstetrical
Ultrasound* (Philadelphia: J.B. Lippincott, 1994), chap. 19.
Courtesy Lippincott Williams & Wilkins.

attitudes in Western culture toward perfect and imperfect human beings
and of searching for scientific and technological ways to delineate and
define them. Modern secular beliefs trace to the eighteenth century, to
Condorcet and the Perfectibility of Man. Wedded to science, medicine,
and the Idea of Progress, this Enlightenment dream of human perfectibility, egalitarian on its surface, had an underside in the grotesque, in the
irrational madness to be contained within Foucault's asylum. In the nineteenth century, perfectibility discourse would be taken up and transformed by the positivists, the Social Darwinists, and the eugenicists into a
selective ideology upending the Enlightenment promise. Science and the
Idea of Progress came to serve a perfectibility discourse to preserve a
Eurocentric "race purity," as Others were marked unfit to procreate. Although the supporting science was discredited and the Nazi excesses made
such views unfashionable, they were alive in less openly biased form—
both among intellectuals and in popular culture—as we entered the biotechnology age at mid-twentieth century. Half a century later it is still
acceptable to view the birth of a child labeled defective as a "tragedy," and
for medical research and practice to relentlessly pursue the defective fetus.

   This is not a Luddite book. Prenatal diagnosis and other reproductive
technologies, and the advances in genetic research, are remarkable achieve-

ments. I wish neither to stop them nor to condemn them out of hand. Rather, my purpose is to look carefully at how the discourse of the perfect child has emerged from within reproductive medical practice, and what its impact may be. I wish to explore how and why we should be concerned about the discourse and how we can modify or seek alternatives to it. I argue that the discourse of the perfect child, as it aggregates slowly, will give rise to a health hierarchy of birth, setting criteria for the imperfect, and for the perfect. These criteria will be imbalanced economically, racially, ethnically, culturally, and by gender.

The research and practices that nurture the discourse of the perfect child undeniably have a material base. This is nowhere more apparent than in the privatized and corporatized health care system prevailing in the United States. Many critics have explored and analyzed the central role of the profit-making structure of research and practice in medicine, as well as in many other areas. But far less attention has been paid to ideology and the role it plays as a driving force. Like all ideologies, that of human perfectibility—of which the discourse of the perfect child is the latest manifestation—has a material base as well. But the strength and staying power of ideologies cannot be reduced to economics. The public may be gulled at times into spending money on the latest technology. But unless that technology meets felt needs, it will not remain viable and profitable for long, even if those needs have in part been induced by its promoters and then exploited. In vitro fertilization and other forms of assisted reproduction are cases in point. They have become a growth industry—despite costs and failures—precisely because they speak directly to people's powerful desires for their own biological children, a sociocultural phenomenon that some would argue has a biological base. So, too, the quest for a "perfect baby" is grounded in people's deeply felt hopes and fears for the children they will bear and raise. When the promise comes in the form of technology—however misunderstood as a guarantor of perfection—it is readily sought and accepted. The technology enables the medical researcher and practitioner to extend their commitment to prevent as well as cure disease in the patient, now extending from the adult to a new patient, the fetus. At the same time, the technology serves the goals of the underside of perfectibility ideology: to discover and weed out the imperfect.

The discourse of the perfect child, therefore, is culturally and technologically constructed, heir to the dream of human perfectibility as it has developed over more than two centuries of scientific, technological, and medical changes, and attendant shifts in belief. The critical development in the second half of the twentieth century was that the means emerged to bring that dream closer to reality. Although the eugenicists sought to control procreation in order to achieve "race purity," their tools were limited to sterilizing the "unfit" and exhorting the "fit" to be fruitful and multiply. Science fiction's utopian visions of genetically engineered futures remained fantasies. But the revolution in genetics and medical technologies that began at mid-twentieth century placed engineering birth in the practical realm, providing the means to give tangible shape to the dream.

Discourse and Deconstruction

The term *discourse,* especially associated with French philosopher and social critic Michel Foucault, suggests a set of actors' cultural and ideological beliefs and practices at given historic moments. Historian Joan Scott has described Foucault's conception of discourse as "a historically, socially, and institutionally specific structure of statements, terms, categories, and beliefs." Discourse is "contained or expressed in organizations and institutions as well as in words; all . . . constitute texts or documents to be read."[8] I use the term in this sense to link the discourse of the perfect child to a historically evolving discourse of human perfectibility. *Deconstruction,* a perhaps overworked and too loosely used concept, derives from *poststructuralism,* and provides a tool to get at these specific structures. Both approaches emphasize language. Poststructuralists channel the postmodernist challenge to universalized canons of knowledge into a critique of language, confining their method to "readings" of "texts" to derive multiple meanings and interpretations. Poststructuralists ignore social context, refuse to give priority to one interpretation over another, and therefore opt out of political or social action. But others within a postmodernist framework welcome the method of deconstruction, finding in language a useful tool with which to engage in social critique. This is true especially of feminist postmodernists, who have adapted deconstruction to a more broadly conceived approach with which to critique received knowledge, drawing on Foucault's use of discourse, his genealogical method, and his concept of power.

Foucault's genealogical method describes history as a series of specific moments in which particular practices reveal dominant values and prevailing norms, and the relations of power that produce and sustain them. Exploring these moments, he traces the origins of the mechanisms and ideologies of control and their influence on later practices, focusing especially on the ways that eighteenth-century science, technology, and medicine have affected human bodies. This new knowledge gave rise to "disciplining technologies" intended to effect control over bodies. In his famous study of Jeremy Bentham's design for a "Panopticon" prison, with its technologically innovative surveillance, he traced the origins of the "perfectly administered ideal" of modern prison systems, designed to control every facet of the prisoner's existence. So, too, the "birth of the clinic" and the asylum mark the rationalized control of the diseased and devious, and their removal from view. Thus, Foucault maintains, bodies are "imprinted" by history.[9]

Power for Foucault is a series of "relationships of force." Rather than characterized as two opposing forces, power, coming from below, arises from confrontations among different and unequal groups and forces in the social body. The major dominations that emerge are sustained by these confrontations. Power viewed in this way always includes resistance, which is located everywhere within the power network: power relationships depend on a "multiplicity of points of resistance." Each of these "resistances" is a special case: it may be "possible, necessary, improbable"; "spontaneous, savage, solitary, concerted, rampant, or violent"; or "quick to compromise, interested, or sacrificial." Resistances are distributed in irregular fashion: "the points, knots, or focuses of resistance are spread over time and space at varying densities"; they traverse "social stratifications and individual unities." The "strategic codification of these points of resistance . . . makes a revolution possible."[10] Deconstruction therefore becomes a tool to get at origins of practices, to break apart the systems and networks of power to reveal the ideological constructs that support them. The deconstructive project dismantles the discourse so as to explore meanings that the discourse masks.

Feminism factors gender into the critique of categories of knowledge and the relations of power. In feminist analysis, *sex* means the biological categories of female and male, while *gender* signifies socially derived constructs of feminine and masculine. Conflated in most cultures, *male* and *masculine* have more power and are more highly valued than are *female* and *feminine* qualities and attributes. In the dualism that has marked Western categories of knowledge since the Enlightenment, science, reason, culture, history, indeed human knowledge itself, are male and masculine. The dualism was and is hierarchic, not least in its gendered aspects. Exploring history and a wide range of disciplines, Simone de Beauvoir a half century ago illustrated how male/female and masculine/feminine dualisms are deeply embedded in the dichotomies of mind/body, reason/feeling, culture/nature, spirit/matter, and self/Other. The male self, representing mind, reason, culture, and spirit, is ranked superior to the female, who is nature, body, matter, and Other.[11] Feminist analysis takes deconstruction further to show the significance of gender in patterns of domination and subordination at specific historic moments.

This book will use this feminist and Foucauldian method of decon-struction and Foucault's genealogical approach to examine the ideology of human perfectibility as it has intersected with medical science and technol-ogy and cultural norms at particular historic moments from the late eighteenth century to today. Getting at origins, we find medicine and biology emerging as "disciplining technologies." Their use by dominant groups has meant the historic "imprinting" of imperfect and perfect be-ings.[12] In today's practice, reproductive science and technology become the tools to inscribe the "imperfect fetus," an "unborn patient" estranged and separated from its "fetal container." As women's procreative role is eclipsed, the discourse is further revealed as a masculinist construct, the postmodern expression of a disembodied, abstracted, technological dream of perfected beings.[13]

The historical and cultural framework of the book is Western Euro-pean and North American, with particular emphasis on the U.S. historical experience. While the technological and scientific research described in part 2 is international in scope, the medical practices and responses to those practices are set almost exclusively in the United States, within the distinctive framework of U.S. medical, social, economic, and political culture.

Transforming the Dream

There is no sinister plot to usher in an era of "designer genes," alarmist warnings to the contrary. Nor are the new technologies and genetic re-search all-powerful and to be opposed. My purpose in writing this book is, rather, to alert us to the impact of hundreds, indeed thousands, of deci-sions about prenatal testing that are made each day in the doctor's office, the context in which they occur, and how they add up to the discourse of the perfect—and imperfect—child. These prenatal diagnosis decisions de-fine the contours of the "imperfect child," as well as the "perfect child," socially, economically, and culturally. Genetic determinism aids and abets the process, and is reinforced.

Most important is to realize that the discourse arises from and is embedded in reproductive medical practice. To transform the discourse, practice must be transformed. Mainstream bioethics, operating at a re-moved and abstracted level, has been ineffective in raising significant questions and bringing about change, and has come to support the status quo. Resistances and questions, however, do arise from within or close to practice. They come from medical professionals, parents, people with disabilities, and feminists. Feminist approaches derive theory and proposals for change from the experiences of women. Feminist ethics and feminist postmodernism, and a relational model of human development and social interaction, provide an alternative view for human behavior in the reproductive medical setting, one which contrasts sharply with the prevailing legalistic and atomized "rights" model. The feminist model offers ways to listen to resistances and to make connections, so that alternative procreative discourses can emerge to change reproductive practice and so transform the dream.

A formidable obstacle to initiating change is the dream's undeniable power. It appeals to parents' deepest desires: to have a normal, healthy child, free from crippling or debilitating disease. Who—even those questioning or resisting prenatal testing—does not share this wish, that every child born have the chance to grow into an able, intelligent, attractive human being? Yet in reproductive medical practice these deep-felt human desires take on the aura of technological promise, the dream distorted into an oppressive discourse, the discourse of the perfect child.

The discourse is oppressive because it masks that the dream is founded on a nightmare. It is founded on the fears of the "imperfect child," who remains hidden and unacknowledged, yet starkly present. The illusion of the "beautifully perfect" child is a cruel illusion, masking its dark underside, and transposing the desire for a "normal," "healthy" child into the dream of a perfect one. The rhetoric's seductive promise widens the gulf between the perfect and the imperfect, subtly imprinting the imperfect as Other. The gap between promise and reality needs to be unmasked, and the discourse transformed. That is the intent of this book.

PART ONE

Origins: Enlightenment, Evolutionary, and Eugenic Discourses

ONE

The Perfectibility of Man

With the coming of the Enlightenment in the eighteenth century, the vision of human perfection took a dramatic turn. Rooted in the Age of Science, Reason, and of Progress, and the ideals of the French Revolution, a new discourse of human perfectibility arose, the Perfectibility of Man. Dynamic rather than static, secular rather than spiritual, human perfectibility meant that it was possible to continuously better the human condition—intellectually, physically, culturally, morally—in this world. Science, not religious faith, was the key.

The search for perfectionism has a long history in Western thought.[1] From the Greeks to the German idealists, from Judaeo-Christian traditions to the utopians, philosophy and religion have offered the promise of a state of absolute perfection for human beings, either in this world or the next. Abstract, often metaphysical, perfection represented an ideal, albeit tuned to particular belief and historical circumstance. Even when held out for all of humanity, the idea of absolute perfection was set within a hierarchically structured universe in which conformity and unquestioned acceptance were articles of faith. Often couched in spiritual terms, the state of perfection was a fixed goal, and once achieved, unchanged.

Absolutist forms of religious and philosophic perfectionism are still with us. But in the eighteenth century came a discourse that articulated a secular, egalitarian, and progressive, and progressively changing, vision. Separating itself from the old idea of absolute perfection,[2] human perfectibility began to speak in the language of freedom, of equality, of rational thought, of scientific progress. Epitomized in the Marquis de Condorcet's "indefinite perfectibility of man," perfectibility discourse was an attainable vision for all human beings. To be realized in the tenth stage of human history, human perfectibility was to be the fruit of progress and science, of reason and knowledge, as they spread far and wide.

Yet the new perfectibility discourse did not fully shed the absolutist and hierarchic trappings of the past. Wedding perfectibility to scientific progress and to a mathematically based ideal, the Enlightenment dream was framed within a new authority, a canon of truths that reflected the norms and values of a Eurocentric, especially Franco- and Anglo-American, intellectual elite. Based on privileging science and scientific method to advance knowledge in every field of human inquiry, the discovered laws of nature would apply not only to the physical world, but also to framing laws for social policy and morality. But this reliance on science could prove to threaten the dream's egalitarian and libertarian promise.

The Enlightenment Vision

Condorcet's "indefinite perfectibility of man," set within the progress of human history, marked the culmination of the Enlightenment vision of Turgot and other *philosophes* before him. In his *Sketch for a Historical Picture of the Progress of the Human Mind,* published posthumously in 1795, the Marquis de Condorcet outlined ten stages or epochs of human history.[3] The tenth and final stage, not yet achieved, would bring equality both within and among nations and the "true perfection of mankind." His vision of equality extended to inequities of wealth and status, to equality for women, and across races. Natural differences, according to Condorcet, should never lead to dependence, poverty, and humiliation,[4] nor be used to claim superiority and to dazzle; natural advantages should be used to benefit others.[5] Although it focused on the human condition and the individual and was nurtured within the Revolutionary idea of the Rights of Man, Condorcet's vision for the progressive improvement of humanity was framed within a social context. More French than Anglo-American in his concept of human nature and the relationship of individuals to society and the state,[6] Condorcet viewed human beings as social by nature. The individual's rights and liberties were realized in civil society, in a freely constituted political state; indeed, such rights and liberties depended on society for their development and realization. Thus, for Condorcet, it was in the social order of the tenth stage, an inclusive society of free and equal human beings, that indefinite human perfectibility would be fully expressed and realized.

Condorcet's progressive social vision for humanity rested on the advance of scientific knowledge. Reason and a science based heavily on the calculus (Condorcet was a mathematician) were the means to dispel ignorance and prejudice, the enemies of progress and of the advance of the human mind. The growth of reasoned and scientific knowledge through the epochs constituted a continuing challenge to vested authority which, especially in the guise of religion, had perpetuated inequality through prejudice and superstition since the very first epoch of human society.[7] The scientific discoveries of the eighth epoch provided the means to make amends for the exploitation of the earlier epochs of exploration and conquest. Such scientific works, however, will repay humanity for their costs only when Europe renounces her "avaricious system of monopoly; . . . when she remembers that all men of all races are equally brothers by the wish of nature . . . [and] only when she calls upon all people to share her independence, freedom and knowledge."[8]

Condorcet credits his own epoch, the ninth, the era of the "Rights of Man," with reason's and science's triumph over the ignorance of the past. Finally, we see the rise of a new doctrine which was to deal the final blow to the already tottering structure of prejudice—the doctrine of the indefinite perfectibility of the human race of which Turgot, Price, and Priestley were the first and most brilliant apostles.[9]

Science meant discovering truths and applying them, especially through education, in all areas—from the natural sciences, to the arts, to human faculties—so as to improve and perfect the human condition.[10] The advance of agriculture and industry through free trade and physiocratic principles—here Condorcet was very much influenced by the political economy of his day—would help to ensure material well-being. Contributing to this goal as well was the art and practice of medicine to bring about physical or organic perfection. According to Condorcet, "[o]rganic perfectibility or deterioration amongst the various strains in the vegetable and animal kingdom . . . one of the general laws of nature . . . also applies to the human race." Preventive medicine especially, in company with better food and housing and a healthier life style promoting exercise and shunning excess, would combine to strengthen and extend human lives. A "more efficacious" medical practice, arriving with the "progress of reason and of the social order," would signal the end of "infectious and hereditary diseases and illnesses" from varying causes, whether known or yet to be discovered.[11] Assuming from observation of animal breeds that perfected physical faculties could be transmitted among humans, Condorcet considered it "probable" that we could "extend such hopes to the intellectual and moral faculties."[12]

But the ideal encompassed still another dimension. The mathematics so central to the scientific concept of knowledge also infused the Enlightenment's aesthetic ideal of human perfection. In a point further developed in her book *Body Criticism,* art historian Barbara Stafford and two physicians writing in a journal of medical ethics have maintained that the attitudes of medical professionals toward "abnormal" and "perfect" babies today reflect the eighteenth century's aesthetic ideal of perfection as imaged and measured by contemporary artists and anatomists.[13] This aesthetic ideal, a "hidden assumption" of M.D.s in their ideal "picture of health," has been largely ignored by ethicists. An aesthetic ideal—in the eighteenth century and our own, and in periods before and between—is a social and cultural product and thus inextricably tied to prevailing racial, ethnic, and cultural standards.

A critical area of the advance of knowledge for Condorcet was the discovery of laws for the social and moral realms, to provide laws for society and human conduct. Scientific knowledge, especially the *diffusion* of knowledge,[14] would improve human behavior and promote virtue.

> [D]o not all these observations [on the influences of the sciences on the perfection of laws] . . . show that the moral goodness of man, the necessary consequence of his constitution, is capable of indefinite perfection like all his other faculties, and that nature has linked together in an unbreakable chain of truth, happiness and virtue?[15]

Here, indeed, was a dynamic, optimistic vision of the Perfectibility of Man in a perfectible human society. For Condorcet, as for other Enlightenment *philosophes,* the "heavenly city" was here on earth, the dream of liberation and equality made possible through applying science and reason in this world.[16] Quintessentially eighteenth-century, the forward march of a science-based Progress, though building on the past, thought to shed that past, as perfectibility was redefined in light of a new vision. But the legacy of natural science and its readings of progress plus Condorcet's own sociocultural milieu dimmed and skewed that vision.

Progress for Whom? The Scientific and Sociocultural Legacy

Turgot, the "Father of Progress" and Condorcet's mentor, had first joined the Idea of Progress to human perfectibility. The course of human history was to be continuously progressive, societies advancing through successive stages "towards greater perfection."[17] Condorcet, as he developed his ten epochs of history, equated progress not only with perfectibility but also with a future of equal human dignity. But Enlightenment progress was heir to a tradition of natural science and philosophy that ordered the universe and its forces into distinct hierarchies that were inegalitarian, and which ranked and excluded people according to set criteria.

In using the term *hierarchy*, I refer to socially constructed hierarchies, or what Garland Allen has termed *rank-order* hierarchies, classifications which rest on value judgments. In biology, notes Allen, there are both *constitutive* and *aggregational* hierarchies. The first describe levels of organization within a system, such as from cells to tissues, organisms, and populations, the properties of the lower levels constituent within the higher levels. Aggregational hierarchy refers to taxonomic classifications, such as phylum, class, or order, the categorizing from lower to higher levels merely a device to classify. Problems arise, as Allen points out, when rank-ordering hierarchies based on value judgments intrude into biological thinking. The biologically based race classifications adapted by the eugenics movement became the most glaring example of this intrusion.[18]

The progressive evolutionism that predated Darwin embraced two forms of value-laden hierarchy: *species* hierarchy and *intra-species* hierarchy. In the ranking of known species from the lower to the higher orders, humans were placed at the top of the evolutionary ladder. As the highest form of life, humans were superior to all other creatures. But rankings were also made among human beings, setting up an intra-species hierarchy. For the naturalists, some humans were better than others. Their classifications depended especially on race, and on ethnicity and culture, extending as well to such attributes as sex, intelligence, and physical endowments. Rankings accorded with degrees and states of perfection.

The notion of species hierarchy goes back to the Great Chain of Being, an interpretation of creation that held sway into the eighteenth century.[19] Fashioned complete and perfect by a divine creator, all of nature's forms were linked in one inviolable system. The order of creation was fixed and hierarchical, descending in stages from an original state of perfection. Humans were at the top of this hierarchy, the highest of God's creatures. By virtue of their intellect, human beings were assured their place over and above all plants and animals. The eighteenth century Idea of Progress upended the Great Chain of Being, interpreting the cosmic process as moving upward, as forward and future-oriented.[20] Yet, as eighteenth-century naturalists began to reverse the order of creation from descent to ascent, offering more progressive and dynamic explanations of origins and change of life forms, humans remained secure in their niche at the top. Created last, they were still the highest and the superior life form.

The Comte de Buffon, a transitional figure in the evolution story at mid-century, illustrates the continuity of the theory of species hierarchy as progressive concepts took hold. Though, as historian John Greene points out, he thought "more in terms of degeneration than improvement," Buffon assigned to "man . . . a unique place in the self-sustaining system of nature," his resemblance to the "higher apes" confined to physical structure. "Man alone" possessed the "divine gift of intelligence." Thought and speech created the immense separation that gave "man" the right to rule "over the brute creation" and to seek control over nature for human convenience.[21] It would be left to others, such as Erasmus Darwin, grandfather of Charles, late in the eighteenth century, and Lamarck, in the early nineteenth, to solidify the idea of upward progression of life forms and to link that progress to the idea of perpetual improvement, with humans as the most complex and highest form. Complexity of biological organization was assumed to be both higher and better. Later evolutionary and then eugenic thought would continue to link perfectibility to humans as the top species in the hierarchy. But it was intra-species hierarchy, the ranking of humans on a perfectibility scale, that would mark the idea and the practice of human progress as blatantly selective. The eugenicists of the nineteenth century had ample precedent for their own racist agenda in the racist discourses of the naturalists of the eighteenth.

Underlying the eighteenth-century naturalists' Eurocentrism was their commitment to White supremacy. The view that Caucasians were superior prevailed whether naturalists held to theories of racial degeneracy or racial progression, or believed that racial varieties of humans belonged to one species (monogenists) or to different species (polygenists). Following earlier patterns, anthropological thought of the eighteenth and nineteenth centuries ranked the races along a spectrum with Blacks at one end and Whites at the other, attaching other physical and cultural attributes along the way. For example, Johann Blumenbach, known as " 'the Buffon of Germany,' " in the late eighteenth century described degeneration from the white Caucasian to the yellow, brown, and finally black Negro.[22] In 1813, British physician James Prichard proposed that the "black races of men" have progressively evolved into the white European, physical as well as mental perfection being embodied in the European racial variety.[23] A "progressive" view of racial inequality meant, in all cases, superior status for White Europeans and inferior status for all others, with the Negro ranked lowest. In the nineteenth century, the pre-Darwinian Robert Chambers and leading scientists, physicians, and educators in the United States would entrench this notion of intra-species hierarchy in evolutionary thought and practice.

Condorcet, thus, was heir to eighteenth-century naturalism's belief in white supremacy, with white Europeans at the pinnacle of human progress. Given the pivotal role of science in achieving the Perfectibility of Man, was it possible to separate Condorcet's vision from the views of progress and perfectibility characteristic of the natural science of his day, even though he did not rely on a biological model? Historian Francesca Rigotti's analysis would suggest that it was not.

> Amusement over the idea of monkey-like Newtons and Leibnizes and ideas such as Robinet's fish-men have often sidetracked us from grasping how great was the affinity between this chain of beings, quivering with life and pointing towards a future perfection, and contemporary philosophies of history focussing on the triumph of mankind in constant progress toward betterment. If the evolution-epigenist movement (Maupertuis-Buffon-Diderot) gave history that dynamic and genetic sense that was to find full development in the nineteenth century, the foundation of that striving towards perfection, or at least the image of a better future than the present, is to be found in the naturalistic movement founded on continuity.[24]

The late-eighteenth-century sociocultural milieu reinforced the legacy of natural science and its ideal of perfectibility, which was less than egalitarian and inclusive. Although Condorcet's France was awash in Revolutionary and egalitarian rhetoric, it contained a discourse at once more selective and privileged. "Civilization" meant Western civilization, Europe and Europeans marked by progressive evolutionism as the most advanced among cultures. (That Europe and its Graeco-Roman roots remain the pinnacle of civilization, with exclusive claim to the world's highest culture, is still defended on both sides of the Atlantic, "multi-culturalism" notwithstanding.) Eighteenth-century elites took the superiority of their own culture as a given. In arts, education, politics, in every institution and all aspects of knowledge, theirs were the models for the rest of the world to follow.

The Marquis de Condorcet, along with other intellectual leaders of his day whether titled or not, was nurtured in this climate. Reason and science had become the primary tools to advance Western European culture to new heights, and to bring its benefits to the un-Enlightened. In what today would be termed cultural imperialism, Condorcet called for the scientific excellence and well-being of the French and Anglo-Americans to permeate other nations; such scientific knowledge was to raise the more backward to a higher level.[25] The title of his "sketch" (or "*esquisse*") for the planned but never written larger work, "The Progress of the Human Mind," suggests that Condorcet's model was the scientifically and intellectually advanced mind of the Enlightenment. This solipsistic model of human perfectibility, framed in the language of equality, was equally a product of a sociocultural milieu whose discourse reflected elitist and selective values on race and culture.[26]

The aesthetic dimensions of the perfectibility model, as revealed especially in the artistic and medical imaging of the day, perhaps best illustrate its inegalitarian aspects. In the article by Barbara Stafford and Drs. La Puma and Schiedermayer cited earlier, the authors point to the importance that geometric models of living forms have had since Greek antiquity. Proportion was the key to predicting character, mental abilities, and beauty or ugliness. In the eighteenth century, in an attempt to establish a direct correlation between facial features and character and abilities, precision was sought through quantification.

> [The] *measurement* of elusive moral qualities became contingent upon a calculus of beauty. What was simple, homogeneous, and ruled by geometrical proportions was considered also to be beautiful, undefiled, "four-square" or "straight." . . .
>
> Conversely, vague, "amorphous" features, i.e., those that were not susceptible to geometrical analysis, and excessive, or conventionally "disorderly" features were deemed sure signs not only of aesthetic deformity but of inner irrationality *and* ethical monstrosity. . . . when translated into the language of geometry, . . . if the ninety-degree angle (equal to rectitude) is identical to proper being, then "obtuseness and acuteness" are deviations erring in the direction of the "more-and-less."[27] (emphasis in original)

Illustrations from Johann Caspar Lavater's *Essays on Physiognomy*, published in German in the 1770s and soon appearing in English and French, relate disproportion in facial features to a range of deformities and abnormalities considered "devilish," "unlovely," or "incongruous," while the comparative anatomical drawings of Dutch surgeon Petrus Camper mark the ungeometrical visages as racially and nationally inferior. In Camper's "Comparative Proportions Distinguishing the Apollo Belvedere from an

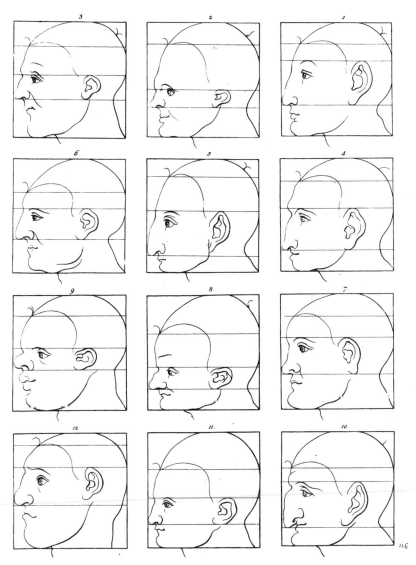

4. Johann Caspar Lavater, "Facial Disproportion," from Essays on Physiognomy, 1792, III, part II, pl. facing p. 271. Courtesy the National Library of Medicine, and as illustrated and cited in Barbara Maria Stafford, *Body Criticism* (Cambridge, Mass.: MIT Press, 1993), p. 32.

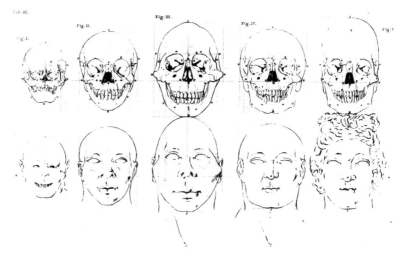

5. Pierre Camper, "From Ape to Apollo Belvedere," also called "Evolution of the Head and Skull" from *Dissertation Physique*, 1791, pl. 3 engraving. Courtesy the National Library of Medicine, and as illustrated and cited in Barbara Maria Stafford, *Body Criticism* (Cambridge, Mass.: MIT Press, 1993), p. 111.

European, a Calmuck, a Negro, and an Oran Outang," appearing in an educational manual published in French in the 1790s, " '[f]acial angles' are calculated in a descending order, dropping from the divine, hundred-degree profile of the *Apollo Belvedere* to the noble, well-bred European (ninety degrees), to the 'scarcely human' Hottentot (seventy degrees) and to the ape (below sixty-five degrees)."[28] In the next century a "measuring mania" would capture science in the attempt to demonstrate racial, cultural, and sexual inferiority.

Significant for the eighteenth century is the fusing of medical practice with a mathematically based model of human perfectibility, as art and medicine were joined. Camper's pedagogical treatise—he was a university professor—was entitled *On the Connection between the Science of Anatomy and the Arts of Drawing, Painting, and Statuary.*[29] Mathematics provided the means to underwrite and promote a highly selective, inegalitarian model of the ideal of human perfection. For Condorcet, mathematics was critical to advancing scientific knowledge and so to achieving the Perfectibility of Man. Did this mean, perhaps, that his ideal could be mathematically defined? Just as we cannot dismiss the Eurocentrism of his cultural milieu when we deconstruct his vision, so can we not dismiss the possibility that a reliance on calculation as a route to scientific knowledge

[22]

could distort that vision, which would present a far more circumscribed model. Reason and science could well be false friends. By the late eighteenth century, science and scientific knowledge had the ideological power to establish and reinforce such social-scientific links.

Uses of Science and Reason

That Condorcet looked to science to bring about the Perfectibility of Man illustrates the degree to which scientific knowledge had become the new faith. The terms *knowledge* and *science* were equated and conflated until they were almost synonymous. Postmodernism and feminist critique today, following on critical theory, have increasingly questioned the Enlightenment view of knowledge, especially its claims to scientific objectivity, and the ways in which the production and use of scientific knowledge are tools of power. Particularly relevant for the current discussion is the questioning of the model of science as it shaped the "imperial categories" of history and human nature,[30] and, by extension, the ideas of progress and human perfectibility.

At the heart of the scientific model is its rationalist premise, rooted in the oppositional categories of Cartesian dualism: reason/emotion, mind/body, self/Other, male/female. The dyad is ranked, the superior category —reason, mind, self, male—subsuming and excluding its opposite. The scientific method and scientific knowledge, resting on reason, on abstracted mental processes, discount the testimony of feeling and of the physical. Knowledge becomes the preserve of the rational male, excluding the female, invalidating the Other.[31] Knowledge, self-defined and self-produced and verified by its own categories and scientific method, claims to be absolute and universal.

Ignored, subsumed, or explained away is one-half of the binary universe. Even eighteenth-century artistic attempts to fuse the oppositional categories, notes Stafford,

> sequentially linked opposites according to a vertical scale of values . . . [which] were predicated on the longstanding sociocultural conviction of the supremacy of the rational, the linear, the geometric, the male. . . . Both in the constructed and in the natural sphere, unruly "animal" elements, shapeless feminine "chromatic" appetites, or "passionate" particulars had to be fused into a general equilibrium. The resulting perceptual union was subservient to the dominion of an underlying or overarching "bodiless" cerebral architectonic.[32]

One irony of subsuming the physical, of relegating the body to inferior status in the construction of knowledge, is that the scientific method itself is grounded in empirical observation of physical matter and a material world. Condorcet's view of human capacities relied on the empiricism of Locke's *Essay on Human Understanding,* as did that of many of his eighteenth-century contemporaries. But it was a selective empiricism. To the degree that their method did indeed draw on the experiential, it still defined and narrowly circumscribed what and whose experience would be observed and how. This classic model of scientific knowledge and its supporting epistemology—I say "classic" because it survives today—offer an account of human history that is, at the very least, distorted and, at the most, highly oppressive. Separating subject from object, and defining who and what are subject and object, the model has operated as a tool to dismiss and suppress knowledges based on feeling, the physical body, and the experiences of "others," as well as varying attempts to transcend the oppositional categories. Persons and groups labeled inferior, including women, are objectified. Scientific knowledge functioning as ideology becomes a means not to liberate, but to oppress and control, as Foucault argues.

What happens, then, to Condorcet's vision of the Perfectibility of Man if its realization rests on this model of science and scientific knowledge? Since the construction of scientific knowledge excluded the experiences and knowledges of females and other Others, privileging a select body of experiences and abstracted rational thought, one is hard put not to read the Perfectibility of Man as referring literally to men. Given the race- and culture-bound interpretations of human progress prevalent in Condorcet's sociocultural milieu, those men are white Europeans. The dynamism and open-endedness inherent in Condorcet's indefinite human perfectibility fall prey to the absolutism of an Enlightenment scientific construct. A scientifically construed and attainable goal, the Perfectibility of Man turns into an elite male construct, absolute and defined by the new scientific knowledge.

Yet the Perfectibility of Man as an optimistic and egalitarian promise of indefinite human progress and perfectibility was a significant discourse. How do we reconcile its coexistence with a discourse and a sociocultural milieu which seemed to upend that promise, especially given that reason and science were the main supports for both discourses? Perhaps the answer lies in a purpose that both reason and science served for the Enlightenment culture that championed them: the control of unreason and of an uncertain future. In this reading, following Foucault, reason and science are disciplinary mechanisms. Replacing religious faith and the

God of the old vision of perfection in an afterlife, reason and science promise an indefinite human perfectibility in this world. The eighteenth-century apostles of reason became the new high priests of this vision. But they ruled uncertainly in a world of unexplained grotesqueries and monsters, one in which the divine order and divine right of kings were toppling and a new class ascending. Intellectual elites' defense of science and reason and their promise for the future can be read as masking their intent to control, to rescue reason from unreason, to bring order out of disorder, and to insure their own position and rule in a revolutionary climate which could threaten their ideals and their very existence. That Condorcet himself was imprisoned as an aristocrat and died in the Terror of the French Revolution is more than ironic, illustrating as it does the contradictions inherent in the intellectual elite position.

The eighteenth century was fascinated by the grotesque, the barbarous, the strange. But it also sought to contain and hide the deviant, the socially undesirable, the mad. For Foucault, this urge underlay the "birth of the asylum." Replacing the old lazar houses for lepers, the asylum became the place where madness was to be confined and controlled, where it was to be defined, but not where it was cured. By the end of the century, the doctors had taken over, medicalizing madness.[33] In the Age of Reason, madness represented a threat to all that civilization had achieved and stood for, the unreason which had to be contained. Controlling and, indeed, hiding and erasing madness from public view, the asylum functioned to suppress and subvert the threat posed by the life of unreason.

Foucault's view of madness in relation to civilization is a metaphor for eighteenth-century attitudes toward the imperfect. In the Age of Reason, *madness* equals *imperfection* equals *unreason*. As reason adheres to the perfect, so are unreason and the imperfect inseparable. For the guardian of science and reason, the Perfectibility of Man offers a defense against and a counter to the unreason of the imperfect. The vision of the perfectible human being, cast in the image of the rational man of science, stands in opposition to the disruption and disorder of the image of unreason: the madman or madwoman. The discourse of the Perfectibility of Man then becomes a means to curb the forces of irrationality by defining and controlling those it can label imperfect.

Social control of the imperfect has continued as a leitmotif in social thought and practice to this day in varying guises, methods, and intensities. In the eighteenth century, Enlightenment scientific elites, defining the perfect in their own rationalist image against the unreason of the imperfect, suggested standards for the scientific "imprinting" of perfect and imperfect humans, which would subsequently occur.

A final way in which Enlightenment uses for reason and science implied social control was their application to framing laws for society and moral conduct. For a number of critics, this prescriptive use of science advocated by Condorcet prefigured the reductionist patterns for "scientific" social and moral laws in the next century. Condorcet, and Turgot before him, clearly linked the advance of science with the advance of society, to be realized in Condorcet's tenth epoch in the Perfectibility of Man. Not only would the new knowledge enhance physical well-being, science would also extend its benefits to the social and moral realms. The diffusion of scientific knowledge would affect human behavior, improving social relations and moral virtue. For both Turgot and Condorcet, mathematics was to be the universal language of science, explaining social phenomena, calculations to become a basis for social and political decision-making.[34]

Frank Manuel and Krishan Kumar suggest that this meant seeking scientific "laws" for society. They link Condorcet directly to Saint-Simon and Comte and their attempts to construct a decidedly un-liberatory, elitist "science of society."[35] Kumar further holds that Condorcet's choice of a scientific elite as the enlightened leaders toward progress and perfectibility translates directly into Comte's scientific priesthood.[36] Charles Frankel, on the other hand, argues against such a clear prescription for Condorcet.

> The practical, political application of the idea that diffusion of knowledge leads to moral progress is not in the development of a "scientific system of morality," but in plans for public education, for the development of a free press, and for the maintenance of civil liberties.[37]

Frankel adds that Condorcet is not to be blamed if things did not precisely work out that way.

Rigotti, however, points out that such applications are inevitably prescriptive:

> The prescriptive aim seems to appear insistently whenever natural or scientific models are applied to the sphere of social behavior. This purely descriptive value when limited to the biological sphere changes into a specifically normative one when grafted onto the social sphere. Description is formalized in norm.[38]

Whatever Condorcet's intent, prescription was indeed on the agenda of nineteenth-century advocates of scientific progress as they applied such natural and scientific models to the social sphere. Condorcet bequeathed a two-sided legacy.

The Enlightenment Vision: The Janus Legacy

The eighteenth-century vision of the Perfectibility of Man presented a Janus-like visage. On one side of the coin, Condorcet's hope for a better life for humanity was indeed a noble vision. In an age when republican values were still the exception and not the rule, and racism, patriarchalism, and ethnocentrism permeated respectable Western intellectual thought, Condorcet's view of human potential was wonderfully optimistic, expansive, and egalitarian.[39] This was so despite the still class-based society in which his dream was formed.

But, on the other side of the coin, his faith in the power of science to speed the inevitable forward march of progress, a faith that reflected the norms of an intellectual elite and their canon of Enlightenment truths, presented a face that was less than liberating and expansive. This face in the next century mapped a route to selectively and scientifically label those who were marked for progress and perfectibility and, more importantly, to label and control those who were not. The first face morphed into the second.

Forty years after Condorcet's *Sketch* was published, Alexis de Tocqueville invoked the vision's original promise in his *Democracy in America*. Explicitly linking American democracy and egalitarian values to human perfectibility, de Tocqueville spoke partly to the class-rooted contradictions implicit in Condorcet's vision. A commitment to equality, he wrote, was a precondition for Condorcet's "indefinite perfectibility of man." An egalitarian society, as opposed to an aristocratic, class-based one, provided such conditions. While "an aristocratic people" do not deny the "faculty of self-improvement, . . . they do not hold it to be indefinite; they can conceive amelioration, but not change." Assuming that "they have pretty nearly reached that degree of greatness and knowledge which our imperfect nature admits of," they will fix things as they are, regulating the destinies of future populations. By contrast, as castes disappear, classes draw together, customs and laws vary, and new truths displace old ones, "the image of an ideal but always fugitive perfection presents itself to the human mind." Those adversely affected by continuous changes will realize no one is infallible and will retain hope, while those whose conditions improve infer "that man is endowed with an indefinite faculty for improvement."[40] In a democratic society, according to de Tocqueville, failure and success both reinforce the possibility of human perfectibility. De Tocqueville had indeed come up with a concrete version of Condorcet's tenth epoch as it might come to pass in the new democracy of America.[41]

But his expansive rendering of human perfectibility in a democratic society also would not prevail.

The contradictions produced by class and cultural milieus placed their own limits on Condorcet's vision of human perfectibility. His commitment to free trade and the scientific advance of agriculture and industry as means to equalize wealth and status also reflected these limits, leading to his failure to predict the double-sided legacy of capitalism, which, along with spreading wealth, brought with it extremes of wealth and poverty. But more important for subverting the vision was the view of science and the central role it was assigned. In believing that science would carry the human race to indefinite progress and perfectibility, Condorcet, and Turgot before him, had a flawed concept of scientific knowledge itself. Along with its power to enlighten came science's power to control. As Enlightenment intellectuals made science the queen of knowledge, hailing it as the supreme authority to explain and prescribe human affairs, they transformed it into ideology. Science as ideology would become increasingly prescriptive as it described and ordered human conduct and society.

In the next century, new sets of scientifically minded elites seized and expanded upon the scientific reductionism latent in Enlightenment science and progress. The biologizing of scientific progress gave rise to a biologically based scientific reductionism that upended the egalitarian and libertarian promise of the eighteenth century. Reinterpreting scientific and evolutionary progress, and calling on hierarchic dualism, the new scientific elites fashioned a science to circumscribe and redefine the origins, nature, and goals of the human condition. As the positivist and elitist elements within Enlightenment science came to dominate in Comte, Social Darwinism, and eugenic thought, the scientific and technological dream of perfectibility for all human beings, attainable in a just and equitable society, was transformed. Under an ideology of scientific and biological reductionism, human perfectibility and progress were selectively ordered and marked by genetic heritage.

TWO

The "Perfect Race"

In the nineteenth century an expansive vision of perfectibility for all humanity gave way to the pursuit of perfection for a select few. Amid fears of "race degeneracy," the new high priests of biological science replaced the goal of the Perfectibility of Man with the goal of the "perfect race." Reproduction was their chief means to accomplish this. But disciplinary tools were limited. The superior specimens designated to carry on the race could only be urged to be fruitful and multiply. To achieve "race betterment," eugenicists focused on the imperfect: labeling the mentally and physically "defective" and instituting coercive measures to isolate and confine them, and to cut off their ability to procreate.

The path to the dominant discourse of eugenic perfectibility lay via the positivists, evolutionists, and Social Darwinists as they biologized science and increasingly explained human progress in terms of biological categories. In the hands of the eugenicists, the emerging science of genetics became the means to rank human beings according to race, ethnicity, sex, character, and economic and professional success, or failure, and to justify use of disciplinary tools—above all, reproductive tools—to gain and maintain eugenic control.

Evolutionary Progress

If the eighteenth century gave intellectual birth to the modern idea of progress, the nineteenth century gave it a solid material base. Especially in the U.S., rapid territorial expansion and industrial growth created a climate receptive to belief in continual improvement for the chosen and unchosen alike.[1] Equating belief in human perfectibility with democracy and equality, de Tocqueville had suggested that Condorcet's egalitarian vision of perfectibility might take hold in America and flourish.[2] But progress, as defined by science, led elsewhere. Evolutionary thought begins the transformation story as it carried through the species hierarchies found in eighteenth-century natural science. Humans, the highest life form, were superior to, and so had the right to dominate, all other species. And, by virtue of race, culture, sex, and other attributes, some human beings were superior or inferior to others.

We pick up the evolutionary narrative with Charles Darwin's grandfather, Erasmus, who anticipated Lamarck's theory of organic and progressive transformation. In 1794, Erasmus Darwin held that "all animals undergo perpetual transformation" and that "all nature exists in a perpetual state of improvement."[3] Originating the idea that forms progress organically in response to their environment, Lamarck in his *Philosophie Zoologique* in 1809 conceived progress "from the simplest animal organization to that of man, which is the most complex and perfect."[4] Robert Chambers continued this line of thought in his influential *Vestiges of the Natural History of Creation* in 1844. Often cited as an important forerunner of Darwin, Chambers described a natural, organic progression of the universe and all life, with humans as the highest, best adapted form. The present race of human beings, who were "rude" and "impulsive," he speculated might be superseded by a "nobler type of humanity" through evolutionary progression and adaptation.[5] Reinforcing eighteenth-century racial hierarchies, Chambers regarded Caucasians as the highest type, while the Negro was possibly of a different origin entirely, being so different and black in appearance and "so mean in development."[6] Monogenists in the United States, who believed that all human races shared a single origin, still maintained that despite a possible equal starting point, Caucasians were now superior and Negroes inferior. The argument, both before and after the Civil War, that evolution had stopped in the inferior races justified relegating the Negro to inferior status.[7]

Auguste Comte, in building human inequality into his positivist idea of progress in the middle decades of the nineteenth century, contributed to this discourse of the hierarchical development of life forms, even though he was not an evolutionist. His biologically based theory of "social dynamics" meant a "natural progression" in the "organic kingdom" from vegetable to animal. Progress came as superior forms succeeded one another, the animal prevailing over the vegetable, and complex animals over the simple. As the organic characteristics retire and the animal prevails "more and more," the "intellectual and moral tend towards the ascendancy." In this way, he connected the "scientific view of human progression" with the "whole course of animal advancement, of which it [human progression] is itself the highest degree."[8] Along with Saint-Simon, Comte held that the belief in equality (which he considered as "erroneous" as belief in liberty) impedes progress. Human inequality, being natural, is essential. Given that inferior forms diminished as superior forms superseded them, Comte held that the progress of civilization tended to widen the gap in intellect. The numbers of intellectually inferior are reduced, while superior intellects prevail.

Herbert Spencer's "law of progress" provided a link between Comtean progress and evolutionary ideas. According to Spencer, forms advanced hierarchically from homogeneity to heterogeneity, increasing in complexity along the way. Applying this theory to humans, he found the physiognomy and nervous systems of Europeans more complex, and thus more advanced, than those of savages or primitive peoples.[9] The struggle for existence that would produce higher skills and intelligence, with the weaker races dying out,[10] meant, in effect, that progress toward better and superior forms was reserved to Caucasians. John Fiske, a popularizer of Spencer in the U.S., cited brain size and development, and longer periods of infancy among the more highly evolved, to show that "psychic evolution" had fixed some types, for example the Negro, outside Caucasian progress and civilization. European civilization represented the highest cultural types to which primitives tend.[11]

Scholars disagree about the extent to which Charles Darwin emphasized a linear evolutionary progression, some holding that he did not,[12] and whether he subscribed to "scientific racism." But there is perhaps less dispute that he was a man of his time and his sociocultural milieu, reflecting prevailing views of race, sex, culture, and the place of human beings in the scheme of things. According to John Greene, Darwin sensed there was "an a priori conviction that man was the highest form of life on earth and that his rank was not dependent on mere ability to survive." Mental capacities were the distinguishing mark, Darwin holding that human beings were not fully human until the mind developed, which then led to social and moral development.[13] Human intellect has advanced through natural selection: those better able to defend themselves, to cooperate, and to develop arts and skills succeeded and supplanted other groups.[14] Greene notes that Darwin, like Spencer and other social theorists, shared the prevailing belief that humans had progressed from savagery to civilization, natural selection tending to favor the most intellectual, and moral, individuals. For Darwin, as well as Spencer, "human progress depended on the rise and spread of ever superior breeds of men."[15] Darwin also did not disagree with his cousin Francis Galton about the impending racial degeneracy of the most fit, though he found it presented a moral dilemma.[16]

Spencer and the Social Darwinists applied the evolutionary struggle of the most fit to survive directly to the social realm. Their hierarchy of winners and losers closely resembled the White supremacist, ethnically and culturally superior models of progressive evolutionism. Eugenicists, opting for hereditary explanations to support their hierarchies, rejected the adaptive, environmental interpretations of the Social Darwinists. But eugenicists clearly subscribed to Social Darwinian ideology and scientific racism in the ranking of individuals and races, and in determining who *should* be fit to survive. To understand how science, progress, and human perfectibility were joined in eugenic discourse, we need to stop the narrative at this point to look more closely at the development of scientific reductionism, the ascendancy of biology, and how such scientific knowledge was applied to human affairs.

Science and Biology

Biological models had been applied to social phenomena in the eighteenth century. But the connections between biology and society were not made fully explicit until the nineteenth. Comte's positivism was key to the process. In placing science at a higher stage than philosophy and abstract speculation, Comte privileged scientific knowledge to the point of scientific reductionism. All other knowledge was inferior, to be subsumed under and explained by science. The sciences themselves were hierarchically ordered, moving progressively through six levels from abstract to natural to physical to social. Biology was the fifth science, and "social physics," or the science of society, the sixth and highest. Social science, maintained Comte, was rooted in biology, its predecessor in the hierarchy. "The subordination of social science to biology is so evident that nobody denies it in statement, however . . . neglected [it is] in practice." For Comte, biology was the starting point for all social speculation because human beings and society were part of organic nature. Organic conditions determined the character of human social faculties. As the human organism was invariable, social evolution would be in accord with the inviolable natural laws of biology and of social phenomena. Positivism's final task was to discover these laws of society so as to usher in the positivist stage of progress, the perfect and highest stage for humanity and society. Since science provided the basis for action, in the positivist state all human actions would be ordered according to scientifically derived social laws.[17] As Gertrude Lenzer points out in the introduction to her translation of Comte, science was a means not only to control nature in the Baconian tradition, but also to control humans.[18]

After Comte, Spencer provided the next step in biologizing progress and human perfectibility, joining them to evolutionary thought. Writes Greene, "Not until we reach Herbert Spencer . . . do we find the idea of social evolution linked to the idea of organic evolution."[19] Here is Spencer in his *Principles of Sociology* (1877): "A social organism, like an individual organism, undergoes modifications until it comes into equilibrium with environing conditions." Combinations of factors that cause structural change and progress for one organism at the expense of others operate in social evolution as well. Progress occurs through race conflict: "the more-evolved societies drive the less-evolved societies into unfavourable habitats; and so entail on them decrease of size, or decay of structure."[20] In Social Darwinist parlance, transferring the biological struggle to human social struggle meant "natural selection" of the most socially "fit." The winners of the struggle for survival—whether individuals, races, or nations—demonstrated by their winning that they had superior adaptation and were marked for progress and continued improvement. Social Darwinists had "adapted" evolutionary science to explain the inequality of the struggle and to justify its winners and losers—on the basis of race, ethnicity, and culture.

> Darwin and Spencer bequeathed to posterity the dream of an evolutionary social science, a science continuous with the science of biology, a science whose concepts were derived in large part from biology, a science that viewed man as distinguished from other animals chiefly, if not solely, by his superior intellectual powers.[21]

A parallel development was occurring in psychology in the work of Franz Josef Gall and Paul Broca, who undertook to biologize the study of the mind. Focusing on the brain as a physical organ, they sought to use scientific observation of its structure and function to locate physical sites for mental activities. While this work, known as craniometry, was criticized in some quarters for tending to support such dubious practices as phrenology, psychologist Robert Young cites the importance of these early practitioners for the development of structural and functional psychology. Spencer was among those who drew on the work of Gall, Broca, and others to integrate it into evolutionary thought.[22] Certainly, as Stephen Jay Gould has pointed out, craniometry gave credence to the racist and sexist views of intelligence prevalent at the time.[23] The methods used in biologizing the study of the mind typified the degree to which "scientific" quantification was sweeping both the human and social sciences in the latter half of the nineteenth century. What has been called the "measuring mania" was to engulf eugenics as well.

The story of this measuring mania, and its uses and abuses in the nineteenth century (and since), has been told many times over.[24] From measuring and weighing brains, to comparing bodies, to "intelligence" testing, numbers were used to measure, classify, and rank human beings on the basis of race, ethnicity, sex, and moral and social behavior, as well as closeness to our ape ancestors. Numbers became the means to prove "natural" inferiority, whether of Blacks, women, criminals, or the poor— and conversely, either implicitly or explicitly, the superiority of European and North American White, successful males. Numbers backed up theories of selective racial progress, with arrested development for the inferior groups, and continued and inevitable amelioration for the chosen rest. Such beliefs were widely supported, not least because science and scientific quantification carried the imprimatur of reputable scientists, physicians, educators, and other intellectual leaders.[25]

In biology itself, the beginnings of the science of genetics would also help to frame eugenic discourse. In the late 1880s, August Weismann, whose experiments refuted Lamarck's theory of inheritance through acquired characteristics, became famous for his "germ plasm" theory of heredity. A German embryologist and geneticist, Weismann demonstrated that inherited traits of somatic or body cells are carried by "determiners" in separate germinal cells, or reproductive germ plasm, in all sexually reproducing species. Only the germinal cells, he held, could be affected by environment and so pass on hereditary traits. A believer in natural selection, he was not a hereditary determinist, though he was misinterpreted as such.[26] Chromosomes had been discovered in the cell nucleus in the 1880s, and their function as carriers of genes was detected at the turn of the century.[27] Mendel's work, originally published in the 1860s, was rediscovered in 1900. Revealing patterns of inherited traits in plants, his work was a final signal for the birth of the science of genetics. Experimental research accelerated in the early decades of the twentieth century, with one of the foremost centers at Columbia University. Thomas Hunt Morgan and his colleagues and disciples, in their research on fruit flies, soon went beyond simple Mendelianism, revealing the multiple factors and complexities of heredity, including sex linkages, cross-over patterns, and environmental influences.[28] American eugenicists, however, applying genetics to human beings, apparently ignored these complexities.

In eugenic readings, the biologizing of science, along with the new genetics and new methods of quantification, produced a reified science that legitimated a highly selective ideology of progress and human perfectibility, and elevated human reproduction to be a central tool of disciplinary science.

Progress, Science, and Procreation

Changing social conditions in the later decades of the nineteenth century and in the early twentieth focused attention on urban crowding, crime, new waves of immigration, and perceived signs of social and moral decay. In striking parallels to the late twentieth century, ideologues sought to fix blame as racism, nativism, and related "isms" intensified. Fears grew that the inferior and undesirable classes would overwhelm or otherwise threaten the worthy—indeed, arousing suspicions among Social Darwinists as to whether natural selection and the struggle for survival were working according to plan. Into this climate of fear and blame stepped the eugenicists. Holding out the specter of race degeneracy and its threat to "inevitable" human progress, eugenicists declared the goal of "race betterment." They proceeded to develop their own version of evolutionary theory and supporting science to reach their goal.

Out the window went the Lamarckism of the Social Darwinists as well as the aspects of Darwin's theory that involved environmental adaptation. In their place came a hereditarian view of human descent, and therefore of all human traits. Called in to support the eugenicists' biologizing of evolution were statistical and quantification methods and the budding science of genetics. Using physical, intellectual, and moral criteria, eugenicists on both sides of the Atlantic assigned rankings to races, and to people within racial and ethnic groups.

In England, Francis Galton, the father of eugenics, began to develop these methods in the 1880s. Using them to "prove" genius among certain families and populations, he also maintained that Negroes were two grades below Caucasians, with the aboriginal Australians below the Negro.[29] Building on Galton's work, mathematician Karl Pearson by the first decade of the next century had developed a sophisticated statistical theory of biometry to demonstrate Galton's hereditarian theories.[30] Pearson, who headed the Galton Laboratory for National Eugenics in London, declared that the "characteristic feature of eugenics" is the "transition from declamatory assertion to statistical proof." We "start from three fundamental biological ideas": 1) in weighing nature against nurture, much more weight goes to nature; 2) there is no inheritance of acquired characteristics; and 3) "all human qualities are inherited in a marked and probably equal degree."[31] Thus armed with "objective" scientific tools, the Galton Laboratory's research proceeded to fix inherited mental, physical, and moral characteristics among populations, according to race, ethnicity, and class. Added in was Pearson's view of progress as a struggle of superior over inferior races and peoples. The White race was superior, the inferiors being the races that lost out: "Chinamen," "Negroes," and "Kaffirs," who had not taken the "narrow path to perfection."[32]

At the center for eugenic activity in the U.S., at Cold Spring Harbor on New York's Long Island, Charles Davenport and Harry Laughlin called on Mendelian unit theory, and Weismann's "germ plasm," rather than on biometry to support their research.[33] They focused on individuals and families, not on populations, an aspect important to British eugenics, although family pedigrees occupied researchers on both sides of the Atlantic. Applying Weismann and Mendel to their own ends, Davenport and Laughlin traced genealogies to show that each family will be "stamped with a peculiar set of traits," depending on its "germ plasm," that distinguishes it and sets it apart.[34] Thinking in terms of separable Mendelian units, they based their research on the inheritance of discontinuous traits, which were isolatable and non-interacting. Thus, there was a "determiner" for feeblemindedness or criminality, as well as for intelligence or morality. Davenport was a trained geneticist whose work on Huntington's chorea and poultry breeding, applying modifications made to Mendelian unit theory made by this time, had contributed positively to genetic research.[35] He was also fully acquainted with the process of fertilization and division in the nucleus of sex cells as it was then known.[36] Yet, at the Eugenics Record Office, intent on finding a genetic basis for human behaviors and ignoring the admitted polygenic aspect of such traits, Davenport and Laughlin applied their own statistical methods to Mendel and Weismann to seek out mental, physical, and, above all, moral deficiencies among the families of suspect persons or groups.[37] Coming up with race classifications similar to Pearson's, Davenport and Laughlin combined them with extensive examination of the hereditary mental, moral, and physical inferiority of criminals, the mentally retarded, southern and eastern European immigrants, and various other social undesirables and degenerates.

For most leading eugenicists, class was inextricably linked to human superiority and inferiority. Davenport, for example, held that wealth and success marked the effective members of society, while poverty designated inefficiency and mental inferiority. Historian Charles Rosenberg comments that for Davenport the "principle of equality was a biological absurdity."[38] Women were no exception. Progressive evolutionary theories that placed women lower on the evolutionary scale, as more primitive and less specialized, squared easily with eugenic thinking. Although women were obviously needed to breed an improved human race, only *some* women could be so favored. Females of inferior races, classes, and mental and physical capacities were ranked similarly to the men—classifying prostitutes among the "unfit" a good example. Even for the "fittest" females, biology remained destiny; their function and calling to improve and perfect humanity could occur only in the way decreed by nature: procreation.[39]

Going beyond Comte and the Social Darwinists, therefore, eugenicists sought to use biology and scientific methods not only to identify the imperfect and perfect, but also to determine the evolutionary process itself. While we breed animals scientifically, declared Davenport, we fail to apply the science of breeding to humans. Following the example of poultry breeding, he wanted to be able to make "any desired combination" and predict the outcome for the "human product."[40] Pearson put it more expansively.

> The time seems upon us when the biological sciences shall begin to do for man what the physical have done for more than a century; when they shall aid him in completing his mastery of his organic development, as the physical sciences have largely taught him to control his inorganic environment.[41]

In their use of a biologized and quantified science to classify the many categories of undesirables and so mark them, eugenicists found a means to separate favored groups and persons from the rest. Sharpening the contrast, even as fears of race degeneracy were exploited, the unworthy served the social and psychological function of the "Other."

The Imprinting Process: Eugenics and the "Other"

Building on Cartesian dualism that split mind from body, reason from emotion, man from woman, and self from Other, the eighteenth century had developed a discourse of hierarchic dualism that privileged certain kinds of knowledge. As a dominant discourse, it reflected the practice of privileging not only selected research methods—notably scientific—but also the kinds of persons suited to engage in that practice. In effect, this meant the northern European or American male intellectual who, in the process of following the paths of reason and science to progress and per-fectibility, defined and excluded unreason, and those who represented it, as imperfect. As I suggested in chapter one, this extreme of unreason and the imperfect could be equated with madness that, according to Foucault, the eighteenth century sought to control in the asylum. The pursuit of the Perfectibility of Man served as a counter to the disruption and disorder of unreason that the Age of Reason could not tolerate. In the language of hierarchic dualism, the Perfectibility of Man cast the Other as social in-ferior and outcast.

Eugenicists of the nineteenth and twentieth centuries had a somewhat different agenda that reflected their social climate. Playing on, as well as promoting, fears of social unrest and decay, eugenicists devised elaborate systems for categorizing and classifying "defectives." These imperfect oth-ers could be blamed, both implicitly and explicitly, for much that was wrong with society and with people's lives. The Others threw the ideal of the perfect into sharp relief, defining the ideal of the perfect race by its opposite. More important, in focusing on the Other, eugenicists could shore up their own position and worthiness, and the worth of their ad-herents.

Naming is a formidable power. To label someone or some group deviant and make the label stick is to have the power to set and enforce societal standards. It is the power to stigmatize not only asocial behavior but also those engaged in it. In extreme form, deviance labeling turns to scapegoating, the deviant becoming the despised Other, a lesser brand of human who confirms what one is not. "Defectives" for the eugenicists were the subordinate Other that both complements and defines the Self. "Defectives" represented negation and evil, through which the eugenicists confirmed their own goodness and very being.

Once commonly used as an adjective, *defective* began to be used as a noun in the 1880s.[42] Substituting the word for the person implies even greater stigma than when used to describe a quality or aspect; the whole person is now seen as wanting. The "defective" is unredeemable, irrevoca-bly incomplete. The eugenicists' adoption of this usage coincided with events in the field of mental retardation at the time. Faced with ineffective treatment programs and mounting societal problems, professionals were growing pessimistic. As they lost hope of improving the condition of their charges, they found Social Darwinism and eugenic ideas increasingly at-tractive. Among those seeking to prevent the mentally deficient from propagating could be counted many who had run mental institutions.[43] Hereditarian theories powerfully supported the view that those labeled retarded or otherwise "defective" were permanently and irrevocably so. By the turn of the century, specific diseases and mental defect were linked. The "three morbid conditions" of alcoholism, tuberculosis, and diseases of the nervous system (e.g., migraine, hysteria, and mild epilepsy) were considered "far and away the most frequent causes of mental defect."[44] In medical practice, almost all forms of social deviance came to have a biological base and were thus included among pathological conditions.[45]

Against this background, eugenicists had taken to classifying "defectives." The unworthy lower orders were everything the eugenic ideal was not. In 1914, Harry Laughlin at the Eugenics Record Office produced a report entitled "The Best Practical Means of Cutting Off the Defective Germ-Plasm in the American Population." Discarding the more general classification of "social misfits," he came up with "5 D's": "Dependent," "Deficient," "Defective," "Delinquent," and "Degenerate." The five Ds, in turn, covered ten classes: (1) feeble-minded, (2) pauper, (3) inebriate, (4) criminalistic, (5) epileptic, (6) insane, (7) constitutionally weak, or "asthenic class," (8) predisposed to specific diseases, or "diathetic class," (9) physically deformed, and (10) those with "defective sense organs . . . the blind and the deaf, or the cacaesthetic class." This "eugenical classification" was for groups whose "traits are hereditary, cacogenic."[46] In contrast to the Greek *eu-*, meaning good, the prefix *caco-* means bad or evil. The Greek *cacogenesis*—literally "bad or evil origin or birth"—means a "morbid or depraved formation; a monstrosity, a morbid pathological product."[47] *Cacogenic* is thus the Other of *eugenic*, "good origin or birth."

In the language of biological reductionism, unfitness automatically meant physical unfitness. The feebleminded, drunk, criminal, epileptic, or deaf-mute alike were weak, diseased. Eugenicists dwelt on disease, on physical deformity, almost obsessively. In a 1909 lecture entitled "The Groundwork of Eugenics," Karl Pearson declared that "everyone, being born, has the right to live, but the right to live does not in itself convey the right to reproduce their kind." In words not unlike those of certain scientists today (see chapter eight), Pearson continued,

> We must say to the diseased and the deformed, to the syphilitic, the epileptic, the feeble-minded and the insane, "Medical progress will do all in its power to make your life easier, but you have no right to be the parents of the coming generation whenever and wherever heredity or contact insures that even a sensible percentage of your offspring will be themselves deformed or diseased."[48]

The popular traveling circus and freak show that paraded the physically different as a sub-species and as objects of ridicule underscored these eugenic sentiments.[49]

Physical otherness carried with it the stigma of being aesthetically Other. Laughlin applied the term *cacaesthetic* to the blind and deaf, who, because of "defective sense organs," would have a "bad" aesthetic; that is, they would be unable to appreciate art, music, or other kinds of beauty. Denied procreative rights on the basis of their low beauty-appreciation quotient, the sightless and the deaf, as well as others physically impaired, were obviously in themselves wanting aesthetically. Common practice of the day consigned undesirables to asylums, poorhouses, prisons, or the family attic, where they could be hidden from view and would not cause harm. Their physical appearance contributed to the opprobrium heaped on such persons. Historically, White Western culture's views of race and ethnicity have reflected aesthetic criteria. Shakespeare's Othello, though praised as the noble and valiant Moor, presents a barbaric mien and "sooty bosom" to Brabantio, Desdemona's father. Shylock and Marlowe's Jew of Malta are unflattering caricatures of the Elizabethan Jew. In the eighteenth century, Blumenbach deemed Caucasians (he coined the term) the "most beautiful" of the five races, while he and fellow naturalists demonstrated the other races' animal-like appearance.[50] Diane Paul notes that Pierre Tremaux, a French traveler, wrote in his widely circulated 1865 book that "[p]erfection in humans is defined largely in aesthetic terms, e.g., Negroes are ugly, not because of their color . . . but because of their shape, while White Caucasians, especially Greeks, are beautiful"[51] (reflecting the long dominance of the Greek ideal in Europe). As anthropometry developed in the nineteenth century, measurements were used to derive standards of beauty, as well as of intelligence and character.[52] The measuring mania carried these comparisons to new lengths, as researchers minutely measured and quantified not only skulls but also such factors as length of limbs and their relation to body stature. Not surprisingly—as illustrated in work with World War I recruits—the skeletal structure of Blacks was found to be closer than other recruits' to that of apes.

Physical and aesthetic othernesses were connected to moral otherness. If you were diseased, and your appearance was unpleasing, or even less than human, somehow, the eugenicists argued, it signified a fault of character. Morality, too, was lodged in the germ plasm. But the otherness went deeper, especially for those such as Francis Galton or Charles Davenport who equated human weakness, and thus the propensity to commit immoral acts, with sin. For Galton, despite man's "lofty aspirations," there was "weakness in his disposition. . . . The whole moral nature of man is tainted with sin," preventing him from doing right. He did not see this as a fall from grace; rather, the development of conscience was moving the race morally forward, which was all the more reason to identify those impeding moral progress.[53] Davenport transposed "free will" into will generally, which he saw as either strong or weak, and thus working for good or bad. An anti-social, i.e. bad, act was therefore due to a weak will.[54] It became critical to name and root out the weak-willed, the immoral and sinful, lest they perpetuate their tainted germ plasm and remind the upright of their own hidden failings. In the "habitual criminal," the drunkard, the prostitute, the pauper, eugenicists saw what they feared lurking just below the surface, an Arthur Dimmesdale, their own repressed underside. Exorcising the depraved Other for the salvation of the race, eugenicists sought their own salvation.

There was a moral hierarchy. The habitual criminal, for example, ranked as one of the severest threats to race improvement. In the U.S., the disciplining technology of forced sterilization was practiced more widely on prison populations than on any other group. But the most menacing Other was mental deficiency, often characterized under the general rubric of "feeblemindedness." Like morality, mental deficiency cut across the other Others. The physically imperfect, the aesthetically imperfect, and the morally imperfect were likely to be intellectually imperfect as well, though in varying degrees. The tie with moral otherness was particularly strong, and therein lay a basis for finding the feebleminded a threat to race improvement, and to the very survival of the fit. In both England and the U.S. it was widely believed that the feebleminded were especially fecund, rapidly populating society with their inferior offspring. Whether they, like the poor and other social irresponsibles, were actually more fertile than the intelligent, responsible classes, the latter's birthrate apparently was declining, while that of the feebleminded and lower classes was rising. That they were supposedly breeding like rabbits represented a distinct moral failing. Feebleminded females especially were seen as debauched, unable to curb their licentious appetites.[55] On the other hand, according to Davenport, sexual morality was more likely to be found among men with the "best blood," who are less prone to venereal disease because "illicit sexual intercourse" is "repugnant to strictly normal persons."[56] The fit curbed their sexuality, indeed they disdained sex. Although Davenport and his colleagues were more obsessed with issues of sex and morals than were their British counterparts, the equating of sexual license and immorality with low intelligence, and sexual reserve and puritanical morals with high intellect, characterized much eugenic thinking on both sides of the Atlantic (Havelock Ellis notwithstanding). That procreation by the fit was urged as a duty reflected this mindset, as did, in part, later eugenic proposals to separate the sexual act from the procreative process.

Mental deficiency or feeblemindedness, the key defect, incorporated the other Others. As the opposite and negation of intelligence, it contrasted the attribute the eugenicists prized most. In claiming for intelligence and mind the foremost quality for racial perfection, eugenicists reflected the dominant cultural discourse. White male Western society held human intelligence responsible for culture, for creating civilization itself. The eugenicists considered their own time an intellectual high point, a scientific and industrial age in which brains were crucially needed.[57] Intelligence was the ultimate standard by which to separate and rank people by race, ethnicity, culture, and gender. Mental deficiency having served to define what the eugenicists were not, they found in intelligence a positive means to counter their social insecurities and shore up their class position.

Leaders in eugenics and its ardent advocates came largely from the middle to upper middle, usually professional, classes, rather than from the top of the social hierarchy. Owing their rank to what they considered intellectual acumen, rather than inherited wealth and class, they prized intelligence and sought to justify the distinctions it bestowed. In acutely class-conscious Great Britain, an important segment of eugenics leadership fell into this category. Its members were mainly from the professional middle classes, whose status rested on their own knowledge and mental abilities rather than on any traditional class position. According to Donald MacKenzie, eugenics appealed particularly to this social group, their ideas and work reflecting their emergent status.[58] Among eugenic scientists on the left, however, notes Diane Paul, those such as geneticist H. J. Muller saw a socialist revolution and a more egalitarian society as a precondition for implementing a eugenic program.[59]

In the U.S., the criterion of intelligence was used to justify class position within the context of class insecurities peculiar to American culture. The American eugenics movement was born at the height of the Gospel of Wealth, when fortunes were being amassed by self-made men, and the scientific and social science professions were gaining power and authority. It drew leaders from both professional and business groups who believed success, and its attendant social status, were due to one's own mental abilities, plus hard work and discipline. Poverty and failure were your own fault. Class insecurity was endemic in this context, the need to prove yourself constant. That sectors of the American eugenics movement went about classifying and stigmatizing the unfit Others with such zeal can be attributed in part to this characteristic of American social mobility and the uncertainties it bred. Historian Hamilton Cravens has pointed out that members of the emerging "semi-professions," such as social work and applied psychology, were among those who "focused their attention on the poor, the criminal, the feeble-minded, or the delinquent members of society whose anti-social behavior, they believed, constituted a threat to the stability of the urban industrial social order."[60] Lower on the social scale than those in traditional professions—or, for that matter, than successful businessmen—these eugenicists could in this way validate their own work and their own social position.[61]

Patriarchal values played into this framework. Some women were a triple Other: their lower class and race combined with their female wantonness to mark them unfit to procreate. Among the fit, class was as important for women as for men, their inheritance evidently precluding the whorish behavior of their lower-class sisters. (Race and ethnicity were not even issues since only certain Caucasian stocks were deemed fit among either sex.) Yet White Anglo-Saxon women of the middle and upper middle classes were still Other by virtue of being women. The prime function for females of "better stock" was their "natural" one: to procreate, imparting the "womanly" qualities that flowed from motherhood to their progeny, and to the race. Eugenic inheritance theories served to further reinforce the widely held belief that gender attributes were rooted in biology.[62] The discovery by the turn of the century that egg and sperm contributed an equal number of chromosomes and presumably an equal number of hereditary traits did nothing to shake the assumption of the gendered nature of each sex's contributions. From the female came the Victorian qualities of "feminine" nurturance, gentleness, empathy, and higher morality; from the male, "masculine" intellect, vigor, and courage. Educated women who ventured into the public arena, who failed to marry, or who otherwise postponed or avoided motherhood were severely criticized. They were failing in their sacred duty to the race, and were even blamed for impending race suicide. Reflecting earlier nineteenth-century ideas about a woman's ability to control prenatal influences on the child she was carrying, the onus was placed on these women not only to reproduce, but to reproduce healthy, perfect babies by following prescribed regimens.[63] Patriarchy defined these influences. Women's intellect, for example, was a sometime thing; a double standard was at work here. Echoing prevalent beliefs that intellectual pursuits would harm women's childbearing abilities—producing prolapsed uteruses and the like—eugenicists in the early 1900s argued similarly against providing the same kind of higher education for women as for men. Neglecting women's special "natures and needs" would result, according to sociologist Colin Wells, in "damage to the individual, the nation, and the race."[64]

Francis Galton had earlier set the stage for the masculinized ideal and for women's subordinate role in contributing to eugenic goals. Rosaleen Love notes that Galton generally overlooked the contributions of women. "[H]is list of qualities for measuring eugenic fitness included 'health, energy, manliness, and courteous disposition.'" On the "rare occasion" when he considered qualities women might offer, he listed "athletic proficiency, fertility, and 'their capacity to pass a careful physical examination.'"[65] Although Galton acknowledged that women can have a role in producing genius, since "eminent men" tend to marry "eminent" rather than "silly women,"[66] he omitted female relatives from his study of families to determine hereditary genius. He argued that, like certain contemporary males, women were excluded because they were not "public characters."[67] Procreators, yes; persons, no.

The eugenics movement nevertheless counted women among its most ardent advocates, including Margaret Sanger and Mary (Mrs. E. H.) Harriman, the latter a major financial supporter.[68] Pearson's laboratory in England included a number of female researchers who enthusiastically pursued the goals of their enterprise, despite the fact that they were underpaid, even unpaid, and generally undervalued.[69] It was neither the first nor the last time that class, race, and cultural beliefs would mask the patriarchal and ultimately destructive nature of the eugenic perfectibility ideology, especially for women. And although certain socialist and politically progressive eugenicists supported women's rights (Pearson included),[70] their practice and their vision of a perfected race belied their professed politics.

The Goal of Reproductive Control

Eugenicists thus sought to promote positive genetics by urging those genetically fit to procreate to do so. But, from a practical perspective, it was hardly an effective means of reproductive control. Proscription directed at the Others, rather than prescription for the fit, offered considerably more chance of success. Negative eugenics dominated eugenic discourse. Mainline eugenicists saw those they labeled defectives as inferior Others whose repression and elimination could be justified. And so they undertook to prevent such defectives from procreating. In the U.S., this meant instituting sexual segregation and, more important, sterilization. In the first decades of the twentieth century, policies from the 1890s that sought to segregate the feeble-minded and to castrate convicted rapists and murderers, and asylum inmates, gave way to laws for involuntary sterilization. Such laws were enacted in more than half the states by the 1920s. Notes Philip Reilly in *The Surgical Solution*, "castration was too brutal to provide a socially acceptable solution to curbing the fecundity of the feeble-minded. In the early 1900s, however, it provided a foil against which sterilization seemed humane and politically more palatable."[71] The first successful vasectomy in 1897, followed by the development of salpingec-tomy (tubal ligation) for women between 1910 and 1920, were two medi-cal technologies that helped to enlist the support of physicians for eugenic sterilization. In addition to physicians who favored sterilization for those in state institutions, major support for the early laws came from a handful of prominent scientists, non-scientist eugenicists, and wealthy philanthro-pists. There was clearly broader popular support as well. After Constitu-tional challenges relying mainly on the equal protection clause of the Fourteenth Amendment overturned several state eugenic sterilization stat-utes in the 1910s, a second wave of more lasting sterilization laws arrived in the 1920s, carefully crafted to meet court tests. The turning point came in 1927 when the Supreme Court in *Buck v. Bell* upheld a Virginia law that had allowed the compulsory sterilization of a young Black woman. Carrie Buck was described as a "feeble-minded woman who had a feeble-minded mother and an illegitimate feeble-minded child." Speaking for the Court, Justice Holmes declared, "Three generations of imbeciles are enough!" echoing the prevailing mindset.[72] Sterilization laws proliferated over the next 15 years, and in 30 states they remained on the books until well into the 1980s, even if rarely invoked.

In the early wave, especially between 1909 and 1913, recorded steril-izations numbered over 3,000, carried out mainly on those incarcerated, either in prisons or in mental institutions. California and Indiana, at the time and into the '20s, particularly invoked hereditarian arguments about insanity. Sterilizations reached their peak in the second wave, with an average of 2,000 or more performed yearly throughout the '30s and into the early 1940s.[73] Over 60,000 persons were reported sterilized in the period between 1907 and 1963.[74] Beyond the numbers, what is interesting are the rationales and supports for the practice, which persisted even as the discourse changed.

At first, both men and women were sterilized. For male criminals the procedure was intended to modify and change their "aggressive" behavior; for the feebleminded of both sexes, it was to prevent them from reproduc-ing, the rationale entirely eugenic. When the courts declared criminal sterilization statutes to be "cruel and unusual punishment" under the Eighth Amendment, the argument shifted to the genetic basis of criminal behavior. Sterilization was justified to prevent criminals' passing on their defective genes. When the sterilization of a feebleminded criminal was upheld in the 1920s, eugenics became the rationale for new criminal sterilization statutes.[75] All sterilization laws now had the same intent: to prevent the birth of defective offspring by depriving certain categories of persons of their ability to procreate. Mental defectives became the main target. In the heyday of the practice in the '30s and early '40s, more than half the sterilizations took place in mental institutions, women undergoing the operation about one-and-a-half times more often than men. Although eugenics was the underlying motif, public rhetoric argued in the language of sociology and mental health. The mentally deficient were being sterilized "for their own good," so they could rejoin society as productive, but not reproductive, members. The aim was social control.[76] Sociologist Stanley Davies spoke out for this goal in his *Social Control of the Mentally Deficient*, published in 1930. Arguing that the mentally deficient could no longer be regarded as a "menace" to the race and that it was unproductive for society to think so, Davies advocated adopting control measures to turn the deficient from "social liabilities" into "social assets." Such measures included education, special training, community supervision, and, for the "feebleminded, including defective delinquents" only, sexual segregation to prevent their procreating.[77] Although he did not advocate sterilization, his book was published just as forced sterilizations approached their peak.

Negative eugenic discourse ranged from this tempered sociological rationale—with its underlying aim of procreative control—to extremes that would do away with defectives, and to continued open advocacy of eugenic sterilization. The latter arguments mixed in positive eugenic rhetoric as well. French-born Alexis Carrel, a Nobel-laureate surgeon conducting research at the prestigious Rockefeller Institute for Medical Research in New York in the 1930s, represented an extreme.[78] In his *Man the Unknown*, Carrel proposed physical coercion and what amounted to a "final solution" for the unfit. Criminals should be kept in hospitals rather than prisons and conditioned with a whip or "some more scientific procedure." Murderers and other violent criminals, and the insane,

> should be humanely and economically disposed of in small euthanasic institutions supplied with proper gases. Modern society should not hesitate to organize itself with reference to the normal individual. Philosophical systems and sentimental prejudices must give way before such a necessity. The development of human personality is the ultimate purpose of civilization.[79]

Carrel advocated requiring a medical examination before marriage, especially for the insane and feebleminded, so as to make health a key criterion for promoting "better human stock." Although not a strict hereditarian,

Carrel sought voluntary eugenic programs for the "best elements" to propagate a "great race." He was highly critical of the "best" women who refused to have children and were deteriorating by indulging in dieting, tobacco, alcohol, and feminism. Only the "newcomers, peasants and proletarians from primitive European countries . . . beget large families." For Carrel, "[t]he establishment of a hereditary biological aristocracy through voluntary eugenics would be an important step toward the solution of our present problems."[80] First published in 1935, *Man the Unknown* went through 56 editions and was translated into several languages. Upon his later return to France, Carrel became a stalwart supporter of the Vichy regime.

Carrel admittedly was an extreme case—a throwback to the blatant rhetoric which was finding fewer supporters among eugenic advocates by the '30s, even as it gave voice to the Nazi atrocities to come. Yet eugenic arguments for sterilization still had a respectable place in the U.S. well into the 1940s. The Human Betterment Foundation in California—the state accounting for 40 percent of the reported sterilizations in the U.S.—vigorously promoted sterilization as a eugenic measure to halt the spread of defective germ plasm. The foundation sponsored detailed studies, keeping close records of state laws and actions, and actively promoted eugenic sterilization laws and education. In the mid-1940s it lost its chief funder, renamed itself Birthright, Inc., and relocated to Princeton, New Jersey, where it confined itself to educational activities, describing itself as a "national organization devoted to fostering . . . a national program of selective sterilization."[81] The former director and chief researcher of the Human Betterment Foundation and a member of Birthright's board, Paul Popenoe, was also a director of the American Eugenics Society. The society's official journal in the 1940s, *Eugenical News,* on which Popenoe held editorial posts, regularly reported on and promoted eugenic sterilization, including materials from Birthright. Commenting on a report on sterilization laws by Birthright's executive secretary in 1946, an editor's note in the *News* stated that although there is "no record of an official vote at annual or directors' meetings . . . [i]t is probable that a decided majority of the present members of AES believe in the general principles of eugenic sterilization."[82] Two years earlier the *News* had noted public approval of "compulsory sterilization of mental defectives," citing rates of 66 percent in a *Fortune* poll and 70 percent in one by the *New York Herald Tribune,* though no dates were given.[83] This, despite the fact that the Supreme Court in 1942, in a case involving sterilization of habitual criminals, had declared procreation a fundamental human right of which no one could be deprived without due process of law.[84]

The sterilization rhetoric, however, had begun to soften in the 1940s. Sterilization was to be "voluntary," to be "compulsory" only for "incompetents."[85] But the requirement of "consent" may have been more moral fiction than practice, since subterfuge and coercion were often the rule.[86] While numbers began to fall off in the 1950s, between 1946 and 1958 almost 16,000 sterilizations were recorded.[87] Even as language changed, "defectives" remained a category apart, whose procreation threatened further human improvement. In a society increasingly emphasizing the importance of intelligence and insisting on its hereditary nature, this category focused on the mentally deficient, who ranged from persons of low IQ to those labeled insane. Assigning a hereditary basis for traits characteristic of other categories of social and physical outcasts had also become decidedly suspect. But class and race discrimination remained constants. Since most legal sterilizations continued to be performed on inmates of state hospitals, prisons, and mental institutions, dispensable "defectives" were disproportionately poor and, depending on the state, Black.[88]

The eugenicists converted genetics into a disciplinary science, using it to define and mark the inferior Other. Combining genetics with sterilization as a disciplinary technology, eugenic practices, while not yet qualifying as genetic engineering in these earlier decades of the twentieth century, suggested a type of biological engineering. However, directed as they were at the imperfect, eugenicists' attempts to use disciplinary tools to control human reproduction applied mainly to negative eugenics. Unable to similarly "engineer" the procreative practices of societal worthies, eugenicists had to make do with exhortations, pep talks, and propaganda to pursue a program of positive eugenics.

Eugenic Discourse and the "Perfect Race"

Social and sociopsychological factors in part explained eugenicists' preoccupation with negative eugenics. Eugenic claims about undesirables in their midst struck a responsive chord in a less than secure middle-class and upper-middle-class public, even as such claims shored up eugenicists' own status. But the limits of technology and the applicability of science contributed at least equally to accentuating the negative. Selective as their science was, it lent itself more readily to marking the bodies of racial and ethnic inferiors, of the poor, the diseased, the infirm, and of the morally depraved. The chosen's sterling qualities remained more elusive. It was far easier to observe, measure, and quantify the characteristics or explore the lineage of inmates of prisons, asylums, or hospital charity wards than to so objectify the purveyors of wealth and success. Further, tracing the forebears of the self-made champions of the Gospel of Wealth might have revealed a few too many thieves, debtors, or horse traders, clearly upsetting eugenicists' hereditary theories. Their uses of science enabled eugenicists and eugenic thinking to exert enough power to engage the tools of law and medicine to try and curb the population of undesirables. Such tools included restrictive immigration, incarceration, and methods of sterilization. Conversely, while eugenicists could urge the "better sort" to procreate, moral suasion had to substitute for legal coercion. Drawn by the eugenicists in their own image and with the qualities considered ideal by the dominant culture to which they belonged, the "better sort" were still harder to delineate precisely than were the inferior "others." It was perhaps more "we know who we are," and proceeding from there.

They expressed themselves in the movement for "race betterment." The movement emerged in the climate of a "euthenics" or health and fitness craze that caught up segments of American society in the early decades of the twentieth century. A series of race betterment conferences in 1914, 1915, and 1928 promoted the eugenic ideal of being physically, as well as mentally and morally, fit. The 1928 conference, in Battle Creek, Michigan, was financed by John Harvey Kellogg of cereal fame, who was also a doctor and president of the Race Betterment Foundation. The conference's, and foundation's, purpose was to apply "science to human living in the same thoroughgoing way in which it is now applied to industry—in the promotion of longer life, increased efficiency and well-being and race improvement."[89] Titling their meeting "Heredity and Eugenics," the assembled physicians, scientists, social scientists, educators, and health professionals focused for five days on achieving "fitter families" and explaining how science, medicine, and education could improve health, well-being, and longevity, and keep one microbe-free. There were even sessions called "The Physics and Therapeutic Uses of Sunlight" and "Physical Education and Play." These positive prescriptions for the desirable members of society contrasted markedly with sessions called "Crime and Sterilization" or "Immigration and the Average Man," which presented medical and moral arguments for sterilization and restrictive marriage and immigration laws. For those having acceptable or superior germ plasm, science overflowed with health prescriptions, laws, regimens, and rules of behavior to be followed to do one's part for the cause. But there were no scientific health advisories for the "others." For them, science provided only the means to mark them as Other, to sharply restrict their freedom, or to exclude or even destroy them.

Yet, exhorted as they were to live up to and pursue a demanding ideal, the chosen, too, were subject to a form of coercion. Scientific principles delineated the "perfect race," prescribing the paths of fitness and behavior that would lead to it. It was nothing less than the duty of the morally upright, successful, intelligent bearers of superior stock to follow the rules, including procreating, and bring the race to new moral and cultural heights. Failure, they were warned, could mean "race suicide."

But whether they sought to further good genes or to stop the production of bad genes, the eugenicists focused their energies on reproduction and its practice. Linking the aim of race perfection to biological science at the point of procreation itself, the eugenicists profoundly altered perfectibility discourse. Transposing the terminology of stock breeding used by Davenport and Pearson to the human animal, they found the language to describe a biologically based selection that would perfect the human "breed."

It may seem contradictory that the eugenicists, who supported an ethic of individualism and the self-made man, set as their goal race perfection rather than individual perfectibility. They rescued a species of individualism by keeping their club exclusive. Redefining "human race," their discourse reserved membership in it to those sterling individuals who, like themselves, could be defined scientifically as meeting certain cultural and moral criteria. The Others, not making the grade, were less than human. "Human betterment," as used by the California-based, pro-sterilization Human Betterment Association, and "race betterment" were euphemisms that masked the new, selective meaning of *human race*. Eugenics' biological reductionism read eugenic social criteria for defining human beings into the new core of perfectibility discourse.

"Class" and "elite" were also recast. Intelligence was less class-based than formerly; it had become a criterion for the newly constituted experts and leaders. Self-proclaimed, the new aristocracy arrived on the wave of business and industry and the professions, whose leaders attributed their success to their own acumen and efforts. Their position was proof of their superior abilities and moral worthiness. What was not explained, however, was how the self-made man's bearing these superior qualities squared with the eugenicists' claim that all human qualities, good and bad, were genetic, inherited from your forbears. For those who rose from humble, undistinguished beginnings to the top of the heap, where did the superior genes come from, and why had they not emerged before? Galton was content to trace eminent men like himself to their illustrious ancestry. But explanations that relied on hereditary upper-class origins, with which some British eugenicists concurred, would not do for newly arrived, or second-generation, business leaders and professionals in Britain, and still less so in the U.S. If superior genes were inherited, why did each self-made man emerge when he did, and not in an earlier generation? Social factors —i.e., the social environment—had been summarily dismissed by the eugenicists as not having anything to do with forming the unfit. Yet if they ruled out environmental factors (which had of course changed markedly in the nineteenth century) to explain the rise of new elites, their own rise to prominence was logically inexplicable. Cognitive dissonance served them well. The eugenic discourse of record ascribed the human condition to "genes"; eugenic discourse in practice bent to conform to its own social and political agenda.

Drawing selectively on evolutionary progress, positivist science, and the privileged place of biology in the nineteenth-century scientific hierarchy, eugenic perfectibility discourse was racist, elitist, ethnocentric, and patriarchal. The discourse intensified patterns of dominance and subordination in Western dualism, the ideal superior Self being thrown into sharp relief by the inferior Other. Biology and the new science of genetics became the tools to "mark" imperfect bodies, to "imprint" the Other, and to identify the worthy elite. These disciplinary tools were to be applied through reproduction. In linking science, medicine, and technology to procreation, eugenics anchored perfectibility discourse to a realm of practice absent from earlier articulations of the dream. Upending the dream, the eugenicists' attempts at reproductive control signaled the rebirth of the eighteenth-century vision of individual human perfectibility, but now as the dream of a purified race.

The racist rhetoric of mainline eugenics met its end with the Holocaust. Abandoning the language of racial inferiority and superiority, eugenic leaders after the war returned to the individual, speaking now of "improvement," of *individual* improvement. The dissent from eugenic racism that had begun in the '20s and '30s among a number of respected scientists, who still identified as eugenicists, was markedly strengthened by the 1940s. Yet the old ideas died hard. As mid-century approached, life scientists from the prewar period continued to reflect the elitist, ethnocentric, and patriarchal values of their professional and cultural milieu, maintaining faith in evolutionary progress and in the role of biological science in achieving such progress. Loftier in tone and more individually oriented, perfectibility discourse at mid-century would continue to look to science to define the human ideal, and to view control of human reproduction as the means to direct the character and course of human evolution.

THREE

Reformed Eugenics and Medical Genetics

By mid-twentieth century, eugenic discourse had shed its racist rhetoric and supporting genetic justification, thanks in part to evolutionary biologists and the realities of a post-Holocaust world. The movement gained a new respectability and was recast in positive terms, as seeking to improve the entire gene pool and de-emphasizing the coercive measures central to the old eugenics. A reformed eugenics rediscovered the role of the environment, which was joined to biology to bring evolution back into perfectibility discourse. But perfectibility discourse, as redefined by the scientists and reformed eugenicists, still sought to use genetics to control procreation, now extended to control of cultural evolution. The new eugenic rhetoric, however, had little connection to medical practice. It was not until medical genetics developed as a clinical specialty in the late 1950s, providing physicians with new tools to identify and help prevent disease, that the door opened to introduce eugenics into reproductive practice. But, by the 1960s, a new generation of doctors did not have a eugenic agenda. The irony was that, just as even a reformed eugenics lost its following, reproductive medical practice gained the tools to mark and weed out the imperfect, according to medically defined criteria. Medical practice was poised to recast perfectibility discourse as a discourse of negative eugenics.

Reconnecting with the Environment and Evolution

The move among life scientists to question the racism and uses of science of mainstream eugenics and to seek to redirect the movement began in the period between the wars. In 1939, on the eve of World War II, 23 distinguished scientists meeting in Edinburgh issued the "Geneticists' Manifesto," written primarily by geneticist H. J. Muller,[1] in which they repudiated the concept of "pure races," the Nazi excesses perpetrated in its name, and the uses of genetics that gave "scientific" support for such beliefs. Yet, as Kenneth Ludmerer notes, even as these denunciations were made, "most geneticists did not denounce the eugenic ideal of working for the genetic improvement of mankind," Diane Paul noting that the "central point of the statement . . . was that the genetic improvement of mankind depends on a radical change in social conditions."[2] In the 1920s, one of the signatories, British biologist J. B. S. Haldane, and Muller had each proposed ideal future societies in which biology has perfected eugenic selection. Haldane's *Daedalus,* published in 1924, envisioned a society 150 years hence in which eugenic selection is achieved through ectogenesis: removing and keeping alive the ovaries from selected women, fertilizing the eggs, and growing the embryos for the requisite nine months' gestation. Projecting the method's first success by 1951, Haldane praised subsequent results of eugenic selection.

> The small proportion of men and women who are selected as ancestors for the next generation are so undoubtedly superior to the average that the advance in each generation in any single respect, from the increased output of first-class music to the decreased convictions for theft, is very startling.[3]

Opting for gestation the usual way, Muller proposed using artificial insemination to create his vision of a eugenically selected world populated with "admirable men." In *Out of the Night,* the 1935 published version of lectures presented in the 1920s, Muller predicted that

> in the course of a paltry century or two . . . it would be possible for the majority of the population to become of the innate quality of such men as Lenin, Newton, Leonardo, Pasteur, Beethoven, Omar Khayyam, Pushkin, Sun Yat-sen . . . or even to possess their faculties combined.[4]

Even though Muller said he purposely included "men" of "different fields and races," and professed to be a feminist, notably absent from his list are Blacks, or women of any race. Observes Kevles, for Muller women's role is "little more than that of conceptual vessels for the sperm of admirable men."[5] In Haldane's vision women lose all power over their bodies, including any right to experience bearing children or to nurture them.[6] Whether gestation was to continue *in utero,* as Muller assumed, or via Haldane's "external" method, woman's role was that of body, a procreative Other. Both scenarios projected a masculinized view of power, using science and technology to control the natural world, including life processes.

The attribute most highly prized by Muller and Haldane—as by most other eugenicists—was mind, a male mind of science and intellect. For Haldane, the male scientist, having freed himself from the womb, is close to achieving a disembodied procreation. In his future, procreative power is usurped by a bizarre, masculinized, yet asexual biology, the ascendant science of the age. The mythic Daedalus is biologist supreme, who is both hero and eugenic ideal.[7] In projecting a positive ideal, Muller's and Haldane's forays into the future upended the negative eugenics of would-be biological engineers Davenport and Pearson.[8] Yet, critically, control was paramount as they kept alive an age-old dream of scientifically controlled procreation, now for eugenic ends. When evolutionary biologists[9] rejoined biology to the environment in the postwar period, the control they desired was explicitly extended to cultural evolution.

Meeting in Chicago in 1959 to pay tribute to Darwin on the hundredth anniversary of the publication of *The Origin of Species,* 46 distinguished scientists sought to refashion evolutionary goals in light of the modern synthesis. The participants constituted a "Who's Who" of evolutionary thinkers in the life sciences, and most had made their mark in the period between the two world wars—some even before—and the years immediately after.[10] From prestigious institutions, they were North American or Western European in origin, or by training, acculturation, or place of research.[11]

Reintroducing the environment into evolutionary thought, from which it had been summarily banished by mainstream eugenics,[12] they sought to demonstrate both the past and future roles of culture in progressive evolution. Sir Julian Huxley's convocation address, "The Evolutionary Vision,"[13] built on his *Modern Synthesis,* which was first published in 1942. He held that throughout evolutionary history biology and environment had interacted to change and improve species.[14] Biological evolution, however, had reached its zenith in the human animal, who then created human culture. Henceforth, human progress would depend on cultural or "psychosocial" evolution.[15] Although some Huxley colleagues disagreed with him about this break between biological and cultural evolution,[16] there was little disagreement on one point: it was time for that evolution to come firmly under human control. Natural selection must give way to artificial selection. Although science was the means, the discourse turned on culture.

Their view of "culture" linked these scientists to the species hierarchies of the past, yet outlined a new role for them. Like evolutionary thinkers before them, both pre- and post-Darwinian, scientists at the Darwin Centennial, asking how human beings differed from other animals, placed humans at the top of an evolutionary hierarchy. This was true no matter how branched and non-hierarchic some believed the earlier stages of evolution to have been. According to Huxley, humans were the latest and highest "dominant type" to have evolved. Arising through "successive patterns of successful organization," human dominance therefore resulted from evolutionary progress itself.[17] "Man" had "now become a trustee of evolution" on whom future progress depended.[18] For anthropologist Gaylord Simpson, an "anthropocentric" view was necessary because "man," dominant and the "highest animal," practices a new kind of evolution: a transmission of learning, or "societal" evolution.[19] For geneticist Theodosius Dobzhansky, human beings represented the highest phase of evolution; "man" was the "spiritual center" of the universe, knowing change and directing it.[20] "Science," wrote Dobzhansky, "should be anthropocentric, that is, relevant to man."[21]

Ascribing the top spot in the evolutionary hierarchy to humans, evolutionary scientists at mid-century also subscribed to the view that human intelligence, or mind, set the human animal apart from, and above, other animals.[22] It was unique in humans and, according to Huxley, the inevitable outcome of evolution.

> The last step yet taken in evolutionary progress, and the only one to hold out the promise of unlimited (or indeed of any further) progress . . . is the degree of intelligence which involves true speech and conceptual thought: and it is found exclusively in man. . . . Conceptual thought is not merely found exclusively in man: it could not have been evolved on earth except in man.[23]

It was not only the particular kind of intelligence that humans possessed that was so important, but also what they did with it. The human mind created "a succession of successful idea-systems" that utilized and stored experience. Termed "psychosocial evolution," this combined cultural and mental evolution carried the species forward and ensured continued human dominance. Simpson termed the process the transmission of acquired characteristics, that is, of knowledge through language to create societal evolution. Although human beings arose partly as an evolutionary accident, the "result is the most highly endowed organization of matter that has yet appeared on earth—and we certainly have no good reason to believe there is any higher in the universe." No other being can arise who can "compete with man in intelligence, socialization, and other unique characteristics . . . as long as man does exist in fact."[24]

The "idea-systems" the evolutionary scientists called on traced their lineage to the Enlightenment, the scientific revolution, and the earlier and classical civilizations that had preceded their own. This cultural legacy, epitomized in Robert Hutchins's "Great Books" curriculum, then in its heyday,[25] was now threatened. Its future, according to the evolutionary biologists, was tenuous indeed.

Although purposeless and unplanned, biological evolution was progressive. Recalling Darwin's view that each creature tends to become more and more improved in relation to conditions, leading to gradual advancement, Huxley maintained that dominant types evolved by developing characteristics that gave them greater control over the environment and greater independence of changes occurring in it.[26] But, he argued, this kind of unplanned, yet progressive, evolution had run its course. "One of the concomitants of organic progress has been the progressive cutting down of the possible modes of further progress, until now, after a thousand or fifteen hundred million years of evolution, progress hangs but on a single thread. That thread is human germ-plasm."[27]

The reproduction of human germ-plasm therefore must be directed and controlled. A blind natural selection must give way, wrote Huxley, to a selection that is "conscious, purposeful and planned."[28] In other words, to artificial selection. According to Dobzhansky, natural selection increases Darwinian fitness, but "not necessarily fitness for social progress." Because of the weakening of natural selection and the need to improve human genetic endowment, biological evolution needs to be managed and directed.[29] At this point, in the name of progressive cultural improvement, the discourse of positive eugenics, as well as of negative eugenics, was recast into the language of the new evolutionary science. Argued H. J. Muller, although cultural and biological evolution might have interacted successfully in the past to select and improve the species, natural selection was now "dysgenic." For humans, the feedback between genetics and culture had become negative.[30] Drawing on Muller, Huxley maintained that differential reproduction of the "less favoured classes," medical advances allowing "genetically defective human beings to survive and reproduce," and atomic explosions causing mutations all illustrated how organized civilization had caused genetic transformation to become regressive. Culture itself was now working against genetic improvement.[31] Categories explicitly singled out by race, ethnicity, class, or moral worth could no longer be blamed solely on faulty germ-plasm. Rather, the procreative habits of the "less favoured classes," while still disapproved of, were but some of a number of sociocultural factors that were out of control. Science, biological science, would restore that control.

Calling for nothing less than a scientifically controlled biological and genetic evolution, evolutionary scientists followed in the positivist tradition that past as well as future progress depended on scientific knowledge. Modern evolutionists described culture and civilization as scientifically defined and scientifically based. Huxley sought to bring science and the scientific method to bear on psychosocial evolution. "Man must take a scientific look at his values, at his ethics, at his art and aesthetics, at his social and economic organization, and at his religion. . . . Above all, . . . [he must] take a scientific look at the historical process in general . . . [seeing it as begun with] biological evolution."[32] Cultural evolution, therefore, was not only a scientific phenomenon. It was necessarily grounded in the science that had the most power to explain current and future human evolution: biology. In this biologically reductionist mode of thinking, despite the invocation of "culture," human improvement could be reduced to genes, and their manipulation.

Muller's *Out of the Night* had proposed using the sperm of "great men" to advance the human gene pool and prevent further genetic deterioration. Although his program was one of positive eugenics—indeed, he opposed negative eugenics—it rested on a decidedly negative analysis of what was happening to the human gene pool. A Nobel prize winner for his work on mutations, Muller had coined the term "genetic load." In his 1949 presidential address to the American Society of Human Genetics, which he had co-founded, Muller declared the human species in biological decline because genetic mutations were now outrunning "genetic deaths." In the past, mutations—occurring in about 20 percent of genes in each generation and mostly detrimental—had died off with those carrying them. The equilibrium allowed the species to survive. But, in recent years, each step in saving lives through medical science and technology has reduced "genetic deaths" and increased the "genetic load," with each mutation surviving and continuing into succeeding generations. Muller predicted that, if no action were taken, in a few million years humans would be "genetic monstrosities," a race of mutants entirely supported by medical technology. Environmental techniques alone would not halt this decline. Hence his proposals for artificial insemination as well as yet-to-be-invented reproductive technologies that sound far less fanciful today.[33]

Although Muller sought so-called positive rather than negative measures to arrest genetic decline,[34] others used his theories of genetic load to support measures to curb further survival of defective genes and "defectives." Huxley, for example, although he found negative eugenics of "minor evolutionary importance," strongly urged that we "reduce the reproduction rate of genetically defective individuals." The "human species is threatened with genetic deterioration, and unless this load of defects is reduced, positive eugenics cannot be successfully implemented." Among the measures he proposed were voluntary sterilization and, especially for the "social problem group," development of effective contraception, preferably to be administered through compulsory injection.[35]

Dobzhansky expressed such concerns as well. To achieve genetic equilibrium, he argued, harmful genes must be eliminated by selection, entailing a 20 percent genetic death rate in each generation. He did not mean deaths of human beings, speaking instead of *genetic elimination,* that is, eliminating harmful genes before conception. He sought to persuade those with "serious hereditary defects . . . to refrain from reproducing their kind." If "they are not mentally competent to reach a decision, their segregation or sterilization is justified."[36] Geneticist James Crow, arguing that mutations had to stop if genetic deterioration was to be halted, stated that the "ideal mutation rate . . . is zero." There was, he suggested, sufficient genetic variability in the species for human evolution to continue into the foreseeable future, with enough combinations to produce a Shakespeare, Newton, or Mozart.[37]

Where the old eugenics had been concerned with "race degeneracy," fastening on a White North American–North European elite, these scientists feared the genetic deterioration of the entire human species. Although they had a clear sense of sociocultural hierarchies and the relative worth of human germ-plasms, mid-century geneticists pointed out that harmful mutations ranged throughout populations. All of us harbor some "bad" genes. But they also saw nothing amiss in focusing genetic research on differentiating bad and good genes—isolating the bad ones was still the easier proposition—and in supporting measures to arrest the bad and promote the good. Here was eugenics by other means.

What had changed was the structuring of the arguments and thus the language of perfectibility discourse. Eugenics was not the problem; rather, the former uses of science and racist language were. The coupling of biology and eugenics had obscured both the need to balance biological and environmental factors, and the values of eugenics. Wrote Dobzhansky,

[T]he eugenical idea has a sound core: human welfare, both with individuals and with societies, is predicated upon the health of the genetic
endowment of human populations. Health and disease, physical and
mental, depend upon heredity as upon environment. . . . [An] appalling
amount of human misery is due to defective heredity.[38]

Muller, who was an early critic of eugenic excesses, pointed out that past
mistakes, which overestimated the speed of genetic processes and under-
estimated the influence of culture, and propounded the "vicious doctrine
of racism," should not throw out the "hard core that is really valid."[39]
Reaffiliating with the eugenics movement, which they had never fully
abandoned, evolutionary biologists lent a reputable scientific imprimatur
to a now reformed movement that would welcome not only the scientists
bearing the new genetics, but also the doctors developing its medical
applications.

Genetics and Medicine: Controlling Hereditary Disease

Up until the 1940s, most American geneticists, shunning human genetics,
concentrated on plants or animals, especially small organisms with short
life spans, such as the fruit fly *Drosophila*.[40] When human genetics did
begin to develop as a science in the U.S. after World War II, it grew rapidly,
becoming a "flourishing field" by 1961.[41] Contributing to this rapid rise
were the increasing involvement of doctors and the emergence of the
science and profession of medical genetics.

The old eugenics movement had tried to woo the medical profession.
But physicians sympathetic to eugenics were attracted to it as a social
movement rather than as a science. Nor were eugenicists helped by those
who criticized doctors for ill-serving the "race" by enabling mentally and
physically unsound persons to survive. A brief and earlier interest in eugenics by medical societies had ended by the 1920s.[42] In the 1930s, Madge
Thurlow Macklin, a physician who taught histology and embryology at
the Medical School of the University of West Ontario, tried to revive this
medical interest. Speaking at the Third International Congress of Eugenics, she urged that training in genetics and eugenics be incorporated
into the medical school curriculum.[43] Further pleas came from medical
professionals in the late '30s and early '40s, still from a eugenic perspective.
Haven Emerson, of the DeLamar Institute of Public Health at Columbia
University's College of Physicians and Surgeons, proposed a eugenics program for the medical profession to include training for genetic counseling,
use of family pedigrees, and health examinations for marriage and parent-

hood. Using the terms "preventive medicine" and "pre-conceptional care," he sought to reverse the trend of "levelling *down*" and eventually "*out*"; he wanted to bring human beings closer to "visionary perfection."[44] Research geneticist Morton Schweitzer at Cornell Medical College, cautioning that medical genetics was not yet developed enough to provide an adequate scientific basis for a "concrete program of eugenic control," urged that medical genetics be "an important ingredient" in the physician's training for understanding and counseling about hereditary diseases.[45]

But for genetics to be meaningful to physicians, it had to speak to the practical, professional aim of treating disease. In the 1930s physicians were concerned with environmentally caused diseases, that is, those due to bacteria or viruses, parasites, or toxins of various kinds, such as tuberculosis, pneumonia, influenza, and enteritis. Consequently, physicians' research interests lay in toxicology, parasitology, and bacteriology. As long as conditions defined as hereditary seemed rare and were apparently incurable, and especially since few severely affected individuals survived for long, physicians found genetics of little relevance for their professional skills.[46] But the 1930s also brought interest in the growing concept of "preventive medicine." At the same time, in the '30s and '40s research in human genetics began to discover the genetic foundations of some hereditary diseases, revealing the Mendelian pattern of the inheritance of Tay-Sachs disease and finding that phenylketonuria (PKU) was genetically determined and caused by a missing enzyme. Medical responses followed. A simple test of newborns for PKU was devised, along with a dietary remedy. Testing newborns for PKU soon was routine; a once fatal disease became controllable. Although Tay-Sachs even now remains incurable and brings early death, discovering how it was inherited allowed physicians to begin to identify its carriers and to associate them with specific populations. Physicians could now predict the odds of its occurrence and, in lieu of cure or treatment, could offer counsel. Genetics had become relevant for medical practice.[47] Even if they could not cure a given hereditary disease—as was usually the case—physicians could use their new and growing knowledge of genetic inheritance to prevent or reduce its occurrence.

Increasingly, preventive action involved genetic counseling, a further reason for physicians to be trained in human genetics. By the early 1950s, more than half of U.S. medical schools included human genetics in the curriculum.[48] "[A] veritable explosion occurred in clinical genetics" from 1958 on, as physicians became involved in research on human genetic diseases.[49] Medical genetics became a field in its own right, its purpose "to learn to control all pathological conditions which are caused by changes in the molecular arrangement of normal genes."[50] The *American Journal of Medical Genetics* appeared in 1977, marking the full recognition of the discipline.[51]

Medical genetics developed as a clinical specialty within reproductive medicine, in a one-on-one setting between doctor and patient. The practice of genetic counseling reemerged in this setting. As genetic counseling followed a contradictory path—breaking from, yet also echoing, its early eugenic roots—perfectibility discourse would be significantly shaped at mid-century and in the decades to follow. The discourse would come to reflect a changed balance of private aims, social concerns, and ideology.

In the clinical setting of reproductive medicine, the decision to bear or not bear a child with a possible birth defect was individual, private, involving only the physician and the parent-patient(s). Although eugenicists had wooed doctors earlier, when the linkup of medicine and genetics finally came it arose out of the professional interests and requirements of physicians themselves. For the physician who focused on the individual patient, the broad sociocultural goals of the evolutionary biologists did not speak to immediate needs and tasks. Yet in the transition period, as doctors became more involved with genetics and hereditary disease and engaged in genetic counseling, the reformulated eugenic agenda continued to play a part in the emerging practice of genetically oriented reproductive medicine.

When genetic counseling developed into a profession in the 1970s and '80s, it called for a "non-directive" model. The counselor meeting with a would-be parent or parents was to avoid "advice" that followed a eugenic, or any other, rationale. But when physicians started to counsel patients in the late '50s and the 1960s they entered a practice derived from and steeped in the eugenics movement. Genetic counseling was then often explicitly directive, with a eugenic aim.[52] Originally called "heredity counseling," it was practiced at "heredity clinics," which were started in the 1940s. The first was established by zoologist Lee R. Dice at the University of Michigan in 1940, the next shortly after at the Dight Institute at the University of Minnesota, headed by geneticist Sheldon Reed. Generally attached to university-based institutes or medical schools, these clinics were usually headed by geneticists who held Ph.D.s and were based in the research laboratory. The roots of these clinics went back still further. In the first decades of the century the Eugenics Records Office at Cold Spring Harbor had "offered premarital, preconception, and postconception heredity counseling" that was "highly directive . . . as to whether or not to marry or reproduce."[53] Although by the 1930s advocates of heredity counseling and medical applications of human genetics had dissociated themselves from this old eugenics model, adopting a "new" or "renovated" eugenics,[54] their approach remained tied to eugenic goals. Their underlying, but explicit, concern was to reduce the incidence of bad genes and increase that of desirable ones. The heredity clinics they established and worked in, starting in the 1940s, reflected this approach and these aims.

In his presidential address to the American Society of Human Genetics in 1952, Lee Dice discussed the importance of heredity clinics in performing a public service for families carrying genetic defects. Although he held that the geneticist-counselor should not advise someone to conceive a child or not (this was well before prenatal testing), Dice clearly indicated that the purpose of counseling was to present probabilities, to provide information that would lead affected individuals, i.e., those known to carry (or suspected of carrying) a hereditary condition, to choose not to have children. Stressing voluntary measures and roundly condemning compulsion, "except only in the most extreme cases of irresponsibility," Dice saw the clinics as the way to halt genetic deterioration in a democratic society. He also wanted attention paid to good hereditary traits, although these were harder to ascertain. To these eugenic ends, he called for geneticists to work with physicians and for physicians to be trained in human genetics.[55] Moderate in tone, and rejecting the old agenda, Dice reflected the newly defined eugenic goals of heredity clinics and the counseling to be practiced in them. This was the climate in which physicians began to practice genetic counseling in the 1950s.

Physicians' individual, patient-oriented approach would not be fully separated from the societal, eugenic concerns of research geneticists until genetic counseling came under control of the medical profession, later in the 1960s. In the transition period, when divisions between the practitioner and researcher were far less sharp, medical doctors welcomed the clinics and the growth of genetic counseling within a eugenic framework. Counseling patients about hereditary disease as a form of preventive medicine appeared compatible with a reformed eugenics.[56] Like the evolutionary biologists whose support helped to legitimize the reconstituted movement, medical professionals lent credence, by their involvement, to the perfectibility discourse of the "new eugenics" movement.

"Reformed Eugenics": Attempted Synthesis with Medicine

After World War II, the mainstream eugenics movement reconstituted itself as "reformed" eugenics, deploring and repudiating "pure race" theories, the Nazi extremes, and the coercive character of former eugenic programs. As reflected especially in the pages of the *Eugenics Quarterly*, successor to the *Eugenical News,* and in other writings of American Eugenics Society leaders, positive eugenics translated into encouraging those with "socially desirable traits" to choose to have large families, while negative eugenics focused on fostering genetic research to learn more about "dangerous defects." The revised creed now emphasized an individual approach, education, and an informed public opinion. Although the accent was on voluntary compliance, sterilization laws and segregation for those too unfit to understand the choices involved were still endorsed.[57]

Most important, as changes occurred in evolutionary biology, and as developments in genetics and medicine accelerated, the new eugenics became both more scientifically and more medically oriented. In the 1950s, the *Eugenics Quarterly,* increasingly began to reflect the society's revised aims to "promote research," "provide authoritative information," and "explore scientific applications of knowledge" about human heredity.[58] An article charting recent developments in cytogenetics, summing up the state of the art, was typical when it was published in the March 1961 issue.[59] Not the least factor explaining the appearance of such articles in the *Eugenics Quarterly*'s pages was the direct involvement of distinguished biological scientists in the society. Theodosius Dobzhansky, one of these contributors, became a member of the board of directors of the American Eugenics Society in 1964, and its chairman in 1969; geneticist F. Clark Fraser joined the board in 1967, as did Dobzhansky's student Richard C. Lewontin (who would later become a sharp critic of the social uses of genetic research). Much of the journal was increasingly devoted to demographics and population genetics.[60]

But if the new eugenics was to have any practical impact, it needed not only the scientists, but also the doctors. Eugenics leaders were quick to bless the marriage of medicine and genetics and to welcome the practice of medical genetics into the fold. A lead editorial in the *Eugenics Quarterly* in 1954 commended the "new appreciation by the medical profession of the importance of hereditary factors in disease and defect," adding that the "base for negative eugenics is being laid by a group of medical geneticists here and in other countries." Applying medical genetics to this end rested on the personal point of contact of physician with patient, and the power the physician could wield. Although the society "may help" spur practical applications by encouraging research and supporting heredity clinics, the editorial continued, "the attitude of the doctor will be the determining factor. . . . [E]ugenic propaganda can be useful chiefly in promoting public support of measures generally accepted by leaders of the medical profession."[61] Emphasizing counseling was an appropriate way to marshal physician support essential to furthering eugenic goals.

A "Heredity Counseling" section became a regular feature in the *Eugenics Quarterly,* to which both doctors and research geneticists contributed. One such contributor was C. Nash Herndon, president of the American Eugenics Society and both an M.D. and a geneticist on the staff of the Bowman Gray School of Medicine in Tennessee. Bowman Gray was the first medical school in the country to offer a course in human genetics, in the 1930s. Wrote Herndon in 1955, the counselor must bear in mind the "possible eugenic or dysgenic effect of any advice he may give." While it is up to the "parties concerned, assuming their mental competence," to decide whether to limit their families, given the possibility of "genetic abnormality," it should be "the responsibility of the . . . counselor to encourage reproduction in families possessed of a high order of socially valuable characteristics."[62]

The American Eugenics Society was now to pin its hopes for the genetic improvement of society at the level of individuals and families. Given the realities of medical genetics and reproductive medicine, eugenics leaders had little choice but to endorse an individual approach. As early as 1951, the movement's leading spokesman, Frederick Osborn, had urged an individual focus when applying genetic research.[63] Eugenicists sought to provide the framework and the terrain on which an individual patient-oriented reproductive medicine and the socially oriented discourse of research geneticists and evolutionary biologists could meet.

At a symposium on heredity counseling at the New York Academy of Sciences in 1957, the American Eugenics Society attempted to mesh these two levels of discourse, the individual and the social. Participants in the morning session, "Genetics in Medical Practice," were doctors (including the well-known geneticist Victor McKusick of Johns Hopkins Hospital), dentists, and two nurses (the only women panelists). The afternoon panel, "Heredity Counseling," included both research scientists and doctors prominent in the field of genetics, most of whom were in some way engaged in genetic counseling. Among them were, for example, Ph.D. Lee Dice and M.D. and geneticist James Neel from the University of Michigan, M.D. and geneticist Herndon from Bowman Gray, M.D. and geneticist F. Clark Fraser from McGill University in Montreal, and Ph.D. Sheldon Reed from the University of Minnesota. Given the practical professional orientation of participants in both morning and afternoon sessions, their focus on specifics rather than the broadly social was to be expected. They were concerned with specialized topics and issues, with the relationship between patient and the doctor or counselor, and their problems. Topics such as genetic screening programs targeting specific populations were discussed in terms of public health measures and health care delivery to families and individuals, not as eugenic goals. The counselor was not to allow personal views about eugenics to influence the patient, even at the risk of the patient's choice increasing the frequency of a disease-causing gene. It was left to the Eugenics Society's Frederick Osborn, who was neither doctor nor scientist, nor a panelist, to reiterate at the close of the symposium hopes for a more explicit eugenic agenda for the society. But it was necessary to wait. "Otherwise, we would again do as eugenics did 30 or 40 years ago, espouse things which were not justified, and would turn public opinion back against eugenics."[64] Although the practicing research scientists and medical professionals at this symposium may have shared such broad eugenic aims, they were not relevant to their work. Osborn's remarks did not speak to medical practice.

The symposium was prophetic. Eugenicists' attempt to synthesize the discourse of the new eugenics with the practice of medicine was destined to fail. But why? Osborn's brand of perfectibility discourse was hardly dead. Race improvement and other eugenic social goals were still shared by many research scientists and physicians involved at the time. But the C. Nash Herndons were a dying breed. The research scientist and physician— sometimes combined in one person—who shared eugenic aims would soon belong to the past. So, too, would the evolutionary biologists with whom early advocates of medical genetics and genetic counseling shared belief in a eugenics agenda. As a newer group of research scientists and physicians emerged in the 1960s, their practice and functions diverged, separating them from each other as well as from commitments to eu-genics. As historian Kenneth Ludmerer has pointed out, by 1970 physi-cians engaged in genetic counseling did not identify as eugenicists.

But generational changes were only one part of the story, reflecting underlying scientific and structural factors that pulled medical genetics and reproductive medicine away from consciously seeking, or even ex-pressing, a eugenic ideology. The rise of medical genetics, along with such discoveries as antibiotics, linked science and medicine still more tightly and highlighted the scientific expertise of the doctor. This new-found expertise helped to legitimate the medical profession's growing control of both genetic counseling and research in medical genetics through the hospital-based setting where both counseling and research took place. Although the research geneticist was of prime importance to the practice of reproductive medicine, "the physician became gate keeper granting entry and co-existence to qualified Ph.D.s whose predecessors pioneered the discipline."[65] The research scientist was increasingly separated from the point of genetic application, from the site of patient care. Power and control passed to the physician. The interests and goals of the practice of medicine became paramount.

That interest focused on the patient, not on some vague societal ends. This was perhaps the most critical factor in dooming the eugenicists' attempt to further their social goals through medical practice.[66] Considering long-range dysgenic or eugenic effects was incompatible with the individualized patient-care setting; the physician's focus was necessarily immediate, not long-term. Equally important—later to become even more so as technologies multiplied medical possibilities—was the incompatibility of such eugenic concerns with the goals of medicine itself, which are to treat and cure disease. Physicians could not yet predict whether a child would be born with a genetic disease beyond offering statistical probabilities. But could eugenicists reasonably expect, in the name of decreasing the "genetic load," that a physician would deny treatment to an affected child once born? (Even today, in the highly charged debates about treating severely deformed newborns, opponents tend to fasten on such issues as the child's and family's "quality of life," not on so-called dysgenic effects.) In the 1960s, the changing practice of reproductive medicine had little room for or inclination toward a conscious eugenic agenda.

And yet the very practice that denied a forum to the new eugenics would itself create the conditions in which to frame a eugenics from that practice. As genetics-based medicine and accompanying technologies would become increasingly able to identify and prevent the birth of "defective" individuals, reproductive medicine would begin to "mark" defectives unworthy to survive. The evolutionary biologist and research scientist had bequeathed to reproductive medicine a legacy that would allow a new, medically based eugenics to emerge.

Evolutionary Biologists and the Technological Dream: The Legacy

If evolutionary biologists and research geneticists were unable, along with lay leaders of the eugenics movement, to implement their particular prescriptions for positive eugenics, their thinking was not without importance or influence. At mid-century they represented a rearticulation of the technological dream—the Enlightenment dream linking science, medicine, and human perfectibility. Rescuing human genetics from the distortions of mainline eugenics and restoring a role for environment in evolutionary theory, they nevertheless reaffirmed the critical importance of biology, and especially genetics, for furthering human progress. That the vision was optimistic tied it to the Enlightenment and the tradition of progressive thought. But that it was set against the threat of genetic deterioration revealed continuities with the race degeneracy theories of mainline eugenics. Departing from the moralistic fervor of the old eugenics as well, the perfectibility discourse of evolutionary biology nevertheless drew distinctions along lines of cultural superiority and inferiority that reflected a set of moral, class, and ethnic- and race-based values.[67] The evolutionary biologists' most important legacy for reproductive medicine lay in the level of scientific analysis and scientific and technological projections, in their commitment to social control of reproduction, and in the sociocultural values that they sought to perpetuate.

The concept of "genetic load," which was central to their discourse, was the work of honored and innovative scientists. Breakthrough research of geneticists such as H. J. Muller on genetic mutations, for example, pioneered the way for research biologists. Their work continues to be recognized and respected in scientific annals to this day. In projecting the deterioration of the human gene pool, evolutionary biologists thus rested their case on a level of scientific analysis far firmer than that which had characterized the old eugenics. But the respect their work was accorded reinforced a continuing tendency to explain almost all human phenomena scientifically, especially through biology. And if biology explained the human condition, it could also be called upon to change it. As they tied biology to human cultural improvement, evolutionary biologists were very much the descendants of the reductive eugenics they had criticized.[68] Science was the key to the future. Projecting new and further uses for science, and for technology, they signaled medicine's growing reliance on the scientific and technological fix. Muller, who had proposed using the sperm of great men to fill the world with superior individuals, in the 1930s also imagined a variety of reproductive techniques that would allow a mature or fertilized egg to be transplanted from one female to the womb of another, or even to that of an animal, and have it develop.[69] And while Muller worried that human beings could become a race of mutants entirely supported by medical technology if genetic deterioration continued unabated, Dobzhansky welcomed the use of technology to manage genetic defects. Citing the use of insulin to treat diabetes successfully—thus possibly increasing the incidence of the disease—he argued that we should accept such technological dependence as part of living in a scientific and industrialized society. "The remedy for our genetic dependence on technology," wrote Dobzhansky in 1962, "is more, not less, technology." He also speculated that some day a method might be "discovered to induce directed mutations, i.e., to change specific genes in desired ways." (This was nine years after the DNA code had been broken in 1953.) Predicting what is now known as germ-line and somatic cell gene therapy (see chapter four), he explained that this "would enable one to alter certain genes in the sex cells or in the body cells, and thus 'cure' hereditary diseases by removing their causes."[70] Seeking technological ways to curb procreation among "social problem" groups, Julian Huxley foretold the development of injectable and implantable contraceptives, such as Depo-Provera and Norplant.

These scientists expected that scientific and technological advances in human and medical genetics would further their eugenic aims through bringing control over procreation. However, they were not situated to exercise this control. The physicians who by the 1960s were incorporating medical genetics into their reproductive practice were. Research geneticists and evolutionary biologists bequeathed to the medical profession a greatly enhanced potential to direct reproductive outcomes, and therefore the potential to shape the contours of future generations. As opportunities to apply genetic knowledge to control procreation slipped away from research geneticists in the heredity clinics, their research enabled physicians to increase *their* control over human reproduction. But it was the evolutionary biologists, more than the research geneticists in the clinics, who envisioned the potential of reproductive science and technology to unlock the genetic keys to specific inheritable conditions, and thus to name, rank, alter, or eliminate them. With the joining of medical genetics and reproductive medical practice in the 1960s, perfectibility discourse was set to be transformed into a medically defined, but socially constructed, hierarchy of acceptable and unacceptable human traits. More powerful than the discourse of the evolutionary biologists and research geneticists because it was rooted in practice, the new discourse signaled the technological birth of the "perfect child."

PART TWO

FRAMING THE DISCOURSE OF

THE PERFECT CHILD

FOUR

The Tools

In late 1955, medical researchers working independently in four different cities—Copenhagen, New York, Minneapolis, and Jerusalem—successfully determined fetal sex by testing cells obtained from the amniotic fluid of pregnant women. A decade later physicians in Britain succeeded in culturing such cells; the availability of more cells to be analyzed spurred the development of more prenatal tests for possible disorders. By the late 1960s, physicians had developed and refined the procedure that became known as amniocentesis. Additional prenatal tests and screens soon followed, and were integrated into established reproductive medical practice.

In parallel development came the unlocking of the genetic code of DNA in 1953. Moving swiftly over the next half century, genetic research identified and located the chromosomal and genetic origins of increasing numbers of human traits and disorders. The completion of the sequencing of the human genome in 2003—ahead of schedule—gave further momentum to molecular biology and efforts to identify and locate genes and gene patterns.

Genetics and prenatal diagnosis were joined when physicians, who initially found genetic research of little relevance to their practice, saw that genetics could reveal useful information about inherited disorders and possibly help physicians prevent them from recurring. At first, physicians could only use family inheritance patterns to calculate the probability that a given couple would conceive a child with a given disorder, the inquiry often triggered by the birth of an affected child. The only way to prevent further cases was to avoid having more children. The development of prenatal diagnosis dramatically changed these possibilities, shifting prevention from before conception to after it. No longer limited to screening parents who were possible carriers, physicians could now focus on the fetus to discover whether the fetus actually showed the trait. A whole new dimension was added to "preventive medicine": the chance to detect a disorder *after* the fetus was conceived and possibly prevent its birth. Together, genetic science and prenatal diagnosis technologies provided the indispensable initial tools with which reproductive medical practice could mark the imperfect fetus, and so begin to frame the discourse of the perfect child.

Even though the "race" to map and sequence the human genome has had wide media attention, offering lessons in the "new" genetics, popular reporting may confuse rather than instruct. The draft sequence published in 2001 surprised many people with the revelation that the human genome comprises a mere 30,000 to 35,000 genes, rather than the 100,000 or more long held to be the case.[1] Genome experts staged a sweepstakes for guesses at the final number, and in 2003 awarded the prize to a British scientist for his estimate of 27,462, while admitting that the exact number was uncertain and leaving the game open for another five years.[2] Our biology textbooks are barely up to date when published and rapidly become obsolete. Similarly, although prenatal testing and screening are part of public discourse, misconceptions abound, even among women undergoing the procedures. Media hype feeds the confusion, conferring "miracle" status on each scientific or technological discovery. Readers well versed in biology and prenatal diagnosis technologies may want to skim this chapter. But if you would like a primer or review of genetics and prenatal diagnosis technologies, I invite you to read on.

The "New" Genetics—and the Old

Genetic research is currently focused on disorders caused by a single gene. But while there are about four thousand such single-gene disorders, most conditions that have genetic origins (and can thus be inherited) are more complicated. The majority are *polygenic,* that is, due to several genes, and *multi-factorial,* meaning that they are caused by complex combinations of genetic and environmental factors at every stage of the individual's development. This is true of most human traits, not just disorders. Further, the term "genetic disease" tends to be used to describe diagnosable conditions generally, even though some arise from abnormal chromosome arrangements (such as three copies, rather than two, of chromosome 21, indicating Down syndrome) and not from gene irregularity. And then, of course, some human traits and conditions may have little to do with our genes. With these cautions in mind, this genetic primer shows how the "new" molecular genetics rests on the old.

The nucleus of each human cell contains 23 paired chromosomes, for a total of 46. (The exceptions are the egg and sperm cells, each having only a single set of 23.) Packed into each cell are the 30,000 or so genes, distinct units of heredity which constitute the human "genome."[3] Several trillion human body cells each contain this genetic blueprint for the proteins to build a human being. The genes are arranged in specific locations (*loci*) on each chromosome. The unlocking of the genetic code in 1953 revealed that the genetic material was composed of deoxyribonucleic acid (DNA), a macromolecule made up of nucleotides arranged in a long, twisted double strand, or "double helix."[4] Nucleotides consist of a phosphate, a sugar, and one of four bases: A, T, C, and G, which stand for adenine, thymine, cytosine, and guanine, the chemical building blocks necessary for all life. They are arranged in precise sequences, each specifying an amino acid, and each gene consists of thousands of these sequences. The genes in turn instruct the cells to assemble chains of amino acids into proteins. Differences and diversity that occur within and among species come from changes in the sequences of nucleotides through mutation and recombination. There are an estimated three billion nucleotide sequences in the human genome; the Human Genome Project, an international consortium, published the sequence in April 2003.[5] The next and larger task is to apply sequencing to locate genes and identify their functions.

Genes come in pairs called *alleles,* one on each of the two paired chromosomes. One allele is inherited from each parent. If the alleles are identical, the organism is called a *homozygote;* if they are different, it is a *heterozygote.* In a heterozygote, one allele may be dominant, masking the other, recessive, allele. Most genetic disorders are caused by recessive alleles: it takes two, one from each parent, to cause the disorder. The affected offspring inherits the two alleles from parents who are heterozygote, carrying the disorder recessively and termed *carriers.*

When the 23 chromosomes in each parent's reproductive cells, or gametes, come together at fertilization to make up the 46 that constitute the genetic makeup of the new individual, they are at the end of a complex process of rearrangement. In this process, called *meiosis,* the 46 chromosomes in the cells of each parent first duplicate and then divide and reassort twice to produce four mature gametes. Each newly produced gamete, containing 23 chromosomes, will have a random assortment of the parent's chromosomes and alleles. The process is thus critical in determining the new individual's genetic profile. A simple example is the sex chromosome pair. The male has an X and a Y chromosome; the female, two Xs. When the male's X and Y chromosomes reassort during meiosis, approximately half the sperm carry X and half Y. Since the female's egg cells all carry Xs, the X-bearing sperm produce a girl, the Y a boy. Most sorting and pairing, however, is more complex. For example, although genes sort independently in meiosis, genes located on the same chromosome tend to end up in the same gamete: their disposition will depend on where they are on the chromosome and how tightly they are linked.[6] Three things that can take place during meiosis can have critical effects on the hereditary material: crossing over and recombination of alleles in a chromosome, chromosomal aberrations, and gene mutation.[7] Although not all such genetic changes are harmful or disease-bearing—indeed, this is how species change and develop—many are, causing the disorders or "defects" that prenatal testing is concerned with.

Adults can be screened for the presence of a known disease-bearing gene. But since their genes sort randomly in meiosis, only testing the cells of their newly forming offspring can reveal if the gene, or some other chromosomal or genetic anomaly, is present. Prenatal diagnosis uses varying methods developed through genetic and medical research to test fetal (and more recently embryonic) cells for possible genetic disorders. Among the most important of these methods are karyotyping of chromosomal material and several methods of DNA analysis.

KARYOTYPING

A *karyotype* prepares a fetal cell so it can be analyzed. The cell's chromosomal material is dyed and photographed through a microscope, then rearranged so that all 23 chromosome pairs can be displayed and inspected in order, from the largest to the smallest. In addition, chromosome banding and recently developed high-resolution techniques allow pairs and their structures to be compared in minute detail.[8] The deviation most readily apparent is an extra chromosome in a pair, or *trisomy.* Trisomies of chromosomes 13 or 18 result in fetal death at or shortly after birth. Trisomy 21 indicates Down syndrome. The sex chromosome is number 23. In addition to revealing whether the fetus is female (XX) or male (XY), the karyotype can also reveal a discrepancy, such as an extra X in a male fetus

(Klinefelter's syndrome) or a missing X in a female (Turner's syndrome). Chromosome *deletions* can show up on the karyotype as well, indicating loss of a chromosome segment and therefore loss of all or part of a gene. Examples are relatively severe disorders, such as retinoblastoma, a tumor causing blindness, and muscular dystrophy that is X-linked and affects males only. The karyotype can also reveal a chromosomal *translocation*, the permanent transference of a chromosome segment to another chromosome belonging to a different pair. Translocations are fairly easy to spot, starting with testing of the parents' cells. A form of Down syndrome is caused by a translocation, the extra chromosome 21 becoming attached to chromosome 14.

DNA ANALYSIS

DNA analysis involves locating specific genes and identifying the genetic defect or mutation responsible for a disorder. More recently, DNA analysis also may be used for diagnosing chromosomal syndromes. It has become so important in prenatal diagnosis that the annual review issue of the medical journal *Prenatal Diagnosis* in December 1996 was devoted to the subject.[9] The work originally drew on recombinant DNA, or "gene splicing," technology, in which bits of genetic material are removed, spliced into that of another organism, and then replicated or cloned for use or experimentation. This process has aided biochemical analysis in detecting what are known as "inborn errors of metabolism," such as a missing or defective enzyme and a resulting disorder. If the gene product, the defective enzyme, is known, the relevant genes or DNA segments can be cloned, using "gene libraries," and the gene isolated. Newborns are routinely tested for such inborn errors, such as lacking an enzyme for digesting foods essential to life.[10] Among the best known and most prevalent of the conditions which are detected through the gene product, the enzyme, and which can be tested for prenatally are Tay-Sachs disease (a lethal disorder mainly affecting Ashkenazi Jews), galactosemia, and related conditions that interfere with metabolizing sugars.[11]

But the gene products involved in most human genetic disorders have not been identified. Among the newer techniques developed to search for gene loci are linkage analysis, an amplification method, and a fluorescent hybridization technique. The indirect method of linkage analysis, using restriction fragment length polymorphism (RFLP), was developed in the late 1980s. Concentrating on the particular region of a chromosome known to carry the gene, RFLPs are genetic markers that provide the means to track genetic material for links to the gene locus. In 1989, researchers used this method to locate the gene for cystic fibrosis.[12] More recently, the polymerase chain reaction (PCR) technique was developed to aid in molecular diagnosis. It involves amplifying a defined region of a chromosome—replicating it exponentially—using the enzyme DNA polymerase. A variety of testing techniques take "advantage of PCR's exquisite specificity" to create an increasingly sensitive diagnostic tool that can detect a variety of diseases, including cystic fibrosis and sickle cell anemia.[13] PCR is also used to analyze the early embryo. The newest technique, fluorescent in situ hybridization (FISH), allows submicroscopic analysis,[14] and is therefore increasingly used in examining polar bodies in the cells of the "pre-embryo" in preimplantation genetic diagnosis (described later in this chapter). Researchers in the '90s gave much of the credit for the rapid advance of DNA analysis to the progress made in the international project to map and sequence the human genome.[15]

Sequencing the human genome and DNA analysis techniques combine to offer a critical set of tools to carry forward the major job of locating specific genes and identifying their functions, and in particular linking specific genes to particular diseases and conditions. These tools will make it possible to diagnose more conditions prenatally, and therefore will spur the further development and use of prenatal diagnostic procedures.

Prenatal Testing and Screening

Amniocentesis is the oldest prenatal testing procedure and still the one most widely used. Of more recent vintage is chorionic villus sampling (CVS). MSAFP screens maternal blood for alpha-fetoprotein, one of three markers sought by the so-called triple screen. Ultrasound is both a diagnostic tool and a procedural aid. Newer procedures include those that test the embryo prior to its insertion into the womb, such as preimplantation genetic diagnosis, and research to extract fetal cells from the mother's blood for analysis.

AMNIOCENTESIS

The story of amniocentesis starts in the 1950s, when physicians in Denmark, the United States, and Israel successfully identified a fetus's sex from fetal cells in the amniotic fluid withdrawn from a pregnant woman. Since the cells could not yet be cultured, the procedure involved testing the cells for X-chromatin, positive for female, negative for male.[16] The physicians' purpose was medical. The women recruited for the still highly experimental procedure were from families with a history among the males of an X-linked disease, such as hemophilia or muscular dystrophy. The pregnant woman therefore was a likely carrier, who might have already borne one or more affected male children. A male fetus had a 50 percent chance of being affected; a female fetus could be a carrier but would not have the disease. In the research cases reported, the women elected to carry the female fetus to term (though in most cases unsuccessfully) and to abort the male.[17]

The two Danish physicians, Drs. Povl Riis and Fritz Fuchs,[18] who pioneered in this research noted that the procedure could be applied to "certain other severe sex-linked recessive hereditary diseases," but that it was "not restricted to determination of the foetal sex." They predicted in 1960 wider use of cells from amniotic fluid, such as to diagnose "metabolic enzyme defects now known to be the cause of severe disorders." Pointing out that the procedure was highly risky, especially for the fetus, since it "requires puncture of both uterus and the membranes" to obtain the fluid, they cautioned that diagnosis of fetal sex "should not be carried out to satisfy the curiosity of the parents." In fact, they added, "in spite of public interest in the method, we have not had a single request for the procedure out of curiosity."[19]

The next breakthrough in prenatal diagnosis research came in the mid-1960s when British physicians discovered how to culture the fetal cells. Replicating the cells enabled more extensive analysis.[20] Techniques had also been refined. In use by the early 1970s, amniocentesis involved inserting a needle through the pregnant woman's abdomen to draw amniotic fluid, and then culturing and analyzing the fetal cells obtained—a process that took about three weeks.[21] Although in the early trials fluid was drawn at any time between 10 and 36 weeks into the pregnancy (a full-term pregnancy is 40 weeks), 16 weeks became the recommended point, "at which time the ease and safety . . . are maximal."[22] The norm remained between 15 and 17 weeks until the late 1980s, when amniocentesis in the first trimester began to be introduced experimentally, and a time of 11–14 weeks became more common as the '90s advanced.[23] Despite the caveats of some, by the mid-1990s it was reported that "amniocentesis performed at 10–12 weeks is feasible, safe, and easy to perform," and that it "provides a real benefit to the pregnant woman."[24] Earlier amniocentesis reflects a continuing and growing trend toward earlier prenatal diagnosis generally.

When first introduced and practiced, amniocentesis was recommended for what were termed "high-risk" pregnancies. This meant women who had previously borne a child affected with a serious disorder, carriers of recessive traits or of chromosomal translocations likely to produce severe anomalies, parents with a poor reproductive history, and women who had been exposed to substances or environments that could cause mutations. These exposures included viral infections such as rubella (German measles), radiation, and certain drugs.[25] Only a small fraction of pregnancies were "high risk" when the term was defined in this way. Yet doctors in this early period, commenting on the future of amniocentesis, predicted that the number and kinds of disorders that would be able to be diagnosed prenatally would rapidly expand. They were right. Less discussed at the time was the way that the range of detectable conditions was expanding to include the mildest disorder as well as the most severe or fatal, nor how a small "high risk" population would swell to include ever-widening groups of pregnant women deemed "at risk." The use of amniocentesis to diagnose Down syndrome illustrates how the procedures themselves contributed to making prenatal screening and testing a growth industry.

In 1960, a French doctor, Jerome Lejeune, traced the cause of Down syndrome to an extra copy of chromosome 21. That same year, researchers in England and Sweden found that a form of Down syndrome could also be caused by a translocation in a parent's chromosomes. People with Down syndrome "have an increased risk for . . . congenital heart defects, respiratory and hearing problems, Alzheimer's disease, childhood leukemia, and thyroid conditions. . . . [They] experience cognitive delays."[26] As recently as 25 years ago facial features of people with Down syndrome were still infelicitously described as "mongoloid," and because of this the condition was called "mongolism."[27] The overall incidence of Down syndrome is one per 830 live births,[28] but it rises sharply with the mother's age. Although this was noted earlier in the century, it was not until the early 1970s that the age correlation was clearly demonstrated and incorporated as a risk factor for recommending amniocentesis.[29] While the assessed risk of bearing a child with Down syndrome for a 20-year-old woman is one in 1,667, and for a 30-year-old one in 952, the risk rises to one in 378 for a woman of 35, one in 106 for a woman of 40, and to one in 38 for a woman of 45. Down syndrome, however, accounts for only about half of the diagnoses of abnormal chromosomes, only some of which are correlated with age.[30] For the most part, the incidence of these other conditions is lower than that of Down syndrome,[31] and most are far from life-threatening.

The net result of Down syndrome's age correlation was to place all pregnant women over a certain age "at risk." The particular age chosen was originally due as much to the limited availability of the procedure as to medical indications, since the "services had to be prioritized to patients considered to be at the highest risk. Initially," noted Dr. Mark Evans of Wayne State University and his colleagues in 1992, a maternal age of 40 and prior history of a child with a birth defect were picked arbitrarily. As amniocentesis became more popular and the number of physicians and laboratories that could participate in the procedure increased throughout the mid 1970s, the age dropped to 38, and for the past decade it has been hovering at 35.[32]

What is now referred to as "AMA" (advanced maternal age) has become the major indicator for a woman to be recommended for prenatal testing. High risk factors of carrier status, previous birth of an affected child, or family history remain indicators, regardless of age, but they have lost their singular status in relation to the more encompassing, yet less targeted, factor of age. Maternal age became neatly separated from these other high risk factors; a woman over 35 was now deemed at risk *regardless of whether any of the other risk indicators were present*. Discussing the acceptability of various criteria for screening for Down syndrome, a '90s text on prenatal diagnosis states, "Maternal age would be rated as a poor screening test, according to established criteria for judging acceptability, primarily because of its low detection rate. It does, however, have the advantage of being virtually cost free and highly reliable."[33] The introduction of the age criterion, by the late 1970s, was the first major step in expanding prenatal testing to cover a much larger segment of pregnant women.

Because women under 35 bear more children and account for more Down syndrome births than do women over 35, there is some support for lowering the recommended age for amniocentesis still further. Amniocentesis is not without risks, however. Estimates are that one out of every 200 amniocenteses results in miscarriage. The efforts to develop and to use other procedures to reduce the risk of prenatal testing have also served to expand the population subject to testing and screening.

MATERNAL SERUM ALPHA-FETOPROTEIN (MSAFP) SCREENING

In 1972, medical researchers found that measuring the alpha-fetoprotein (AFP) levels in amniotic fluid could reveal neural tube defects (NTDs). The incidence of NTDs in the U.S., which ranges from one in 600 to one in 1,000, "varies markedly," depending on the pregnant woman's ethnic group, geographic location, and socioeconomic status. Incidence varies as well for race within a given locality: for example, the highest incidence in the U.S. is among Appalachian Whites.[34] The term "neural tube defects" refers to a range of conditions that include anencephaly (severe brain malformation) and spina bifida, in which the spinal cord fails to close. Although previous birth of an affected child is the best predictor of recurrence, 95 percent of affected children are born to families with no previous history of an NTD, and there is no correlation with parental age.[35] Using amniocentesis to test for NTDs was therefore indicated only for the very small high-risk group who had previously borne affected children. But when researchers discovered that alpha-fetoprotein levels could also be determined from a maternal blood sample, testing for neural tube defects changed dramatically. Screening for NTDs could now be extended potentially to every pregnant woman.

The procedure that developed and came to be widely practiced is MSAFP, the "MS" standing for "maternal serum." It is best performed between the 14th and 20th week of pregnancy. If alpha-fetoprotein levels in the mother's blood are elevated, a neural tube defect is possible. Since elevated levels could be due to other causes, such as twins or multiple fetuses, fetal death, impending miscarriage, or a problem with the abdominal wall, a second test of the mother's blood is made, followed by ultrasound, to image the fetus. Ultrasound can, for example, reveal anencephaly, since the deformed brain is visible on the screen. For those cases still "suspect," the final backup is amniocentesis, since the only accurate way to measure alpha-fetoprotein levels is by testing the amniotic fluid itself.[36]

By the mid-to late '70s, MSAFP had been adopted as a mass screening technique in the United Kingdom and much of Western Europe. It was not introduced on a wide scale in the U.S. until 1983, when the Food and Drug Administration approved the release of test kits for MSAFP screening. Though not as widespread as in countries where prenatal care is part of government-administered health services, MSAFP screening came to be increasingly offered in the U.S. in private prenatal care and much clinic care as well. In the mid-1980s, California mandated offering MSAFP screening to all pregnant women statewide, and the program has become a model for other states and localities. Such screening has the support of medical and health personnel involved in genetic services.[37]

MSAFP screening received a big boost in 1983 when it was discovered that low AFP levels in maternal serum could indicate Down syndrome and other chromosomal anomalies.[38] The same protocol for elevated levels for NTDs could be followed. Here, it was argued, was a simple, safe, noninvasive procedure that could screen every pregnant woman for fetal neural tube disorders, regardless of whether she was at high risk. In particular, the procedure could be performed on women under 35, who bore the most children and were not considered to be at high risk for chromosomal disorders.[39] Included in screening would be the 996 or 997 out of every thousand women in whose fetuses no sign of either chromosomal disorders or neural tube defects would be found.[40] The effect of introducing mass MSAFP screening was to extend the "at risk" category to encompass virtually the entire population of pregnant women.[41]

THE TRIPLE SCREEN

This screen has in part come to replace MSAFP screening because it includes measuring AFP levels. The triple screen is a three-part analysis of maternal blood which measures the levels of alpha-fetoprotein, human chorionic gonadotropin (hCG), and unconjugated estriol (E3), all of which are produced by the fetus or placenta and enter the woman's blood. Abnormal levels of these can indicate Down syndrome. Use of the triple screen has become increasingly routine. Its growing popularity rests on three factors: it offers a further marker for Down syndrome, which is more prevalent than NTDs; it requires only a safe blood test; it can therefore reduce the number of riskier amniocentesis procedures recommended and performed. A less obvious reason is that the triple screen, like the MSAFP screen alone, makes every pregnancy a candidate for prenatal screening for "defects." Since blood tests are done routinely in prenatal care to monitor the health of the woman, the fetus's health can be tested without the woman being properly informed that tests of substances are being done.

ULTRASOUND

Ultrasound is a technique used to assist other procedures, and it is also a diagnostic tool in itself. As such, it has helped to expand the screened population and to enable earlier diagnosis. Derived from sonar, a technique to use sound waves to detect submarines that was developed in World War I, ultrasound first came into obstetric practice in the late 1950s and early 1960s.[42] Sending sound waves through the amniotic fluid in the womb, ultrasound, or sonography, reflects an image of the fetus onto a screen, either as a still picture or as a moving "real-time" image. Ultrasound has enabled the physician to "see" into the woman's uterus, so as to guide a needle or other penetrating instrument. Ultrasound soon became integral to amniocentesis, and then to CVS and rarer procedures such as fetal surgery or drawing fetal blood.

As a tool in its own right, ultrasound is particularly used to detect structural anomalies of the fetus. Refined to provide higher and higher definition, by the late 1980s the technology was powerful and sensitive enough not only to detect malformations of major organs or skeletal development but also to visualize structures "as small as the lens of the eye and the semicircular canals of the ear."[43] Thus a facial disfigurement might be detected, or the presence of an extra finger or toe. In the 1990s, as operator experience and improved imaging capabilities markedly increased the numbers and kinds of disorders that could be identified, ultrasound gained further diagnostic importance. Working in conjunction with other screens and tests, such as the triple screen, ultrasound has emerged as a critical diagnostic tool, with far-reaching impact on efforts to detect fetal anomalies.[44] Although the optimum time for routine screening for anomalies has been placed in the second trimester, at 18 to 22 weeks, when fetal structures become large enough to be studied,[45] increased and varied diagnostic use also occurs in the first trimester.

Ultrasound has also become routine at varying stages of the pregnancy, not only to monitor a pregnancy that needs watching, but also to reassure the woman that her fetus is developing properly. Claims are made that ultrasound promotes mother-fetus "bonding."[46] A moving, real-time image is held to create an emotional bond like no other between the woman and her fetus—long before she has even felt movement inside her. Pictures of the fetus are reproduced, put in baby books, and faxed to distant relatives. The procedure is held to be non-invasive and safe, even though questions have been raised about its possible long-term effects.[47] Medical professionals have also questioned how effective ultrasound is as a diagnostic tool, and whether its use is cost-effective.[48]

Another type of imaging is fetoscopy, or embryoscopy. It allows direct visualization, using an endoscope to view the fetus or embryo through the intact amniotic membrane. Originally developed in the 1970s, but rarely used, the procedure has become more feasible due to "technological leaps" in the early 1990s that offer "the potential for extremely clear images." However, it is still recommended only in special cases of risk for certain malformations, and its "role . . . in the overall armamentarium of prenatal diagnosis remains to be seen."[49]

CHORIONIC VILLUS SAMPLING

The technique known as chorionic villus sampling (CVS) is the most recently developed of the main diagnostic procedures now used. CVS, performed between the 9th and 12th weeks of pregnancy, when first introduced could be done much earlier than traditional amniocentesis. It involves inserting a needle into the uterus, either through the cervix or through the abdominal wall, and drawing tissue for analysis from the chorionic villi, which later become the placenta surrounding the fetus. Test results can be known within a week. Like amniocentesis, CVS provides fetal cells for analysis, so it can detect most conditions that amniocentesis can detect, except for NTDs. Also, like amniocentesis, it was used early on to identify fetal sex—with very different intent, however. The goal of the research leading to amniocentesis was to discover X-linked diseases; but for the earliest CVS discovering the sex of the fetus was an end in itself. Performed in Tietung Hospital in Anshan, China, in 1975, the first successful withdrawal of tissue and identification of the sex chromatin served the purpose of "a family planning tool." A reported "30 pregnancies were electively terminated for sex preference."[50] Although aborting solely for sex is far more controversial in the West, use of CVS along with ultrasound early in the pregnancy may allow parents to circumvent this cultural taboo.

Except for attempts by some Scandinavian researchers, there was little interest in villus sampling in the West until the early 1980s. Amniocentesis had become an accepted prenatal testing procedure in the 1970s and CVS research did not receive much publicity until late in the decade. Interest in first-trimester testing grew in part because of mounting concerns and controversies over the late abortions that occurred when test results from then current procedures were not available until four to five months into the pregnancy. Improved technical aids and advances in genetics, however, may have been more important in stirring interest among researchers and practitioners. CVS is technically more difficult to perform than amniocentesis and is extremely dependent on the skill of the operator. In its early years, without ultrasound, the procedure posed unacceptable risks for both woman and fetus. But, by the early 1980s, "[r]eal-time ultrasound visualization had progressed sufficiently so that indirect visual guidance of tissue retrieval became possible."[51] Physicians gained the important tool of sight. At the same time, DNA analysis methods were rapidly making it possible to locate genetic factors for a widening range of genetic disorders. The chorionic villi, it turned out, could provide enough uncultured fetal tissue to make such analysis. Molecular biology offered the potential for extending the numbers and kinds of disorders diagnosable prenatally. All that remained was to perfect a procedure that could test for these conditions early in the pregnancy, and with a faster method for culturing of cells than in amniocentesis, providing more tissue for further analysis. CVS provided this technological response.

Because CVS allows both DNA and biochemical analyses to be done on the fetal tissue, it has certain diagnostic advantages over amniocentesis. Not only can the procedure be done earlier, but results can be obtained in one week or less instead of three. Even medical personnel with strong reservations about CVS agree that CVS is particularly well suited to these two kinds of testing methods, biochemical assays and DNA analysis.[52] Leading researchers and practitioners in the field point out that the "development of molecular biologic techniques has opened the door for a tremendous addition to the armamentarium of prenatal diagnosis."[53]

This genetic research is disease-specific. It has so far concentrated on conditions that are deemed particularly severe or debilitating, perhaps bringing early death. Among the most prevalent of these now genetically diagnosable are Duchenne muscular dystrophy ("an X-linked recessive lethal neuromuscular disorder that affects one in 3500 males");[54] blood diseases such as hemophilia, sickle cell anemia (which primarily affects Blacks), and beta-thalassemia (a form of anemia affecting mostly Mediterranean peoples);[55] fragile X syndrome (second only to Down syndrome in causing mental retardation, and more frequent in males than in females);[56] and cystic fibrosis (one of the most common recessive genetic disorders, affecting one in 2,000 live births among Caucasians in the U.S.).[57] DNA analysis can detect a great many more, much rarer, genetic disorders as well.

There is, then, a particularly felicitous marriage between these DNA techniques and CVS as they are applied to diagnosing genetic disorders in the fetal tissue obtained from the chorionic villi. In 1996, researchers reported a still experimental technique of testing cells from the coelomic cavity, moving CVS back to 7–9 weeks.[58] The explosion of genetic knowledge is resulting in an explosion of diagnosable disorders. These methods of genetic analysis are also used to test carriers, including tracking whole families expressing an inherited disorder. As more detectable conditions are identified, the population for genetic testing widens as well, extending to parents or prospective parents who are possible carriers of the newly located disorders.[59] In the early '90s increasing questions were raised about CVS's possible detrimental effects on the fetus,[60] thereby limiting its use. Nonetheless, because it is compatible with the fastest-growing area of reproductive genetics, CVS itself can expand the numbers of candidates for prenatal testing, adding to the pregnancies labeled "high risk."

Newer technologies are of two types: prenatal diagnosis procedures or techniques that allow earlier detection and/or are less invasive and risky, and procedures that can act upon genetic material at the very earliest stages of human development. Obtaining fetal cells from the mother's blood and preimplantation genetic diagnosis are the first type. Prenatal gene therapy is the second.

FETAL CELLS FROM MATERNAL BLOOD

In 1996, a team of doctors and medical researchers at Thomas Jefferson Medical College in Philadelphia, one of the leading centers of prenatal diagnostic research, reviewed the history and prospects of research to isolate fetal cells from the mother's blood: "One of the most promising, non-invasive sources of fetal cells is peripheral maternal blood, and perfecting techniques to isolate these cells for prenatal diagnosis has been an area of intense research in the past decade."[61] With the exception of fetal imaging, which can show structural anomalies, detecting other possible disorders depends on examining the fetal cells themselves. Amniocentesis and CVS—the main procedures to obtain these cells—are invasive and not without risk. Isolating fetal cells from the mother's blood, drawn from a simple blood sample, has neither drawback. Blood samples are taken routinely, and there is no risk to either woman or fetus.

The Philadelphia research team, while cautioning that retrieval of fetal cells from maternal blood was "still only in the investigative phase," found that the "outlook for noninvasive prenatal genetic testing in the future is optimistic."[62] Five years later researchers in such widely dispersed venues as Hong Kong, Madrid, London, Memphis, and Boston were reporting progress in isolating fetal cells obtained in this way and identifying disorders through their analysis.

Among fetal conditions successfully identified at the University of Tennessee were fetal sex, trisomies of chromosomes 13, 18, and 21, and the blood disorders sickle cell anemia and thalassemia.[63] Researchers in Madrid reported that the number of fetal cells in the mother's blood increases from the first to second trimester of pregnancy, but declines in the third trimester. "It appears that the optimum week in which to perform a reliable non-invasive prenatal diagnosis is around the 15th week."[64] Pressures are great to perfect the procedure, and to make it feasible early in the pregnancy.

PREIMPLANTATION GENETIC DIAGNOSIS

Preimplantation genetic diagnosis (PGD) introduces diagnostic testing at almost the earliest point possible: at the "pre-embryo" stage. *Pre-embryo* is the name given to an embryo up to 14 days old (when it has 64 or fewer cells), a term coined in England in the mid-1980s by researchers seeking to gain government approval of early embryo research. Since embryonic cells do not differentiate in the first two weeks, they argued that the pre-embryo had no moral standing, and therefore that research on this undifferentiated mass of cells could not be opposed on moral grounds.[65]

Preimplantation genetic diagnosis, originally called preimplantation diagnosis, is performed on embryos produced outside the womb by some form of assisted reproduction, most commonly in vitro fertilization (IVF). IVF was developed by the British team of Drs. Steptoe and Edwards and made famous by the birth of baby Louise Brown in 1978.[66] Candidates for PGD are prospective parents who are known to carry a particular recessive single-gene disorder, such as cystic fibrosis. After a process called super-ovulation, in which the woman is given drugs to stimulate the production of multiple eggs, the eggs are removed surgically and fertilized with her partner's sperm.[67] Removing a cell from each of the pre-embryos produced, the researchers biopsy, or test, its genetic material for the disease-bearing gene. Those embryos not having two copies of the gene are transferred to the woman. More than one embryo is tested and inserted because it is difficult to get a transferred embryo to implant in the uterus and develop into a successful pregnancy. (Failure to implant is one of the main reasons that IVF itself has relatively low success rates.)[68]

PGD had its first success in 1990 when a team at Hammersmith Hospital in London, the major center for pre-embryo research, led by Dr. Alan Handyside, removed cells for analysis without damaging the developing embryos. Testing cells from women who were carriers of X-linked diseases, the team determined the sex of the embryos, transferring only female embryos to the womb. Two women became pregnant with twin girls.[69] Since then, the predictions that PGD would soon be able to diagnose specific diseases have been fulfilled.[70] In September 1992 the same team at Hammersmith Hospital reported that they had tested three-day-old embryos from three couples for cystic fibrosis, and that a girl free from the disease had been born to one of the women.[71] Diagnosis of several further single-gene defects followed, including fragile X, Duchenne muscular dystrophy, Tay-Sachs, and hemophilia. Two main methods of genetic analysis are used: polymerase chain reaction (PCR), a type of gene amplification,[72] and the newer fluorescent in situ hybridization (FISH), which is becoming more widely used because it is more successful in detecting abnormal embryos.

Surveying the field as of 2000, Drs. Delhanty and Harper at University College London reported more than 40 centers worldwide carrying out PGD, and 150 babies "born after genetic testing on day 3 of development, at the cleavage stage."[73] These figures represent a doubling of the number of centers reported three years earlier in 1997, with "more than a hundred unaffected children . . . born." [74] Figures reported the year before, in 1996, by Dr. Harper cited 68 babies born to 149 patients at 14 centers world-wide.[75] A major center for PGD in the U.S., for well over a decade is the Reproductive Genetics Institute at the Illinois Masonic Medical Center in Chicago, headed by Dr. Yury Verlinsky.[76] The numbers it reports are particularly high. A study of the risks and pregnancy complications associated with PGD, published in 2000, was based on 102 consecutive pregnancies after preimplantation genetic diagnosis at the center, which resulted in 114 live births. The study concluded that PGD itself did not seem to increase the risk of any particular pregnancy complication except one, and certain risks were comparable to those of patients undergoing IVF in general.[77]

The critical interconnection of preimplantation diagnosis and IVF has become increasingly evident as PGD research has accelerated. In 1996, Dr. Harper had noted the need to have "a successful IVF clinic with experience in embryo biopsy" and "highly specialised molecular and/or genetic expertise" in order to perform single-cell diagnosis.[78] Established centers in the U.S. specializing in IVF, such as the Genetics and IVF Institute in Fairfax, Virginia, have added PGD to their work in fertility. Such centers possess both the requisite expertise and unused "extra" embryos available for research.

In some sense, the interdependence of PGD and IVF helps to keep the numbers small within the overall picture of prenatal diagnosis. IVF and other methods of assisted reproduction are not the preferred methods for procreating by most women and men.[79] It is the inability to conceive the old-fashioned way that drives them to IVF. It is their last resort to conceive and produce their own genetic child. The procedure is expensive, painful, psychologically trying, physically dangerous, and of limited success, even after several attempts.[80] Infertility is the motivator. Those at high risk of bearing a child with an inheritable disorder, however, have a different motivation. Their concern is a particular disease. They come to fertilization in a petri dish hoping to conceive and bear a child who does not suffer from it. However, even when offered the possibility of doing so through PGD and IVF, they do not necessarily jump at the chance. In a study in Britain, women and men who were carriers of recessive disorders supported preimplantation diagnosis, seeing the advantages of early reassurance if the news was good and not having to decide whether to terminate a pregnancy if it was bad. But PGD did not displace prenatal diagnosis performed after conception *in utero* as the most useful reproductive option for them.[81]

Research is also underway to carry prenatal diagnosis to an even earlier point, before fertilization, to the gametes themselves. While analyzing sperm and egg cells is primarily concerned with identifying deficiencies or characteristics that may impede the success of assisted reproduction, the practice is diagnostic as well. Dr. Verlinsky's Reproductive Genetics Institute has used the FISH method to probe for chromosomal anomalies in the egg cells of women of advanced maternal age. Evidently, such anomalies as extra copies of the 13, 18, 21, or X chromosome "contribute considerably to the low pregnancy rate" in IVF. In the work described, those egg cells found free of abnormality were fertilized and transferred, resulting in a small number of "healthy deliveries" and "unaffected" pregnancies and births.[82] Similar research into chromosomal deficiencies in sperm is also being done.[83] Such work is part of growing efforts to look for genetic and chromosomal causes of infertility in women and men.[84] The recent discovery that it makes a difference which parent contributes a defective gene and that, in particular, the extra chromosome for Down syndrome is usually in the woman's egg could increase efforts to screen eggs especially, a more invasive process than screening sperm.[85]

Medical researchers frequently suggest that an important reason to pursue PGD is that it eliminates the option of abortion. But given the frontier mentality that pervades this area of medical research, the moral argument may be only a backup rationale.[86] Prospective parents carrying inheritable disorders list avoidance of abortion as only one of the reasons for supporting the procedure, according to early research. The disadvantages of *ex utero* conception can outweigh the advantages. But, if IVF techniques and success rates were to improve and if methods for retrieving embryos from women who have conceived, such as embryo flushing, were to become more feasible, preimplantation diagnosis could become more widespread. The possibility of diagnosis before a pregnancy has begun, and even before egg and sperm have met, coupled with the rapid advances in molecular genetics, raise expectations for finding and selecting out a widening variety of diseases and so-called disorders. As diagnosis and selection become doable at this very early stage, there could well be less questioning about criteria for choosing the "good" embryos from the "bad." And, as genetic research goes forward, the possibilities grow of altering that embryo or cell. Prenatal gene therapy is one means to do this.

PRENATAL GENE THERAPY

Gene therapy modifies, deletes, or otherwise changes the genes themselves. Controversy over gene therapy arose originally over somatic vs. germ-line therapy. "Somatic" refers to body cells: treatment of them affects only the individual and cannot be passed on to future generations. Germ-line therapy, however, takes place in the germ or reproductive cells: changes to the individual are permanent, to be passed on to offspring. As early as the mid-1980s, animals were successfully treated with germ-line therapy: a blood disorder was eliminated in one strain of mice and infertility corrected in another.[87] In 1986, the U.S. National Institutes of Health (NIH) published guidelines restricting human gene therapy to somatic cells.[88] Therapy has been directed mainly to individuals with severely crippling and lethal diseases; the first success, reported in 1990, was treatment of a four-year-old girl with severe immune deficiency.[89]

The possibilities for prenatal gene therapy build on this and subsequent research. Introducing a review article on prenatal gene therapy published in 1995, Eugene Pergament and Morris Fiddler at Northwestern University School of Medicine noted that, with increased research, clinical trials, support, and investment, "[g]ene therapy for the treatment of human disease is rapidly becoming a reality in clinical medicine." Prenatal therapy involves diagnosing the early embryo, including pre-conception. Pergament and Fiddler argue that "the rationale to seek early prenatal diagnosis is the opportunity for early intervention, to apply therapeutic interventions to those conditions for which postnatal treatments will be too late." They also point to the prospect of therapy rather than the choice of terminating the pregnancy. Their article reflects growing changes in the language of the ethical debates: from somatic vs. germ-line to "corrective" or "therapeutic" vs. "enhancement," their argument being that correcting a genetic flaw may be acceptable, even if doing so affects the germ-line and is therefore permanent, while therapy to "enhance" an individual would not be. (I explore the ethical dimensions of this issue further in chapter eight.) Noting concerns over eugenics, Pergament and Fiddler state that the line between therapy and enhancement may indeed be blurred for the individual, but not on a population basis. Declining to predict a time frame, they support continuing research to apply somatic gene therapy prenatally and bring it into "accepted medical practice."[90]

Numbers, Limits, and Labels

As genetics and prenatal diagnosis technologies work together, they increase the numbers of conditions that can be detected prenatally. The pace of this process is an important part of the story. In 1981 Drs. Sharon Stephenson and David Weaver published a list of prenatally diagnosable conditions that totaled 182.[91] In an article Dr. Weaver published in June 1988, based on data as of September 1987, the number had jumped to 380.[92] In his book that followed in 1989 the number of prenatally diagnosable conditions rose to 445.[93] Yet in May 1990, the head of a diagnostic laboratory in Boston pointed out to me that these figures were already out of date, particularly for those conditions detectable using DNA analysis. Referring specifically to DNA and biochemical techniques used in CVS for single gene disorders, a 1989 medical text on fetal diagnosis and therapy noted that the "list of diseases for which diagnoses are now available is expanding geometrically as normal baseline levels are documented for many enzymes in chorionic villi or cells cultured from villi."[94] By 1992, Weaver's list had grown to 601.[95] In the third edition of his book, published in 1999, the numbers of diagnosable conditions had reached 940. As Dr. Weaver shows in his introduction this edition, the biggest increase occurred in the 1980s, from 182 in 1981 to 445 in 1989, for a percentage gain of 244%.[96] The sequencing of the human genome will accelerate further increase.

In addition to sheer growth in numbers, the kinds of conditions detectable will grow as well. Until now, research has concentrated mainly on single-gene conditions which are classed medically as diseases and which are lethal by early adulthood. Gene sequencing and development of new technical capabilities will facilitate diagnosing *polygenic* conditions (those caused by interactions among several genes) and locating the genes involved. By far the majority of genetically traceable common human traits have such multiple origins.

Thus tools will be available to expand prenatal diagnosis more widely to further segments of the population. The question then arises, relevant now as well as in the future: given the growing array of prenatally detectable conditions, how do we decide whom to test and for what? What are the directions, what are the limits? Criteria can include the condition's prevalence in particular populations, the costs of testing, the judgments and decisions of medical personnel and parents, as well as the ideological and sociocultural frameworks in which decisions are made. These criteria will be taken up in the chapters that follow.

Perhaps the most critical effect of our growing ability to identify and locate genetic and other conditions and to detect them prenatally is the way the concept of "defect" expands and is reinforced. The term "defect" is, of course, loaded. In his catalog of what can be diagnosed prenatally, Dr. Weaver uses the neutral term "condition." Classified by type and using medical descriptions, his listings do not evaluate or rank these conditions. But in most of the medical literature, the main word of choice for such conditions is "disorder." Also used are "disease," "defect," and "anomaly." All these terms are linked to "diagnosis." Although I prefer "condition," it is difficult to avoid using the prevalent, value-laden terms, thus inadvertently contributing to the judgments embedded in this language.

Several factors cause the term "defect" to be applied more loosely and more widely. One is the limited information that a positive diagnosis conveys. With some exceptions for fetal imaging, tests reveal only whether a particular condition is present or not—and even here there are errors. The diagnosis cannot indicate how the condition will be expressed or how severe or mild it might be, even as the symptoms of many conditions vary widely. For example, when the karyotype shows trisomy 21, indicating Down syndrome, there is no way to know what this means for the child's mental and physical potential. The same is true for findings of Klinefelter's syndrome (an extra X chromosome in a male) and Turner's syndrome (a missing X in a female); the diagnoses say nothing about how the sex organs, secondary sex characteristics, and intelligence might be affected. When spina bifida is diagnosed by amniocentesis, the test results do not show whether the lesion is high or low; a low lesion is far less severe and can be surgically corrected after birth. Discovery of the gene for cystic fibrosis is complicated by our growing ability to treat the condition and alleviate its symptoms. In chapter six I will discuss how the issue of severity affects decisions to continue or abort a pregnancy. The point here is that all these conditions are called defects, regardless of their severity; their characteristics and prognosis are limited to textbook definitions of their symptoms.

Fetal cell karyotyping, which can reveal a range of chromosomal characteristics signifying lethal to non-life-threatening conditions, can also reveal others which may or may not have clinical significance. Sex is a prime example.[97] Further, while a missing chromosome segment might indicate, for instance, a tumor causing blindness, the deletion might not correlate with any discernable condition at all, or might indicate only a minor vision impairment, slight enough to ignore or correctable by glasses or surgery. As sophisticated high-resolution techniques continue to increase the amount of information a karyotype can provide, will these newly identifiable conditions, too, be classified as "defects"?

Fetal imaging, usually done with ultrasound, is also becoming increasingly refined. Used as a diagnostic tool, it can reveal a wide range of conditions and characteristics, from brain malformations or displacement of organs such as the intestines, to the shape of a foot or hand, to the number of toes or fingers, to male sex organs, which are visible as early as nine weeks. Unlike other prenatal diagnostic procedures and methods, fetal imaging has the potential to add an entire spectrum of categories and qualities to the list of conditions diagnosable prenatally. Each characteristic, whether lethal or cosmetic, or whatever is in between, could come to be medically classified as a "defect."

In this way, the growing ability to identify genetic conditions through sequencing research combines with refinements and advances in detecting techniques to extend the list of "defects." Diagnosable conditions of widely varying kinds can be absorbed into the defect category as they are discovered, regardless of whether they constitute an actual, let alone severe, disease. The language of prenatal diagnosis, sweeping a broad range of detectable conditions into the defect category, can be used to label each of them undesirable and unwanted.

Tools for Use

The practice of prenatal diagnosis unites two fields of research: genetic science and medical technology. Together, they provide a powerful set of tools to function as disciplining technologies in reproductive medical practice. For the gatekeepers of reproductive medicine, they are tools to name and search out the defective embryo and fetus. For parents, they become tools to realize the child they dream of, free from feared disease. As these tools of medicine and science, medical practitioners, and parents meet in clinical practice, the decisions made add up to a process of naming and ranking defects and the defective, a process that imprints and defines the imperfect and perfect fetus.

FIVE

The Doctors:
On the Trail of the Defective Fetus

Building on the work in the 60s, reproductive medicine in the 1970s stepped up development of prenatal diagnosis and applied it in reproductive clinical practice. Led by the gatekeepers focusing on a new patient, the fetus, the search for the defective fetus was underway. Gatekeepers' aims were and are two-fold: to apply prenatal diagnosis as early, safely and in the least invasively ways possible, and to extend prenatal diagnosis to all pregnant women. Several factors have contributed to gatekeepers' ability to influence physicians and other medical personnel in reproductive medicine to support and extend use of prenatal diagnosis. Among them are an increased reliance on scientific expertise and sophisticated technologies and the corporatization of U.S. medical practice, both of which have diminished the practicing physician's autonomy and sense of control. A further contributing factor is in the shared goals for patient care within medical culture.[1]

The Gatekeepers

By the end of World War II the profession of obstetrics was fully in control of pregnancy and birth, completing a process begun at the turn of the twentieth century.[2] In 1955, nine out of ten births in the U.S. took place in hospitals, a proportion that would rise to almost 100 percent by 1970.[3] Doctors had come to treat pregnancy and birth as a pathological condition, to be medically "managed."[4] Noting the degree to which birth procedures had been technologized, Wertz and Wertz have characterized birth during the 1940s, '50s, and '60s as "the processing of a machine by machines and skilled technicians."[5] William Arney describes obstetrics as entering a "Monitoring Period" after 1945. Added to the use of forceps, anesthesia, and various operative procedures were practices such as fetal monitoring, designed to keep both pregnant woman and fetus under surveillance.[6] And in the 1970s, a leading obstetric textbook recognized the fetus as a "second patient."[7]

When prenatal diagnostic technologies began to emerge in the 1960s, they did so in this context of disciplining technologies in obstetric medical practice. Produced by physicians, the early research findings for the new procedures appeared mainly in professional journals of obstetrics or related medical subjects. As genetics research intersected with the new technologies in clinical reproductive practice, prenatal diagnosis became a new form of preventive medicine to be applied to the pregnant woman, her fetus, and later the embryo.

Leading the research and practices in prenatal diagnosis are the "gatekeepers" of reproductive medicine. Mostly located at large medical complexes, usually attached to universities, that are at the forefront of research and practice,[8] the gatekeepers are top-ranked physicians whose specialty is obstetrics-gynecology, and who may be medical geneticists as well. Their primary professional activity, like that of almost all ob/gyns, is patient care. But, unlike most of their colleagues, they are based in hospitals rather than offices, their gatekeeper status enhanced by their position in the hierarchy of ob/gyn medicine. Often heading departments or units concerned with reproductive medicine, they are the top layer of the 6 percent of obstetricians in hospital staff positions. They are likely to come from the established ranks of middle-aged and older obstetricians, among whom seven out of ten are over 45, and they are likely to be male. Therefore, gatekeepers outrank their ob/gyn colleagues on the basis of age, sex, length of service, and professional positioning. Although women ob/gyns now constitute just over 50 percent of the specialty, as newer entrants they remain in the lower ranks of the medical hierarchy.[9] Whether women obstetricians attaining higher rankings would behave any differently about prenatal diagnosis is an open question, which I'll take up in part 3.

In patient care, the obstetrician/gatekeeper may head a three-person team of obstetrician, medical geneticist, and genetic counselor. Regina Kenen has ranked the relative status of team members using interdependent criteria such as claimed expertise, monetary reward, organizational setting, public perception, and sex. Close behind the front-ranked obstetrician is the medical geneticist, a research genetics expert who holds a doctorate. The genetic counselor belongs to a profession for which formal training began only in 1969. She holds an M.S. degree and is usually female. Unless she is also a medical geneticist and has a doctorate, she is the lowest-ranked member of the team. She is in close contact with the female patient, or the couple.[10]

Supplementing and supporting their role in patient care, gatekeepers set standards and programs for research and practice in their profession. The seminars and professional meetings they sponsor clarify and pinpoint the latest research, pointing the way to new trends and projects. Their many articles fill the key professional journals in reproductive medicine and related fields. They write the definitive textbooks, which are regularly updated. Maintaining their presence in the professional and public eye, gatekeepers have become the recognized authorities for their profession and for the public alike.

Among their professional goals is to increase obstetricians' and family practice physicians' levels of expertise in genetics, prenatal diagnostic procedures, and counseling. Since the early 1980s, voicing continuing concern that levels of knowledge are inadequate, gatekeepers have been instrumental in calling for more attention to genetics in the medical school curriculum, and for programs to educate practicing physicians.[11] At the same time, some leaders in the field have sought to reserve specialized procedures and genetic services to the experts, rather than letting them be performed by obstetric practitioners and general practice physicians. In the late '90s, however, changes in medical practice appeared to make it urgent to educate practitioners more widely. In their preface to *Invasive Outpatient Procedures in Reproductive Medicine*, published in 1997, Dr. Mark Evans and his colleagues at Hutzel Hospital at Wayne State University noted that with the "rapid pace of change in the practice of medicine," specifically citing managed care, "many physicians are now performing new procedures in their own office they would not have done previously." Residents

can be taught the new technologies within the confines of their training program; [but] older, established physicians often find it more difficult to find appropriate ways to learn new procedures. The purpose of this book is to present, in a very detailed fashion, the techniques for a number of increasingly common procedures that are being performed on an outpatient basis. . . . The determination of those that are done routinely and those that will still be specialized will be dictated by practice location. Certainly no single physician would be expected to be expert at all of these procedures.

The authors go on to "hope this book will be a teaching guide for those . . . specifically learning . . . these procedures, and a more general reference guide for all physicians who need to know how they are done." The obstetric procedures described relating to prenatal diagnosis specifically include amniocentesis, CVS, embryoscopy, plus "selective termination" and "pregnancy reduction" (i.e., abortion). Gynecological procedures are covered in the book as well.[12]

As the corporate structure of U.S. medicine increasingly tends to undermine the position of individual practicing physicians, authoritative voices that bring scientifically and technologically based approaches to patient care become more attractive and desirable to them. In reproductive medicine, this has meant bringing the full force of science and technology to bear on relieving the patient's pain and suffering, and, indeed, preventing that pain and suffering.

Perhaps the most critical development in such patient care is the shift from the pregnant woman to her fetus as the object of attention. Prior to the advent of prenatal testing, the pregnant woman had star patient billing. As the object of care, the woman was monitored for such conditions as anemia or rubella which could endanger her fetus. Producing a healthy child depended on *her* health and well-being; the fetus's health was contingent on *her* health. Prenatal diagnosis reversed that focus. With the new technologies, the physician could in effect bypass the woman and go directly to the fetus. The pathologic view of pregnancy, now trained on the "unborn," took as its object the defective fetus. Every fetus was potentially defective, every pregnancy suspect.

The Fetus as Patient

It was not until the last half of this century that the prying eye of the ultrasonographer rendered the once opaque womb transparent, letting the light of scientific observation fall on the shy and secretive fetus.

. . . the sonographic voyeur, spying on the unwary fetus, sees the fetus kicking and rolling, . . . swallowing enormous quantities of amniotic fluid, . . . [e]ven the beautiful rhythmic motion of the heart and its valves.[13]

Waxing rhapsodic as they penetrate forbidden territory are the three male authors of *The Unborn Patient*. Dr. Harrison, a pediatric surgeon, Dr. Golbus, an obstetrician-geneticist, and Dr. Filly, a sonographer, are co-directors of a fetal treatment program in San Francisco. Published in 1984, *The Unborn Patient* marks the start of a shifting trend toward the fetus as patient.

> The fetus has come a long way—from the biblical "seed" and mystical "homunculus" to an *individual* with medical problems that can be diagnosed and treated: that is, a patient. Although the fetus cannot make an appointment and seldom even complains, this patient will at times need a physician. (emphasis added)

As the future of fetal diagnosis and therapy unfolds, the fetus needs not only "an advocate or protector," but also "a healer."[14]

The First International Symposium on the Fetus as a Patient was held in 1984, the papers published as *The Fetus as a Patient,* edited by Dr. Akim Kurjak from the University of Zagreb. Similar publications followed subsequent symposia of the society into the next decade, with Dr. Kurjak and Dr. Frank A. Chervenak from Weill Cornell Medical Center co-editing *The Fetus as a Patient* in 1994, and *Current Perspectives on the Fetus as a Patient* two years later. Having shed the colorful language of Dr. Harrison and his colleagues, the fetus had fully arrived at patient status.[15]

Much of the new attention to the fetus as patient derives from the growing specialty of fetal medicine and the emergence of fetal treatments, and especially fetal surgery, within that specialty.[16] The objectives of fetal medicine are therapeutic. Yet the route to therapy is diagnosis. As described by Drs. Chervenak and Kurjak, the International Society of the Fetus as a Patient is "an interdisciplinary group of physicians dedicated to improving all aspects of fetal diagnosis and therapy."[17] Fetal diagnosis, which casts the fetus as patient, is an extension of the long-prevalent view of pregnancy as pathological, which originally cast the woman as the primary patient. New technologies can now make the health status of the fetus the primary concern. The representation "unborn patient," as both language and concept, permeates reproductive medicine, most particularly the research and practice of prenatal diagnosis. Monitoring a pregnancy means monitoring the fetus, and searching for the defects it may have.

Supporting and promoting this quest, gatekeepers seek the earliest, safest, least invasive prenatal diagnosis methods possible, and to extend testing and screening to all pregnancies. Introducing a symposium titled "Prenatal Diagnosis in the '90s" in 1992, Drs. Mark Evans and Mark

Johnson observed, "First-trimester diagnosis is rapidly becoming the mainstay in prenatal diagnostic centers."[18] As described in the previous chapter, amniocentesis and CVS practices bear this out. Amniocentesis can now be performed successfully at 11 to 14 weeks, that is, in the first trimester instead of the second. CVS, in wider use since the late '80s, is a first-trimester procedure. CVS also has limits, being unable to diagnose neural tube disorders such as spina bifida. There is also lingering controversy over its safety. A massive study of women undergoing CVS, published in the *New England Journal of Medicine* in 1989, claimed the test to be safe,[19] as did a worldwide study reported at an international conference five years later. Published in 1996, the latter study concluded that "chorionic villus sampling is a safe procedure with an associated fetal loss rate comparable to that of amniocentesis."[20] Earlier reports of damaged limbs in babies born to tested mothers, however,[21] plus the procedure's high dependence on operator skill, have kept some physicians skeptical. Yet its use is increasing faster than that of other major procedures.

Amniocentesis and CVS meet the criterion of earlier use, in this case first trimester, for a prenatal diagnosis procedure. Both tests, however, are invasive, and still pose some risks for woman and fetus; thus they do not fully satisfy the safety criterion. As for the aim of extending use, these tests still concentrate on only a small percentage of pregnant women: mainly older mothers—women over 35—or those in special high-risk categories, such as carriers or those who have given birth to an affected child. Limits on the facilities available and costs of administering the tests also preclude wider use, even though some medical professionals urge lowering the testing age, especially to detect Down syndrome.[22]

The triple screen, requiring only a sample of the woman's blood to screen it for three markers, is non-invasive. It has become increasingly routine in prenatal care, particularly because it can indicate possibilities of NTDs such as spina bifida, and most especially for Down syndrome. A positive result calls for a follow-up ultrasound, and then amniocentesis, to take place in the second trimester. Use of the non-invasive triple screen among women who are ordinarily recommended for amniocentesis, by screening out unaffected pregnancies, reduces the number of invasive procedures performed. In the long run, however, extending the triple screen routinely to more and more women would mean increasing the numbers of women requiring invasive testing procedures as the numbers of positive findings inevitably increased.

Advocacy of wider use of blood screening started with MSAFP in the 1980s, which had then become more widely applicable. Even though anomalies were ultimately diagnosed in only .3% to .4% per thousand women screened and then tested, medical support was building for extending the MSAFP screen to all pregnancies. Four physicians argued in the early '90s, "Fetal malformations affect 2–3% of pregnancies," imposing "serious ethical and medical dilemmas" on the "parents-to-be." Since most of these abnormalities occur in "low-risk pregnancies," prenatal screening procedures are needed to identify low-risk patients who are really high-risk. Procedures targeting certain "ethnically linked genetic disorders," such as Tay-Sachs or sickle cell anemia, cover only specifically limited populations. And so, these physicians continued, MSAFP screening "should be offered to *all* pregnant women" (emphasis in original).[23] Yet they readily acknowledge advocating screening for the vast majority of pregnant women who are "patients *without a recognized genetic risk*" (emphasis added)! Since then, and despite the mixed picture, extending the triple screen has been strongly advocated, the goal of discovering more defective fetuses apparently overriding.

Ultrasound, in its role as a diagnostic procedure, is also a non-invasive procedure. It was originally used to image the fetus to make sure that the pregnancy was going well. But then the focus shifted from assuring what was right to discovering what was wrong. In the early '90s two obstetricians from the UCLA School of Medicine noted the change: "Ten years ago recognition of what is normal was the dominant concern of the ultrasound community. That has now been replaced with detailed reports and observations of the abnormal." Pointing to the number and kinds of disorders that could be identified, indeed "described in detail," as a result of "increased operator experience and remarkably improved imaging capabilities," Drs. Carlson and Platt found ultrasound opening "new windows into the antepartum world." They concluded, "the careful prenatal ultrasound examination of the fetus is now the cornerstone of genetic counseling, recommendations for prenatal karyotyping and possible management decisions in labor."[24]

During the '90s, controversy developed over ultrasound's effectiveness as a diagnostic tool. In 1993, for example, the RADIUS study asked whether it was cost-effective to extend the procedure more widely, since its use did not change pregnancy outcome. The study's sampling, procedures, and cost estimates, and therefore its conclusions, were questioned in turn, although even the study's detractors cautioned that ultrasound might not be an especially good diagnostic tool for the "low-risk patient."[25] By the end of the decade, however, ultrasound, especially when combined with the triple screen, had regained its stature as an important diagnostic tool. "Whether used alone or in conjunction with additional biochemical or molecular serum markers," claimed researchers at the UCLA School of

Medicine in 2001, "ultrasound is an important and powerful tool in pre-natal genetic evaluation."[26] They were referring to ultrasound in the second trimester, the usual practice. A study at the University of Washington, also published in 2001, reported successful use of ultrasound in the first trimes-ter to detect Down syndrome, the fatal trisomies 13 and 18, and Turner's syndrome.[27]

Whether referring to ultrasound, the triple screen, or such screens combined, medical advocates argued that use of these non-invasive screens would reduce the need for invasive procedures such as amniocen-tesis for detecting fetal anomalies. Yet, as suggested above, if these screens were extended to all pregnant women in an effort to identify more fetuses with defects, then more women would be subjected to the invasive pro-cedures required to confirm the diagnosis. A major goal of medical advo-cates continues to be to search for alternative, non-invasive ways to detect more fetuses with anomalies. The University of Washington researchers noted,

> If fetal karyotype analysis could be performed without sampling through the uterus, prenatal diagnosis could be offered to all pregnant women, and screening would be unnecessary. Despite its limitations, ultrasound will have an important role in prenatal diagnosis at least until isolating and testing fetal cells from maternal blood or other sources becomes practical and widely available.[28]

As pointed out in chapter four, obtaining fetal cells from the mother's blood is the ultimate goal of prenatal diagnosis research. In 1992 Dr. Wolfgang Holzgreve and his colleagues could already say that "there has been a strong motivation for many years to develop the least invasive technique for prenatal diagnosis, ideally through the isolation and analysis of fetal cells in the maternal circulation during pregnancy."[29] Within less than 10 years researchers from around the globe, from Hong Kong to Madrid to Boston, were coming closer to attaining the goal. Among the fetal conditions they identified with some success were sex, trisomies 13, 18, and 21, and various blood disorders.[30]

Obtaining fetal cells from maternal blood for testing fulfills all the criteria for the ideal prenatal test. It is non-invasive, performed early, and virtually without risk to the pregnant woman or her fetus. It would enable prenatal diagnosis to be extended to all pregnant women. A diagnostic test, not a screen, it could test the fetal genome, precisely and accurately, for any number of genetically based disorders, as molecular genetics re-search reveals and locates them.

Not sufficiently discussed, however, is what will happen as the number of defective fetuses detected increases, which is inevitable if this procedure is successfully applied. Would treatments or cures be available, given the likely increase as well of the kinds of conditions detectable? Most physicians are reluctant to talk about the fact that medicine offers virtually one way to respond to a positive prenatal diagnosis. With the exception of still rare, and costly, fetal and neo-natal therapy, the only "treatment" for the fetus diagnosed as defective is to prevent its being born, to abort it.

The disjunction between diagnosis and treatment arises in part because prenatal diagnosis falls within the category of preventive medicine. Ideally, the goal of prevention would best be served if detection could precede pregnancy. Preimplantation genetic diagnosis (PGD), which biopsies a cell from the early embryo before the embryo is transferred and implants in a woman's uterus, is just such a procedure. Only an embryo free of diagnosable defects is transferred. Advocates of PGD generally agree that the same onus does not attach to eliminating an embryo found defective as to aborting a fetus inside the womb. In 1981, when research on PGD was in its very earliest phases, embryologist Dr. Robert Edwards, of "test-tube baby" fame, speaking at an IVF conference, noted that the " 'abortion *in vitro*' of a defective preimplantation embryo, still free-living, minute and undifferentiated, would be infinitely preferable to abortion *in vivo* at 20 weeks of pregnancy." (At that time, amniocentesis and CVS in the first trimester were not yet possible.) It would be "less traumatic," he added, "for parents and doctor to type several embryos and replace or store those that are normal."[31]

Yet PGD is not yet a significant option for non-invasive prenatal diagnosis. It is still reserved for high-risk cases, such as known carrier status, and it is not widely offered or practiced; it has resulted in fewer than 200 successful births worldwide. That it depends on fertilization outside the womb, by IVF or other forms of assisted reproduction, rather than by "normal" and generally preferred means, makes it less appealing, and further limits its use. Another drawback is that obtaining eggs requires the woman to undergo a highly invasive surgical procedure, although there has been little comment on this in the medical literature.

Decision-Making and the Doctor-Patient Relationship

Decisions about prenatal diagnosis take place within the individualized and privatized clinical setting. The physician-patient dyad extends at most to include relevant medical staff and the patient's immediate family. This restricted sphere for decision-making reflects the U.S. cultural norm, which views people's actions as isolated rather than in social context.

Cultural commitments to individual privacy, autonomy, and free choice are further embedded in law and the political economy. As high-status members of society, physicians may well share the values of the dominant culture, such as prevailing negative views of disability.[32] The "medical model" that in the early twentieth century replaced one that had marked a person with a disability as incompetent, to be segregated for special protection and care, has both reflected and influenced public discourse. When physicians use the word "tragedy" to characterize the possibility of a child with a birth defect, they shape and reflect disability discourse in reproductive medicine.

The image of the doctor-patient relationship has undergone substantial change in the past few decades.[33] The traditional paternalistic pattern, in which the doctor's judgment and authority went unquestioned, has given way to a more reciprocal model. A better educated, more questioning health care consumer wants quality care, information, and greater autonomy in decision-making.[34] Although race, gender, and class differences between physician and patient can still serve to enhance the physician's mystique and power over the patient,[35] the reciprocal model is the norm invoked.

Addressing the Pacific Coast Obstetrical and Gynecological Society in 1985, its president Dr. Edward Hill closed his remarks this way:

> In our fascination with the science of medicine and rapidly advancing technology, we must never lose sight of the fact that we profess to care for patients. It means that we must communicate with the patient and her family, respecting the sovereignty of her desires, her beliefs, and her aims and goals. It means that we must weigh all decisions first according to patient benefit, for, in general, what's good for the individual patient is good for society. It means, also, that we must realize—and discuss openly with our patients—the uncertainties that make obstetrics and gynecology an art. Finally, it means that we must be wary of moral extremists who believe that there is one morality that fits every situation, acknowledging that only those whose medical decisions allow for individual differences are meeting the deeper demands of the ethics of our profession.[36]

Dr. Hill's words reflect medicine's positive ethic to confer benefit, to alleviate suffering, and relieve pain, extending the Hippocratic Oath's injunction to, above all, "do no harm." In chapter eight I will explore medical professionals' ethical responses to prenatal testing and screening within the context of the field of bioethics. But the pressures to universalize prenatal diagnosis raise particular issues within reproductive medicine itself among professionals performing or researching prenatal diagnosis. The tenor of their concerns is marked as much by the issues they do not explore as by those they do. Typically, ethical commentary from within reproductive medicine has only selectively sought to question the value of prenatal diagnosis itself and of extending its use much more widely. The focus is usually on the effectiveness of a particular diagnostic tool, and especially whether its use is cost-effective. Still, supporters of prenatal diagnosis do offer more stringent cautions and caveats,[37] some of which I will discuss at the end of this chapter and in chapter nine.

Class and ethnicity issues surface as physicians express the need to widen underserved populations' access to testing and screening. Writing on ethics and prenatal diagnosis in the late 1980s, Susan Johnson and Thomas Elkins, obstetricians at university-based hospitals, recommended using public resources to provide greater access to diagnostic services so that "poor fetuses" would not be discriminated against. Among other issues for Drs. Johnson and Elkins were safety of procedures, the availability of facilities and trained personnel, and quality control.[38]

Medical professionals also must consider when and under what circumstances to recommend prenatal diagnosis. Johnson and Elkins favored voluntary testing, and not forcing any patient to undergo a diagnostic test that is not considered "standard practice."[39] They do not spell out their criteria for "standard practice" in this context but, like many of their colleagues, they caution against routine use of a procedure still under study or development. How do the role and status of woman and fetus affect decisions about prenatal diagnosis? Johnson and Elkins found that four paramount ethical issues are unique to prenatal diagnosis: "1) the moral status of the fetus; 2) the use of selective pregnancy termination; 3) the need for bodily participation of the mother in the performance of procedures; and 4) the need for the use of proxy decision makers for the fetus." Their phrasing clearly implies the adversarial relationship between woman and fetus that characterizes medical ethics discussions. Whose rights have a greater claim? What are the criteria and circumstances for deciding between two patients vying for attention, the struggle taking on aspects of a zero-sum game?[40] The "need for bodily participation of the mother in the performance of procedures" suggests that while the woman's wishes cannot be ignored, her body impedes access to the real patient, the fetus. In turn, the fetus may "need" a "proxy decision maker," presumably to protect it from the body that sustains it.

The image of maternal-fetal conflict, as a contest of "rights," permeates the literature. This is so even where physicians explicitly reject "the language of fetal rights," as do Dr. Chervenak and his colleagues, who see the fetus as a patient but not as an autonomous being possessing rights. In deciding whether to intervene to treat the fetus, they weigh the benefit to the fetus against the autonomy of the woman.[41] But in fetal medicine the mother-fetus conflict arises when a therapy is proposed that is designed to benefit the fetus. Terminating the pregnancy, and therefore the fetal patient, is beside the point as "treatment," unless perhaps therapy were unable to correct a lethal condition.

Abortion, however, is a central issue for the field of prenatal diagnosis. As noted earlier, "treatment" to "correct" or "prevent" a disorder detected in the fetus almost always means one thing: abortion. Expressed euphemistically as "pregnancy termination," or "selective pregnancy termination," abortion is not a choice that physicians and other medical professionals in reproductive medicine feel comfortable with. Even physicians who perform abortions acknowledge that it contradicts their training, the very goals of medicine: to care for and cure patients, to try and preserve their lives. Above all, it seems to contradict the fundamental ethical principle of medicine: "do no harm." A variety of studies and interviews with doctors indicate that they are increasingly unwilling to do abortions, especially late abortions, even when they are pro-choice. Their reluctance is apparently not solely attributable to pressures from militant anti-abortionists.[42]

What happens, then, if the fetus is regarded as a patient? Raising the fetus to the status of an "individual" with "rights" could compound the moral dilemma. Should the physician assume the role of fetal protector, as Dr. Harrison and his colleagues have suggested?

Part of the rationale for seeking earlier prenatal diagnosis is so that, if abortion is indicated, it will happen in the first trimester, when the procedure is safer and less traumatic—not only for the woman, but also for the doctor. Preimplantation genetic diagnosis, of course, performed before there is an actual pregnancy, would make the question of abortion moot, given medical consensus that the "pre-embryo," less than 14 days old, has no moral standing. But PGD, as discussed above, is not likely to become a widespread and routine procedure in clinical reproductive practice in the near future. Even if an affected fetus is to be aborted in the first 13 weeks of pregnancy, the physician's qualms remain.

If, then, the fetus has the status of a full-fledged patient, how do or can physicians reconcile their support of prenatal diagnosis with the "treatment" that is likely to follow diagnosis of a defect in the fetus? As physicians strive to locate each defective fetus, and are likely to diagnose more and more, will the responsibility for deciding the fate of what is now a defective patient shift? The pregnant woman once again becomes significant.

In their introduction to the "Prenatal Diagnosis in the '90s" symposium, Evans and Johnson noted, "In the '80s and '90s the offering of prenatal diagnosis is no longer linked to abortion," as it had frequently been in the mid-1970s.

> There is an ethical and practical separation between information and action. The focus of the '90s is making prenatal diagnosis more readily available earlier and more privately. . . . [The] trend toward early diagnosis will probably be accelerated both by personal desires and the need to keep the pregnancy private until fetal status is assessed.[43]

The person who has the most "need to keep the pregnancy private" is the pregnant woman. She is the one who wants to know the "status" of her fetus before her pregnancy is obvious. She then will be the one to take "action," that is, the one to decide about abortion, once she has the "information." The professional norm of patient autonomy means that responsibility for moral decisions lies with the patient. But not the patient who cannot call for an appointment or complain. Rather, responsibility falls on the living patient whom the physician has otherwise eclipsed in the interest of the "patient within." The goal of relieving pain and suffering is refocused on the pain of the woman, or parents, facing the possibility of a defective child. Citing the "[t]remendous burden" placed on families by the birth of a retarded child, the Council on Scientific Affairs of the American Medical Association has stated that "prevention of this event is one of the principal goals of antenatal screening."[44]

The Dominant Discourse: Inscribing the "Imperfect Fetus"

The discourse that emerges in reproductive medicine characterizes the birth of a child with "defects" as a tragedy, to be avoided by every means that science and technology can muster. The gatekeepers express an almost unbounded enthusiasm for the scientific and medical techniques they develop and promote to this end. "Prenatal Diagnosis in the '90s" celebrates "some of the remarkable leaps that have occurred in the past few years." Evans and Johnson write approvingly of how the "explosion of technology makes possible the development of new genetic procedures—preimplantation diagnosis, fetal cells in maternal blood and the opening of the door to gene therapy."[45] Speaking at an NIH conference to a combined professional and lay audience in May 1990, two years before preimplantation diagnosis would be successfully performed, Dr. Joseph Schulman, director of the Genetics and IVF Center in Fairfax, Virginia, used slides to illustrate the "very exciting" research then current at Hammersmith Hospital in London, including cell biopsy and egg retrieval. Among other procedures he extolled, which were still on the drawing boards, were attempts to obtain fetal cells non-invasively from the mother's blood. "This type of approach," he predicted, "could open the door to universal screening of pregnant women for a large variety of genetic diseases in the future." He concluded that it "may well become the prenatal genetics of the 21st century."[46]

Dr. Schulman is enthusiastic about not only diagnosis but also possibilities for gene therapy. While their intent may not be explicitly eugenic—indeed, they may skirt the issue—Dr. Schulman and others find the prospect of modifying embryonic genes exciting and welcome. In 1985 Dr. Schulman, with co-authors Dr. Andrew Dorfmann of the National Institutes of Health and Dr. Mark Evans, predicted that the technical difficulties of transferring genes into human embryos (as had already been done in mice) "will largely be overcome in the near future." As to "ethical problems," they foresaw instead "ethical uses." Their "most telling example" of such "ethical use" was a situation in which both parents suffered from a "recessive disorder, such as sickle cell anemia," and thus had "a 100% chance of having a defective child with the same disorder." "It seems probable," they concluded, "that within the lifetimes of many of us, experiments of this type will, after scrupulous scientific and ethical evaluation, be performed to the benefit of the unborn patient."[47]

A few enthusiasts of the technologies have an explicit eugenic agenda. Since the 1970s, Dr. Aubrey Milunsky, director of the Center for Human Genetics at Boston University School of Medicine, in books and articles aimed at both medical professionals and popular readers, has steadily advocated the supreme importance of genes and the need to act to maintain "quality" offspring. By 1986, he could write, in the second edition of his *Genetic Disorders and the Fetus,* that the "tide of medical and legal opinion in North America has steadily forced recognition of a genetic standard of care."[48] In a 1975 text on the prevention of genetic disease and mental retardation he had declared, "In a heavily populated world beset by increasing, serious problems, parental wishes for healthy 'quality' offspring have become paramount. It is my fervent hope that *prospective* parents will realize their wishes through programs based on principles and approaches elaborated upon in this volume" (emphasis in original). The book supported the idea of a national registry of genetic disease, although Dr. Milunsky did warn that it was necessary to "maintain absolute privacy and confidentiality." He emphasized that parents should be educated about early prenatal care so that they would act to prevent genetically caused conditions, and outlined "strategies" to develop such "attitudes."[49]

Dr. Milunsky's books for a lay audience have carried such titles as *Know Your Genes* and *Choices Not Chances*. The subtitle of the 1986 *Choices Not Chances* was *How to Have the Healthiest Baby You Can,* and of the 1989 version, *An Essential Guide to Your Heredity and Health.* In the preface to the latter, he argued for making "choices" about genetic inheritance, since "every facet" of health is regulated by genes.[50] Dr. Milunsky, who is also professor of human genetics, pediatrics, obstetrics and gynecology, and pathology at Boston University's medical school, regularly counsels patients at the center. In the preface to the fourth edition of *Genetic Disorders and the Fetus,* published in 1998, he wrote, "I hope this book will pilot us into the next millennium, when we will soon see more intensive and wide-ranging preconception risk determination, extensive voluntary screening of *all* pregnant women, recognition of susceptibility genes, predictive diagnosis of monogenic disorders, and therapeutic intervention" (emphasis in original).[51]

In her presidential address to the American Society of Human Genetics in 1983, Dr. Margery Shaw predicted that "parental rights to reproduce will diminish as parental responsibilities to unborn offspring increase."

> No longer are we playing genetic roulette. . . . [T]he medical geneticist is rapidly changing from a bookie to a fixer. Future generations will be the beneficiaries of our increasing predictive powers and therapeutic tinkering. Parenthood may become a privilege to be cherished rather than a right to be exercised even when a child is harmed.[52]

Dr. Shaw, who holds a law degree as well as an M.D., is on record as a firm advocate of each advance in prenatal diagnostic technology and the interests and rights of the fetus. For her, control of genetic disease is a matter of public health. Although she states that women should have the right not to abort a defective fetus, she also upholds the right of children to sue parents over genetic defects that were preventable; further, she states that a woman should be held accountable for negligence toward her fetus during pregnancy.[53] A well-known and outspoken practicing physician for many years, Dr. Shaw has alluded frequently to the late Rev. Joseph Fletcher, a theologian and bioethicist whose strong advocacy of eugenic selection is discussed in chapter eight.

Although Dr. Shaw was no longer actively practicing by the late '90s, she and Drs. Milunsky and Schulman were never fringe players. Despite the extreme tenor of their views, they were and are not entirely unrepresentative of their colleagues' thinking. They may simply go further, their extreme language revealing what underlies the physician's commitment to "help the patient." Dr. Milunsky's highly directive, genetically deterministic views are a stronger rendering of the physician's need to maintain professional control. Dr. Schulman's unbridled enthusiasm for new technological developments is medical professionals' fascination with these technologies writ large. And in her explicit condemnation of "genetically defective" offspring, Dr. Shaw bares the negative attitudes toward disability found in reproductive medical practice, and which reflect prevailing societal values.

The increasingly routine use of prenatal testing and screening procedures attests to their support by practitioners of reproductive medicine. But obstetricians and family physicians differ in their attitudes toward and use of these procedures. For example, a study published in the *American Journal of Obstetrics and Gynecology* in 1996 found that obstetricians were more likely than were family physicians to offer the triple screen under an expanded state program in Iowa. The obstetricians favored offering the screen to all patients, while family physicians were more likely to offer it only to women perceived to be at risk or who requested it.[54] Although obstetricians also question the use of prenatal diagnosis,[55] it seems more problematic and controversial in the pages of family physicians' journals.[56] This may partly reflect a greater influence of gatekeepers on practitioners within their own specialty.

Physicians' growing use and support of prenatal diagnosis is, however, more than a response to gatekeepers'—and parents'—pressures. In the changing structural climate of medicine, the new procedures, while bringing further challenges, can offer physicians new mechanisms for control. Prenatal screening and testing came on the scene just as the physician's status was changing. "Managed care" is now the norm in U.S. health care coverage, largely eclipsing the traditional fee-for-service system.[57] From individual entrepreneurs, in the sense that they could set the terms of and criteria for services rendered, physicians, along with other medical professionals, became in effect employees of the corporate enterprise.[58] The result has been to erode the physician's highly valued autonomy and independence, an erosion which had started even before managed care became pervasive. Philosopher of medicine John Ladd finds that physicians in the twentieth century have become more like engineers. Instead of setting their own standards, they offer a product which is judged by their clientele. The very successes of medicine have helped to transform medicine into a commodity in which the client, i.e., the patient, judges and evaluates the outcome.[59] A national survey of physicians conducted in 2001 by the Kaiser Family Foundation found that "three-quarters of physicians say managed care has had a negative impact on the way they practice medicine

(76%) and on the medical care services available to their patients (75%)," attitudes that have grown "somewhat more negative since 1999." Eighty-seven percent of physicians in the survey say "the overall morale of physicians has decreased in the last five years."[60]

In the past few decades the practice of medicine has also come to rely increasingly on science, on research-based scientific expertise, and on sophisticated technologies. This is especially true in reproductive medicine as practiced in much of the developed world. At the 1996 annual meeting of the European Society of Human Reproduction and Embryology, a keynote lecturer put it this way: "A new paradigm called evidence-based medicine has emerged, which places less emphasis on intuition and the clinical experiences obtained in a non-systematic manner as being sufficient grounds for making clinical decisions."[61]

In the increasingly negative environment of medical practice, the demands for scientific and technical expertise can further erode the physician's status. But the new technologies can also provide a new source of power. Enabling the obstetrician to closely monitor the pregnancy with enhanced technical skills, the new procedures function as disciplining technologies to offer an opportunity to exercise control and regain lost status. New mechanisms of control carry their own risks, however. In the climate of an altered doctor-patient relationship, the autonomous patient judging the "product" may expect, even demand, perfection, assuming science and technology can deliver. The physician is in a double bind: in the event of a bad outcome, malpractice suits for "wrongful birth" may be brought regardless of whether the physician sought to encourage testing or did not.[62]

Most physicians in reproductive medicine do not subscribe to a eugenic agenda, and will explicitly reject one when asked.[63] They do not see prevention and control of genetic disease as eugenically inspired. Yet, in their support and use of prenatal diagnosis, practicing physicians serve to shape genetic outcomes. As they use prenatal diagnosis to relieve parents' pain and suffering and to search for defects in the "unborn patient," their focus is on the immediate, the patients at hand. When Dr. Hill states that "what's good for the individual patient is good for society," his is a peculiarly American rendering of the relationship of society and the individual. Starting from the individual, this view precludes discussion of social contexts which shape physicians' professional actions, and of possible societal consequences of many individual reproductive decisions. Unrecognized is that decisions are cumulative. One by one, each decision serves to mark the imperfect fetus. As the numbers of diagnostic decisions ratchet upward, imperfections, and undesirable fetuses, are inevitably selected and ranked. In this way, physicians' individual professional actions contribute to framing a genetically based health hierarchy of birth. Operating within medical culture to fulfill the goals of medicine, reproductive medical professionals inscribe the imperfect fetus to underwrite a form of genetic selectivity far more powerful than under the old eugenics.

Medical professionals are clearly responding as well to clients' desires, though they do so with cautions and mixed views. Some physicians have expressed concerns over parents' unwarranted expectations. Writing for the general reader in the *New York Times Magazine,* Boston pediatrician Dr. Perri Klass, for example, has cautioned that prenatal testing does not bring certainty; it reveals only the absence of certain conditions. There is no way, she writes, to guarantee a "perfect baby."[64]

Addressing a professional audience, Dr. Laurence Karp was concerned that some parents do indeed seek perfection. They are under the illusion that prenatal testing can produce the perfect child. He recalled "one particular patient, an elegantly coiffed, flawlessly made-up woman who smoothed her silk dress over her crossed knees, and said, with a chilling little smile, 'Doctor, I don't want to have this baby if it's not going to be perfect.'" Pointing out that such parents were a "minority" but one "whose numbers seem to be increasing," Dr. Karp attributed this "expressed intolerance of imperfection in offspring" to a number of causes. Seen as an extension of the parent, the defective child suggests that the parent is defective, "less than perfect." The perfect child is a ticket to immortality, but "produce a child with Down syndrome, and you're dead." The "current wave of consumerism" insists that if a product is not "shiny and clean," perfectly packaged and defect-free, "the manufacturer should take it back in exchange." The child is also seen as an investment, the money spent on a child with a learning disability "seen as 'dollar bills flushed down the toilet,'" as one of Dr. Karp's patients is quoted as saying. Concerned less about the fate of the imperfect, Dr. Karp wondered about the expectations for the children who *are* born to such parents. "After all, they will have been certified products. Will many of them suffer . . . all their lives being forced to measure up to an idealized conception of perfection?"[65]

Not all parents support prenatal diagnosis without question. Those who do, however, contribute powerfully to the discourse that inscribes the imperfect fetus. Pregnant women, and their partners in effect exhibit a range of reactions to prenatal diagnosis as they face the changing and confusing "choices" in current reproductive practice.

SIX

The Parents:
Only the Best and the Brightest

"If I had a child like that," said the dentist's wife to my mother, "I'd ask the doctor to kill it." We were in the dentist's waiting room. I don't remember my mother's response. I only remember those chilling words. For I knew.

A child "like that" meant the boy who smiled and played placidly in front of the apartment house where we lived, with a nursemaid always by his side. I knew he was called a "mongoloid." Sometimes we children would stare. But mostly we walked quickly by, and we never invited him to play with us. But now I knew something else. I knew the depth of a woman's fear of bearing such a child.

Today, we argue, women have "choice." They need not give birth to a child with Down syndrome. Women can choose prenatal diagnosis and terminate the pregnancy if the tests are positive. But fear still motivates. Attitudes toward children with Down syndrome or other birth defects have little changed in the intervening decades. Only the ability to act and the timing of our actions have changed.

But what does having choice mean? It means, to start with, deciding whether to be tested or not in the first place. It also means being pressured

[111]

to do so if one hesitates. Choice means having virtually only one option to avoid a diagnosed defect: abortion. Choice means deciding, often on the basis of ambiguous information, whether to terminate or continue the pregnancy. Parents want to know: Will the child's mental capacities be impaired? What about physical abilities? What will the child look like? Their decisions, although made individually, become cumulative, defining and ranking undesired—and by default desired—qualities of children to be born. As they participate in prenatal diagnosis, parents become complicit in inscribing the imperfect fetus and in designating which fetuses are acceptable and which are not. To regard children as special is not new. But the value placed on them and the attention paid have reached a new level of intensity today.

The "Priceless Child"

As the nineteenth century turned into the twentieth and the U.S. became an urbanized society (the 1920 census marked the population shift from rural to urban), children lost the economic value they had had on the farm. Rapid farm mechanization also reduced the need for agricultural workers of any age. Child labor laws—to the extent they were obeyed— reduced the opportunities for children's wages to contribute to urban poor or working-class families. Children became expensive. Parents sought to limit their families for economic reasons, even as women sought to have fewer children for the sake of their own health and survival. Fewer children became both a necessity and a cultural norm.

As their economic value declined, children's emotional value increased. Viviana Zelizer describes the " 'sacralization' of children's lives" that invested children with sentimental meaning. Instead of being seen as an economic asset, the "new normative ideal of the child" was an "exclusively emotional and affective asset."[1] Although advocates of an economically useful childhood fought this emerging ideal, Zelizer claims that the "economically 'worthless' but emotionally 'priceless' child" prevailed by the 1930s, and that this norm transcended class.[2] The irony was that this "exclusively emotional valuation" placed children back in the cash nexus. Parents became willing to pay any price to secure their children's love or their health and happiness, and expected to receive monetary compensation for their loss.[3]

Although ethnic, religious, racial, and class patterns diverged from the new norm in various ways, the ideal of smaller families and the image of the child as a priceless emotional investment were dominant cultural values when reproductive medicine began to change so dramatically in the

1960s. Investments need to be protected; people want to direct and control what happens to them. Prenatal diagnosis offered parents a means to ensure that control even before the investment was made, before the child was born.

The medicalization and technologizing of childbirth, well in place by the 1960s, also helped set the climate for parents to seek and accept prenatal testing. With almost all deliveries taking place in hospitals, women were accustomed to accepting drugs and technical procedures. Now such procedures were becoming available prenatally, perhaps increasing the chances of bearing a healthy, normal baby. Earlier in the century it was women themselves who sought out and welcomed medical procedures that would reduce the pain of childbirth and promote safer delivery. Deaths of women in childbirth markedly decreased in the twentieth century, as did infant mortality. Faith in reproductive medical science and technology and in the physician's expertise was part of the White middle- and upper-middle-class woman's experience.[4]

It was among these women that prenatal diagnosis was first accepted and began to be used at high rates. Even though prenatal diagnosis is increasingly being offered to poorer and "minority" women, its use in the U.S. is still skewed by class, race, and ethnicity. This is partly because poorer women more often refuse it, even when financial barriers are removed. Still, better access to genetic services has somewhat increased prenatal diagnosis among women in these groups. For the far too many women who have minimal access to prenatal care, however, prenatal testing is not even an option. With laws and regulations on the delivery of health care, and prenatal care in particular, varying from state to state, publicly funded access to abortion is often restricted. Cultural and class gaps between medical practitioner and patient are among other social and cultural factors which operate to limit marginalized women's use of prenatal testing.[5]

The mainly White and relatively privileged women who were the initial and frequent users of prenatal diagnosis share other characteristics as well. Their class position is marked as much by education as by income, their own as well as their husbands'. Since the most important indicator for prenatal testing is maternal age, these women tend to be 35 or over, and are often professionals who have put off childbearing. Their age, jobs, expectations for their offspring, and resources incline them perhaps more than any other group to want to limit their families to one or two children. They are more likely to be pro-choice and to accept abortion as an option if a defect is diagnosed. Even if opposed to abortion, they may accept it in their particular case, reflecting the widely held view that legal abortion

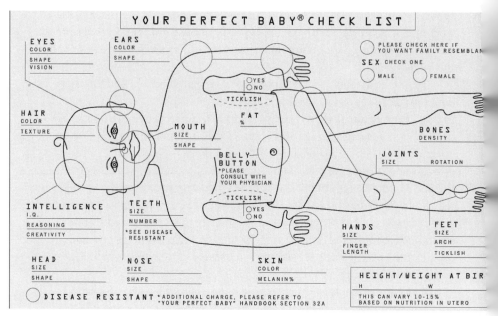

6. "Your Perfect Baby Checklist," January 24, 2003, *The New York Times.*
Courtesy M. K. Mabry/*The New York Times.*

should be available for serious fetal defects. As to broader class and cultural norms, these women are likely to feel positive about the benefits of science and technology, and to subscribe to the ethos of individual choice and patient autonomy.[6]

Although research patterns have changed to increasingly cover more diverse segments of populations undergoing prenatal diagnosis, the decisions and experiences of the more privileged group have so far been more widely studied. Because of their class position, their decisions provide some measure of prevailing social and cultural attitudes toward science and technology, and toward disability and disease. Their decisions also can have an impact disproportionate to their numbers and so perpetuate such values. If we look at their decisions, condition by condition, as to which pregnancies they choose to end and which to keep, we can begin to get a picture of how diagnosed defects are ranked. Further, we can discover how earlier diagnosis—in the first trimester, or even earlier—may affect their decisions and thus the ranking of particular conditions.

CHOOSING AMONG "DEFECTIVES"

"I've never seen a pregnant woman who wasn't anxious about her baby being normal," a genetic counselor told me. Through prenatal screening, women seek assurance that their baby will be healthy, if not necessarily perfect. Even though physicians and genetic counselors caution that tests can't guarantee a normal, completely healthy child, that results are limited, anxiety is regarded as a form of suffering to be treated.[7] (Some physicians, however, do refuse to test just to relieve a woman's anxiety if there is no other medical indication.) Women express relief when no defect is found. Indeed, "reassurance" is the term that crops up most frequently in discussions of pregnant women's feelings about testing. But misperceptions persist among women and parents[8] that "reassurance" means guaranteeing a normal, even "perfect," baby, and that the "choice" to test, and to abort or not, brings control.[9]

Prenatal diagnosis procedures can also increase anxiety, producing what Barbara Katz Rothman has called the "tentative pregnancy."[10] When amniocentesis is performed at 15 to 17 weeks, with results coming as late as the 20th week, as was the norm until the early '90s, it means that the woman of 35 or older, with no other "risk" besides age, is in suspense for fully half her pregnancy. Even though these women are at higher risk for birth defects than are younger women, only about 2 percent of their fetuses will be diagnosed with a defect. As the triple screen is extended to increasing numbers of pregnancies, regardless of risk, women under 35 (who are the majority of pregnant women) will join their older sisters in anxiously waiting for results well into the second trimester.[11] The social and peer pressures to test in the first place lest she bear a "defective" child that women report experiencing can also add to a woman's anxiety—as will be discussed further in chapter nine.

By far the point of highest anxiety comes when a woman must decide whether to abort or not if a diagnosis is "positive." Even for those women most supportive of testing, the decision is not an easy one. Tension is often heightened because the decision usually involves a much-wanted child.[12] To help parents make decisions, including whether or not to test initially, counselors sometimes borrow from statisticians' risk assessment methods, such as decision trees.[13] The mother's age can be weighed against the probabilities of certain defects, or the risks can be assessed for prospective parents belonging to a population group with a higher than average incidence of a particular condition. Yet, when the time arrives for parents to make a decision, statistical probabilities are often of little help. It becomes a matter of "either-or." Parents ask simply and straightforwardly, Will my child be affected or not? They want a yes or no answer. But counselors or doctors frequently can answer only with probabilities. A Belgian researcher has commented on the "potential inadequacy of assumed total rationality of the decision maker."[14] Rather than implying that parents are irrational, his statement suggests that an abstract statistical model cal-culating the odds of bearing an affected child does not fit the needs of the parties involved. The "rationalized" model indicates a communication gap between patients and medical professionals, even when they are not other-wise separated by class or culture.[15]

Through each stage of the pregnancy, deciding whether to test, wait-ing for results, and deciding whether to keep or abort the pregnancy if a defect is found, the anxiety escalates. Women's fears and tensions are directly related to both personal and social and cultural views of disability and disease. That most women in the so-called high-risk category—defined mainly by maternal age and the class indicators I have outlined—opt for testing illustrates the strength of prevailing negative attitudes to-ward the imperfect. The reassurance that a woman seeks is precisely so that she will not have a child "like that." Implicit in women's willingness to test and the growing acceptance and routinization of prenatal diagnosis is the message that children labeled defective are not wanted.

Ranking and classifying defectives was an important preoccupation of the Eugenics Record Office in the first decades of the twentieth century. Less overtly and without deliberate intent, today abortion decisions per-form the same ranking function. When studies show a woman less likely to take a fetus diagnosed with Down syndrome or spina bifida to term, but more likely to keep a pregnancy showing Klinefelter's syndrome, we learn how these particular conditions are ranked. At the same time, looking at abortion decisions over time can reveal changing patterns, such as in-creasingly positive views of Down syndrome. Improved treatment and prognosis for some conditions, such as for cystic fibrosis, may affect whether or not such pregnancies are kept. The timing of screens and tests—early or later—has become another critical factor in assessing and ranking diagnosable conditions. We need to consider as well what will happen as genetic research dramatically increases the numbers of genet-ically based diseases identifiable, as a result of the completed sequencing of the human genome.

"SERIOUS" OR "SEVERE"

In most instances, when the condition is regarded as "serious" or "severe," the decision will be to abort. National studies since the early 1970s show "consistently high levels of support (75% to 78%) for making legal abor-tion available for serious fetal defects."[16] But what is "serious" or "severe"? In the late 1980s Abby Lippman called "serious" a "physician-imposed criterion for testing" even though the term was "never rigorously de-fined."[17] In 1990, Dr. Arie Drugan and his colleagues at Hutzel Hospital at

Wayne State did present two categories called "severe" and "questionable," grouping various conditions in each. In the "severe" category they included trisomy 21, that is, Down syndrome, and certain types of Turner's syndrome (a sex chromosome anomaly), along with trisomies 13 and 18.[18] What is startling about grouping these conditions together is that the tripling of chromosome 13 or 18 is almost always fatal—rendering choice effectively moot—while the prognoses for Down syndrome and the particular forms of Turner's syndrome are decidedly mixed, and hardly fatal. Abortion decisions in these cases are not open and shut. A follow-up study published in 1996, assessing the bases of abortion decisions of a much larger sample of parents after "positive" diagnoses, adopted the same classification, even though the authors acknowledged that "[t]hese categories were defined, somewhat arbitrarily, several years ago" and that "there have been some modifications about counseling for certain conditions . . . over the 8-year period." Nonetheless, "for consistency and to keep the data sets from being too small to be meaningful, the original definitions have been maintained." The only change was to rename the "questionable" category "mild to moderate."[19] In addition to revealing the persisting negative attitudes toward so-called defects, such groupings also obscure whether parents distinguish among conditions in making their decisions, and therefore how "severity" might be ranked.

Down Syndrome
For example, some changes have occurred in decisions about Down syndrome. Throughout the late 1980s the termination rate for fetuses diagnosed with Down syndrome hovered at about 90 percent. In the 1990 study of Drugan and colleagues the overall termination rate for "severe" conditions was 93 percent, with most of the 7 percent not aborted attributable to Down syndrome pregnancies. But when the 1996 study showed a drop in termination rates for "severe" conditions, such attribution was not clear. Among diagnoses confirmed by amniocentesis, termination rates for "severe" conditions fell from a high of 95 percent in 1986–88 to 75 percent in 1989–91, and then rebounded somewhat to 81 percent in 1992–94. Because this study did not distinguish among "severe" conditions, we cannot know for sure whether this drop was due to Down syndrome. It seems likely, however, that the almost one in five women now continuing their pregnancies were carrying Down syndrome fetuses. This conjecture is supported by the fact that Down syndrome is much more common than the other chromosomal anomalies included in the "severe" category.

While attitudes toward people with Down syndrome have been changing during the past decade—as I will discuss in the following chapter—the overall rate of abortion for a Down syndrome diagnosis continues to be relatively high. When, as reported in these studies, CVS rather than amniocentesis was used to diagnose a "severe" condition, termination rates remained consistent between 1986 and 1994, at 88–89 percent. Although both studies maintained that differences between CVS and amniocentesis rates of termination were less important than what the condition was and its perceived severity, the figures show that earlier diagnosis, by CVS, is more likely to lead to abortion. This discrepancy was more marked for "mild to moderate" conditions, which had a considerably higher rate of pregnancies continued when diagnosed later in the pregnancy. The growing move toward earlier diagnosis—including earlier amniocentesis—may serve to arrest trends toward dropping rates for Down syndrome, which would keep it in the "severe" or "serious" category.

Sex Chromosome Anomalies
With one exception—a form of Turner's syndrome—the studies discussed here placed discrepancies in sex chromosomes in the "questionable" or "mild to moderate" category. There are a number of variations: an extra X or Y chromosome, or a missing X for females, for example. Symptoms vary widely, but can include lowered intelligence compared to siblings (though not usually retardation), problems in sexual development, infertility, and some physical disabilities. Consequently, abortion rates have shown a mixed picture. Studies in the late 1980s ranged from as many as two-thirds of pregnancies terminated following amniocentesis to only about half. By the mid-1990s rates had dropped to about one-third, which meant that about two-thirds of pregnancies diagnosed with sex chromosome discrepancies were being taken to term. Dr. Arthur Robinson, head of the National Jewish Center for Immunology and Respiratory Medicine at the University of Colorado School of Medicine in Denver, has attributed the shift to effective counseling by well-trained professionals.[20] The 1996 Wayne State report clearly showed this trend for conditions classed as "mild to moderate," which included the sex chromosome discrepancies. But, again, the failure to distinguish among the chromosome anomalies in this category impedes attempts to rank the conditions that parents consider more, or less, acceptable.

Physicians report that high on the list of parents' concerns about sex chromosome anomalies are problems with mental development and learning abilities. Following this, they ask, Will the child look peculiar, that is, as one doctor put it, will it be a "freak"? Boys with Klinefelter's syndrome (an extra X chromosome) may develop breasts and other secondary female characteristics, while girls with Turner's syndrome (a missing X chromosome) fail to do so. Parents are also very worried that their child will be sterile. Although each chromosome anomaly tends to have a certain cluster of symptoms or characteristics, the specifics vary enormously. The karyotype cannot predict which symptoms will be expressed, nor how severe or mild each may be. Physicians and counselors, hard-pressed to convey these ambiguities to parents, can deal only in averages. They can offer only a general prognosis, which parents, wanting clear-cut yes or no answers, may find less than satisfactory.[21] Parents' ambivalence and uncertainties are reflected in the mixed but lower abortion rates for sex chromosome anomalies than, for example, for Down syndrome and spina bifida. But earlier prenatal diagnosis could have an effect on rates, as it does for the more "serious" conditions. The 1996 report showed that while termination rates for "mild to moderate" conditions diagnosed by both CVS and amniocentesis did drop over time, the rates remained appreciably lower when diagnosis was later in the pregnancy, with more women continuing their pregnancies.[22] But, again, because the study does not distinguish among "mild to moderate" conditions, further refinement of preferences is not possible.

Neural Tube Disorders

Neural tube disorders (NTDs) are generally classed as severe. They occur less frequently than Down syndrome, but have a similarly high termination rate. Level of severity is the critical factor. At the high end is anencephaly, in which all or most of the brain is missing. There is no chance of survival; abortion is almost always the case. For spina bifida, in which the neural tube fails to close, level of severity depends on where the lesion occurs. The higher the lesion is on the spine, the more critical the condition is; lower lesions are more amenable to corrective surgery after birth to reduce physical disabilities and considerably improve the individual's prognosis. In one study, 21 of 27 women carrying fetuses with spina bifida elected to terminate, while six continued their pregnancies. None of the six had fetuses with high-level lesions, while several of those terminated did.[23] Sonography (ultrasound) has greatly aided in identifying particular types of neural tube defects and their possible severity (which cannot be done for chromosomal anomalies). A much larger study of 53,000 terminations (on the grounds of NTDs and other anomalies of the central nervous system) ranked severity on a scale of 1 to 4. The scale was developed by a "sonologist-geneticist, whose knowledge of severity had provided the basis for the genetic counseling" for the pregnancies evaluated. While some forms of spina bifida ranked only 2, "an anomaly expected to have little or no impact on the quality of life but which might require surgical or medical treatment," others, such as hydrocephalus (water in the brain cavity), were ranked 3, "an anomaly with the potential for serious impact on quality of life, even with optimal medical or surgical treatment." Rank 4 was for "an anomaly incompatible with life." As expected, termination rates were much higher for grades 3 and 4 than for grade 2. But the study, which focused on demographic characteristics, also found that older women with more education were much more likely to abort a grade 3 fetus than were younger women with less education. The researchers attributed these differences to communication difficulties between counselors and younger, less educated women, the older and better educated women's higher aspirations for their children, and the younger ones' possible skepticism about medical information.[24] The class implications of these findings are reinforced in other studies of women's attitudes toward testing and abortions.

Conditions Affecting Special Populations
Some women are tested, not because of their age or other specific indicators, but because they belong to populations prone to certain conditions, or because they have a child or other family member affected. Because they differ from the general population of women recommended for testing, we cannot be sure, without careful investigation, how their decisions about testing and abortion might apply to those of other women. Reactions of parents to diagnoses of less frequently occurring conditions—even if occurring randomly—and to carrier screening also need to be assessed and questioned in this way.

Fragile X Syndrome
This chromosome anomaly, which is the most common inherited cause of mental retardation, results from a fragile site on the X chromosome. The syndrome affects approximately one in 4,000 men and one in 8,000 women; a woman with only one impaired X chromosome does not manifest the condition, although she is a carrier.[25] Previous birth of an affected child is a prime indicator. In one study, women of normal intelligence who were deemed at risk said they would choose prenatal testing, but were ambivalent about abortion. The issue they were most concerned about, however, was the risk of having a mentally retarded child. Those who already had such a child were more likely to choose to terminate the pregnancy.[26]

Cystic Fibrosis
Since the gene accounting for about 70 percent of cystic fibrosis (CF) cases was discovered in 1989,[27] close to 1,000 different disease-causing muta-

tions have been discovered,[28] increasing the chances of detecting carriers and affected fetuses. Affecting one out of 2,000–2,500 Caucasian births, CF is characterized by a buildup of mucus in the lungs, pancreas, and sweat and other glands, seriously impeding breathing and a variety of other bodily functions. While CF has been labeled "the most common serious genetic disease among Caucasians,"[29] steady gains in treatments are serving to alleviate symptoms and to prolong life. In 1938 the median age of survival was less than one year. Median survival age in the U.S. is now 32,[30] which means that half of persons with CF will live beyond their early thirties, although half will not.

Abortion rates for CF have been relatively high, although changes have occurred over time and there are differences between parents with CF children and those without. Studies in the 1980s of parents of CF children, when markers but not the gene had been found, had mixed results. In one study, one-third of the women who intended to have more children or who were already pregnant said they would abort if the marker appeared, 43 percent said they would not, and one-quarter (24 percent) were undecided.[31] But another study showed that of those women who said they would have prenatal diagnosis, 68 percent said they would abort an affected fetus, although many would test only so they could prepare for the birth of an affected child.[32] When all respondents in the first study, whether they intended to have more children or not, were asked about testing criteria, "more would abort for severe mental retardation, conditions causing death before age 5, or severe physical disability than for CF." Their criteria for an unacceptable fetus were similar to those of non-CF parents, although they considered CF less severe than the other conditions mentioned.[33]

With the discovery of the gene and its mutations came increased attention to the benefits of carrier screening and more studies of responses of parents both with and without family incidence of CF. In Rochester, New York, the more than half of the pregnant women who accepted offered screening for CF, when compared to decliners, "regarded having a child with CF as more serious, . . . would be more likely to terminate a pregnancy if the fetus were shown to have CF, and more strongly supported offering CF screening to women of reproductive age."[34] A cystic fibrosis center in England found very high support among CF families for prenatal screening and the option to terminate the pregnancy, and for offering screening to parents without any history of CF. Carrier-screening programs were deemed cost-effective in a study published in 1998. The cost of screening the woman and then the fetus was measured against the lifetime cost of raising a newborn with CF. Effectiveness rested on the extent to which screening could prevent such births, that is, prevent through abortion. Since "therapeutic abortion rates" were 50–100 percent, the program was deemed to be cost-effective.[35] Discovery of the gene and its mutations has helped to bring better understanding of the disease and to spur advances in treatment. Yet it has also spurred the promotion of screening and testing programs, which appear to be gaining wider acceptance among pregnant women and their families, whether or not there is a family history of CF. Even as the condition becomes more treatable, it become less acceptable in a prospective child.

Neurofibromatosis
Unlike CF, which is recessive (to be affected, a child must inherit the gene from both parents), neurofibromatosis (NF) is a neurological genetic condition with autosomal dominant inheritance: only one gene or allele is needed for symptoms to appear. This means that, if one parent carries the gene, each child has a 50 percent chance of being affected. Incidence is not affected by race or sex. Of the two genetically distinct forms, NF-2, the far more debilitating, occurs only in an estimated one in 50,000 births. The gene is located on chromosome 22. NF-2 is characterized by tumors in the brain or spinal cord. NF-1, the more prevalent form, is estimated to occur in one out of 3,500 births. Isolation of the NF-1 gene was announced in August 1990.[36] NF-1's most obvious symptoms are multiple café-au-lait spots on the skin and tumors of varying size on or under the skin. There can be nerve tumors as well, freckling, and vision impairment from nodules or tumors.[37]

Two studies among NF families, made shortly before but anticipating discovery of the NF-1 gene, showed similar results. Of 100 respondents with NF-1 in Texas, 62 percent said they would use prenatal testing, but only 19 percent would terminate an affected fetus.[38] In a larger study in the Washington, D.C., area of almost 300 persons in NF households—that is, people who had the condition themselves or had an affected family member—64 percent indicated they would test prenatally if a test were available, but only 16 percent would elect to abort.[39] Researchers in the Washington study noted that respondents were not fully representative of the area's population in that they belonged to an NF support group, were predominantly White, and had a relatively high level of schooling and yearly income. They added, however, that the sample did contain a "diverse mix of the population" of the "cosmopolitan" Washington area. They cautioned as well that when a relatively quick and accurate predictive test was actually available—which was not then the case (but is now)—the views reported might change. For example, they compared attitudes toward NF with those toward Huntington's disease, which is also an inherited autosomal dominant condition, and found a much greater willingness to abort a Huntington's fetus if accurate predictive testing were available.[40] Respondents in the Washington study reported that disfigurement was one of the "worst aspects" of NF. Given the importance parents attach to appearance and their probable wish to avoid such stigma for their offspring, more parents at risk for NF children might opt to prevent their birth if there were a sure test. There is no known cure for either NF-1 or NF-2, only treatment to alleviate symptoms. As is the case for other prenatally diagnosable conditions, severity and expression vary widely and cannot be predicted before birth.

Conditions Compared
Patterns like those found for NF and CF are also found in families with children or other family members having other diagnosable but nonlethal conditions. While those surveyed may favor testing, most studies show that relatively few women choose to terminate the pregnancy if the condition is found. Some will refuse testing altogether, while others decide not to have more, or any, children. Mothers of children with spina bifida follow the same pattern. In one study, three-quarters (74 percent) of the mothers said they would test for SB. But only 11 percent would terminate an affected pregnancy. Forty percent definitely would not end the pregnancy, and about half (49 percent) were unsure. Mothers of more severely affected children were more likely to terminate, as were women who saw raising an affected child as a greater burden, although clinical severity did not correlate with the level of burden perceived.[41] Again, relatively few women said they would terminate their pregnancy, even though many SB mothers would want to be tested. On balance, therefore, women or families with direct experience of a particular condition may show greater acceptance of that condition than does the general public.

Such women are the exception, not the rule. Although prior history of a condition is a prime indicator for recurrence, most cases occur much more randomly. Indeed, most children with neural tube disorders are conceived by women with no such history.[42] NTDs occur in one to two of every 1,000 births, and apparently without correlation to age, race, or ethnicity; their cause is not known. Thus most women being tested and who may be positively diagnosed have had no family experience of such conditions. As noted above, more than three-quarters of women will abort after a diagnosis of SB, and the rates are much higher for the most severe NTDs. Although severity is the major criterion, terminations are performed for the less severe forms of SB, now discernible through ultrasound.[43]

Termination rates remain high for the more prevalent Down syndrome and SB. These two major diagnosable conditions account for most pregnancy terminations in the second trimester. As the rates drop for other conditions, what do parents' decisions tell us about ranking of what is acceptable and what is not? What are the criteria? A roundup of the literature by researchers at King's College, London, showed termination rates for five conditions: Down syndrome the highest at 92 percent, Klinefelter's syndrome the lowest at 58 percent, and spina bifida, anencephaly, and Turner's syndrome in between.[44] The perceived severity of the condition is still the main rationale, and as presented in the medical setting in which the decisions are made. As I have argued in the previous chapter and will develop further in the next, medical and cultural cues reinforce choices which result in a higher proportion of pregnancies with sex chromosome anomalies being continued than of those with Down syndrome or spina bifida. Parents' overriding concerns, especially for the "milder" or "questionable" conditions, are mental retardation, followed by abnormal physical appearance or functioning.

But this analysis of abortion rates according to condition applies mainly to second-trimester diagnoses and abortions which take place in the fifth month, halfway through the pregnancy. Studies show that as the option of first-trimester diagnosis, by CVS or earlier amniocentesis, grows, distinctions about relative severity of the disorder tend to get erased. When given the possibility of terminating the pregnancy within the first three months, parents appear to be increasingly unwilling to tolerate any unacceptable "defect" in their fetus that testing may reveal. As the numbers of diagnosable conditions grow, and the label "disease" or "defect" is applied to a widening range of these conditions, the "severity" argument disappears along with the medical rationale. In their place appear criteria that are less and less medically defensible and increasingly socially defined.

Socially Defined Selection Criteria

SEX AS "DEFECT"

When the genes for the most common X-linked diseases, muscular dystrophy and hemophilia, were discovered, making it possible to diagnose both adult carriers and affected (and carrier) fetuses, the medical rationale for testing for sex all but disappeared.[45] But the practice of testing and selecting for sex is alive and well in many parts of the world, such as China, India, and Korea, even though laws have been passed against it. As ultrasound became sufficiently refined to detect male genitalia as early as nine weeks, it began to replace the more invasive amniocentesis, although use of the latter continued. This prompted China in late 1994 to forbid using ultrasound for this purpose.[46] After more than two decades of prenatal sex selection, China had a serious sex imbalance, as increasing numbers of young men were unable to find wives.[47] As in India, where sex selection is also still practiced (though it was declared illegal earlier than in China),[48] China's strong cultural preference for boys meant that female fetuses were almost always aborted after testing, as is the case in many Asian countries.[49] China's enforced one-child policy accelerated the dramatic drop in the number of females in the population. Many groups—led originally by feminists—have been understandably alarmed about the practice and its social implications. But in the U.S. and other Western countries, the issues are not that clear-cut. Parents do not always favor boys over girls; they vary, sometimes showing preferences for a child of each sex. Furthermore, the practice is often opposed, or at least not considered socially acceptable. Yet the possibility of testing for sex selection, especially if invasive procedures need not be involved, and the fact that it does take place—though its extent is not easily measurable—presents us with an example of a "defect" that is not a defect at all. Its status is purely socially defined. Sex identification and selection therefore offer a template for considering the nature and possible impact of diagnosing traits when the only rationale for doing so is social.

Sex identification is often a by-product of prenatal testing for other fetal characteristics. Some parents want to know, others do not, and physicians will comply with their wishes. Testing solely for sex is another matter, for the clear implication is that the parent will abort if the fetus is the "wrong" sex. A Hastings Center report in 1989 indicated that many physicians who were unwilling themselves to perform prenatal diagnosis for sex selection would be willing to refer the patient to someone who would do so.[50] Because of social taboos, which would cause parents to be reluctant to make the request openly and physicians hesitant to comply, information is scarce about incidence of the practice, and about parents' motives and actions. A woman or couple may well mask their reasons for seeking testing, perhaps explaining that they wish to relieve "anxiety" about the health of their future baby.

The development of preimplantation genetic diagnosis (PGD) in conjunction with IVF has pushed detection of disease back to the "pre-embryo" stage, before the embryo is inserted and becomes implanted in the womb. PGD can include sex identification in cases where parents fear one of the rare X-linked diseases for which no gene or other marker has yet been located. The medical rationale is clear. But PGD also opens up the possibility of parents' requesting sex identification for other than medical reasons. The Ethics Committee of the American Society for Reproductive

Medicine has come down strongly against such use of PGD. "Preimplanta-tion genetic diagnosis used for sex selection to prevent the transmission of serious genetic disease is ethically acceptable." Requests for sex identifica-tion for non-medical reasons are not.[51] However, when safe and effective techniques for separating X- and Y-bearing sperm become available, the Ethics Committee will not deny approval for their non-medical use, out-lining conditions and recommendations for physicians, such as for gender variety in a family.[52]

Because PGD depends on the costly and invasive IVF procedure, it is unlikely to be used for sex selection, even though it would mean discard-ing an embryo a few days old rather than aborting a several-weeks-old fetus. Separating X and Y sperm prior to conception, however, would allow achieving the desired sex without any qualms about destroying a potential life. Not only is the decision removed from the medical realm, it is removed from the moral one. It is an isolated, privatized decision in its purest form.

Until the presorting of X and Y sperm becomes more reliable, this asocial, amoral stage of decision-making will not be fully in the realm of possibility. We remain in an ambiguous, more controversial realm. In testing for sex when the intent is to terminate the pregnancy for the "wrong" sex, the parent is in essence labeling the sex a defect, even though it is not one medically. How will parents react when conditions with marginal medical significance for the health and well-being of the future child are diagnosable early in the pregnancy? It might be a missing finger or toe, or a minor facial disfigurement, perhaps revealed through ultra-sound. As these conditions are added to the "defect" list, decisions about whether to abort for them could begin to depend more heavily on social criteria than on medical. At what point will the social criteria become fully acceptable?

While arguments may be advanced against terminating pregnancies for morally unjustified and "trivial" reasons, earlier prenatal diagnosis methods will increasingly make it possible to hide such decisions. A deci-sion to abort for sex or a minor imperfection taken early in the first trimester (at two months no one need know you're pregnant!) is one that is increasingly privatized, one that can evade cultural and moral taboos. Parents' "personal" choices, made privately, in this way can in turn rein-force purely social criteria for the imperfect, and the perfect, child.

THE "PERFECT" PARENT?

Social criteria loom especially large when choices involve parent selection prior to conception. Extending now from donor sperm to egg donation to choosing suitable wombs, the practice seeks to match and select for desired traits. Sperm banks in the U.S., which supply donor sperm, may be part of a physician's practice, based in a hospital or clinic, or commercial corporations, which have become a huge business. According to a study of "artificial insemination" (only the process is artificial; real sperm is used) in the U.S. by the Office of Technology Assessment (OTA) in 1988,[53] of 172,000 inseminations reported each year, about half use the husband's sperm, the other half use a donor's. While the husband's sperm is generally not screened (unless there is a specific reason to do so), donor sperm is screened for certain diseases and conditions, although criteria and procedures are by no means uniform and have come in for considerable criticism on that score when evaluated.

Shortly after the OTA report appeared, the American Fertility Society established a new set of guidelines for donor insemination, supplementing those published in 1980, 1986, and 1988. Among the chief additions was a recommendation that donors be intensively screened for sexually transmitted diseases, particularly HIV.[54] By 2002, the guidelines, published by the renamed American Society for Reproductive Medicine (ASRM), had expanded to cover egg and frozen embryo donation. While the guidelines had become more detailed and explicit, they also included minimal recommendations for screening of gamete donors. In addition to being "generally healthy and young," donors and their first-degree relatives should be free from major Mendelian disorders, major malformations, significant familial disease with genetic component, known karyotypic abnormality, membership in a high-risk group for a disorder, and should be evaluated for current tests for CF.[55] Like those of the past twenty years and more, the carefully spelled out 2002 guidelines remain recommendations, not requirements. Commercial sperm banks, for example, which handle the largest volume of sperm donations, are under no obligation to follow guidelines other than regulations enforceable by the states in which they operate. Evaluations of donor screening indicate that donor facilities repeatedly fall short of and vary considerably in meeting ASRM guidelines, as well as those issued by the Centers for Disease Control and the American Association of Tissue Banks.[56]

Public health and safety are clearly served by monitoring donor practices, especially to prevent the knowing transmission of lethal inheritable conditions. The fact that the list of conditions not to be passed on is medically defined, however, masks the fact that they reflect medical and cultural norms, the latter presumably shared by prospective recipients. Choosing a prospective donor is an individual and personal act, the criteria spanning the medical and social spectrum. The 1988 OTA report also asked physicians and sperm banks about donor screening for other than medically defined traits. About two-thirds of women seeking donor insemination specify certain characteristics, and between 78 percent and 88 percent of the physicians said they were willing to meet those requests. While the report did not show how often each type of trait was asked for, some pattern is suggested by the qualities that physicians were willing to match. Physicians most readily matched characteristics such as race, ethnic or national origin, and physical attributes, including hair and eye color, complexion, and body type.[57] As in requests reported by sperm banks, women want the donor to match their husband, or male partner, as closely as possible.[58] Although more than half (57 percent) of the physicians in the OTA study were willing to select for I.Q. and two-thirds (66 percent) for "educational attainment," the report pointed out that a "substantial portion" who were willing to select for some characteristics were unwilling to match for I.Q. (37%) or education (29%). Intelligence is apparently very high on recipients' list of requested donor qualities.[59] A majority of physicians in the OTA study refused to match for hobbies or income and were about evenly split on whether or not they would select for special abilities.[60] Although donors typically have been students, especially medical students (who are readily available and welcome payment), increased demand for sperm donors—reflecting a rising rate of infertility —and more use of frozen sperm have broadened the sperm donor pool. Perhaps because sperm donation is still generally anonymous, little systematic information is available about who sperm donors are. Partially breaking this rule was the so-called Nobel Sperm Bank, the popular name given to the Repository for Germinal Choice in Escondido, California, because it counted Nobel laureates among its early and publicized sperm donors.[61] That many sperm banks apparently look for "intelligent" men as donors no doubt reflects recipient demand.

Parents hope for brainy offspring regardless of sex. Smart girls are wanted as much as smart boys. But intelligence in donors appears to be gendered. Compare the qualities wanted in "surrogate mothers" and donor fathers.[62] Judith Lasker and Susan Borg, studying infertility, found that while donor fathers are to contribute brains, "special abilities," and physical characteristics matching the husband's, donor mothers are to be warm, caring, and beautiful. In screening applicants, surrogate programs consider "qualities such as stability, warmth, openness, physical attractiveness, strength of character, and compassion . . . more important than intelligence." Surrogate programs screen women for "psychological make-up," although sperm donor programs routinely do not do so for men.[63] Whether or not contracting parents specifically seek such attributes, they accept them and have a stake in the donor mother's "maternal" qualities while she is gestating their child.

Rene Almeling revealed the same patterns in her study of the operations and recruitment policies of both egg donation agencies and sperm banks in California. Pointing out the extent to which these agencies are part of what has become a multi-million-dollar for-profit infertility business, she found that donor screening for both eggs and sperm conformed very much to gendered stereotypes, clearly satisfying client demand.[64] The growth of egg-selling and more recently of embryos further raises questions about the role and impact of patriarchal values, of other kinds of socially selective criteria, and of ethical values, as the ideal parent becomes part of the quest for a special, if not perfect, child.[65]

Framing the Hierarchy

Although some parents opt out of prenatal diagnosis, the majority of those recommended for testing choose, rather than refuse, to be tested. It is their decisions that help to frame the new perfectibility discourse.

When women elect to end a pregnancy for Down syndrome, but not for CF or Turner's syndrome, their individual decisions add up to a grading of "defects," thus ranking children's levels of acceptability. Underlying and extending the perceived seriousness of the condition are the qualities or traits on which parents base their selections. Intelligence, above all, is the most desired trait; mental impairment is to be avoided at all costs. Not only is a fetus with a prognosis of mental disability rejected, as in Down syndrome or fragile X; intelligence is a sine qua non in the sperm donor as well. Almost as troubling for parents are abnormal appearance and physical and developmental problems, as, for example, the disfiguring aspects of neurofibromatosis, or female characteristics in a boy with Klinefelter's syndrome. Conversely, parents seek attractive appearance and good physical health both in donors and in the future child.[66]

Parents' selection criteria do not necessarily add up to a "perfect baby." But the possibility of refining the selections they can make as more and more conditions become diagnosable, and at earlier points in the pregnancy (and even prior to conception), makes trying to influence the outcome more tempting. That each decision is seen as a matter of individual choice, taken privately, masks its wider implications and effects. For the selection process takes place in "real time." Within the privatized setting of reproductive medical practice, parents' individual decisions aggregate to frame a hierarchy of disorders. The criteria that select out the undesirable, and desirable, children reflect the class, racial, and cultural values of those making the decisions: parents who seek to perpetuate their own kind. The "superior" product envisioned by the White and middle- to upper-middle-class parents who predominate will be economically privileged, perhaps male if firstborn, a child of each sex, and as defect-free and gifted as money and technology can buy. Even though there are no assurances that their child will be beautiful, brilliant, a Mozart, or a de- cathalon champion, the very existence of the technologies in the practice of reproductive medicine seem to perpetuate this illusion, despite dis- claimers to the contrary. Responding to the technologies, to the climate of medical practice, and to peer and community pressures, parents perpetu- ate the values of their socioeconomic and cultural milieu. Patriarchal attitudes and prevailing views toward disability are among them.

The Onus of "Bad Genes"

Although prospective fathers' attitudes are not studied as much as are mothers', men appear to react more negatively to the diagnosis of an imperfection and are more willing to reject the fetus. Both genetic coun- selors and pregnant women report that men see lowered intelligence, or another defect, as a blow to their self-image. The man reacts through denial: rejecting the fetus and blaming the woman for the cause of the defect.[67] Not only are women blamed, women also then internalize the blame for producing a defective offspring. A genetic counselor described the case of a couple who had not married until their mid-thirties and whose fetus was diagnosed with Down syndrome. The result was "a severe blow, especially to the husband. He had waited to marry until he found the 'perfect wife' and could not accept the fact that she was carrying an 'im- perfect' child." He was sure his wife was at fault, despite the counselor's explanation. His wife was "all too willing to accept the 'blame' . . . proof of her inadequacy as a wife and female." The husband insisted on an abortion and avoided sex thereafter; by the end of the year the couple had separated and planned to divorce.[68]

Gendered responses aside, both parents who have produced an af- fected child or are themselves diagnosed with a disease-bearing gene often feel unworthy. Genetic counselors and social workers report that parents feel stigmatized, apart from others. Writes former social worker Joan Weiss, "One may feel defective, just like the gene. 'A part of me is bad,' the individual might think. 'Therefore I am a worthless person.' That is a frequent response, although not always verbalized."[69] Physician Neil Schimke finds denial is a recurrent pattern. Parents will try to blame an outside factor: " 'I am not abnormal; if my baby is, it must be due to something external to me.' "[70] But there is guilt as well, especially if the child is malformed. Couples blame themselves, and each other. Dr. Schimke has also noted that medical personnel can be insensitive, referring to a "funny-looking kid" or to "mental retardation" or a "defective child" in front of the parents. People often confuse being the carrier of a recessive trait with actually having the disease, so that stigma attaches to the carrier.[71] When patients learn they are carriers, says medical geneticist Jessica Davis, they experience this stigma, feeling "unclean."[72]

Genetic problems "undermine self-esteem by exhibiting to the rest of the world demonstrably flawed reproductive capacity."[73] Parents who have produced an affected child or who have had a birth defect diagnosed pre-natally frequently "need" to have a "normal" child. Counselors explain that this is a way for parents to prove they are not damaged, not unworthy. These needs and feelings are particularly strong when there is mental retar-dation, as for some parents of children with Down syndrome,[74] again illus-trating the high social value accorded to intelligence and low esteem for those labeled deficient. For parents of children with spina bifida, hydro-cephaly and the possibility of mental handicaps as a result can bring an "acute distress level."[75] That some parents feel so strongly about the pres-ence of a trait or condition labeled defective in themselves or their off-spring, attributing it to "bad genes," means they have internalized pre-vailing societal attitudes toward disability, which, as the next chapter illustrates, still bear some startling resemblances to those in the heyday of eugenics.

Parents' attitudes, and more importantly their decisions made in the privacy of the family and the medical setting, help to rank prenatally diagnosable conditions which are medically defined as serious or severe. As the numbers of diagnosable conditions grow, and as they increasingly include those of minor medical significance, the social bases for parents' "choices" gain importance. Early diagnosis, first-trimester abortion, and even preimplantation diagnosis increase the likelihood that a pregnancy will be terminated for almost entirely socially based, "trivial" reasons, further shaping the discourse of the perfect child.

SEVEN

Discourses of the Imperfect

Why do parents feel "imperfect" if they carry a disease-bearing gene or if their fetus is diagnosed with a defect? Why is such an event "devastating"? Our language has changed. Just as it is no longer socially acceptable to use racial and ethnic epithets, so is there a new vocabulary to describe people with disabilities. But does substituting "Down syndrome" for "mongolism" mean a change in attitudes?[1] Are so-called "normals" now better disposed toward the "physically" or "mentally challenged"? Introduction of the term "African American" has not meant that racism in the U.S. has gone away. More socially acceptable language may merely mask that old attitudes persist. Perhaps we need to look more closely at what we do, as well as at what we say. As the language of disability emerges and changes, newer discourses of the imperfect may remain embedded in the old.

People with disabilities, cultural and social critics, and reproductive medical practices themselves are witnesses to changes in both rhetoric and practice. Classifications and treatment of the "imperfect" have changed, at times markedly. But the new discourses produced bring with them a sense of déjà vu. Remedicalizing and rebiologizing disability, reproductive medicine lodges "defect" once again in the individual's genes. Literature and popular culture show us that the thinking behind the "old" eugenics dies hard.

The Shape and Character of "Difference"

In the foreword to John Gliedman and William Roth's *The Unexpected Minority: Handicapped Children in America,* psychologist Kenneth Keniston writes,

> What makes the handicapped "special" are the attitudes and reactions of others who are not handicapped; and the greatest harm to the handicapped child or adult stems from this socially engendered impairment of daily life, self-concept and future—not from functional impairments themselves.[2]

For disability rights movement activist Marsha Saxton, born with spina bifida, the "pitying stares, the smiling condescension mostly from adults" were more oppressive than the leg braces she wore as a child. "The *oppression* is what's disabling about disability."[3] Sociologist Barbara Altman, reviewing studies of attitudes toward the handicapped, comments, "It is the subtle but pervasive influence of public attitudes that governs the day-to-day interactions of handicapped individuals and affects (either by support or rejection) the lifestyles they develop."[4] For policy analyst Harlan Hahn, the greatest obstacle for the disabled lies in " 'attitudes,' " in the discriminatory and "destructive process of stigmatizing."[5]

Social critics and activists describe three characteristics of such attitudes, which they find rooted in the culture and its social systems: (1) the disabled are defined by their disability, (2) a functional limitations model, which rests on a biological and medical model, is applied, and (3) the impairment is inherent in the individual and is that person's "problem."

DEFINED BY DISABILITY

It is more than a century since eugenicists began using the word "defective" as a noun. Reflecting then current values, the term could conveniently encompass those who already bore the mark of their socially defined defect, whether they were labeled "criminal," "drunkard," or "cripple." We no longer use the term in this way and have discarded some of the social categories, but the labeling persists, though in an altered form. People with disabilities are defined by their membership in the suspect category.[6] Someone who is blind becomes "the blind woman," as if blindness were her only characteristic. The label "deaf man" similarly marks someone who cannot hear. The child born with Down syndrome is described as a "Down's child." Using stigmatizing terms in discourse "as a source of metaphor," writes Erving Goffman, "[w]e tend to impute a wide range of imperfections on the basis of the original one." Whether the handicap is referred to or avoided, an underlying heightened awareness "causes the interaction to be articulated too exclusively in terms of it."[7]

A FUNCTIONAL LIMITATIONS MODEL

Categorized and defined in these ways, people with disabilities are labeled inferior. A functional limitations model, and its companion, a medical model, support inferiority labeling. According to "biological inferiority theory," a person's physical or mental impairments cause the problems the individual may face.[8] There are parallels here to the use of biological differences of sex or race—whether real or construed—to rank and discriminate among individuals. Similarly, the biological difference of the disabled is socially and politically constructed to mark them as inferior.[9] Focusing on the impairment and its departure from a norm (also socially constructed) allows any limits to disabled people's activity to be socially labeled "handicaps." Considered functionally limited because they are biologically inferior, people with disabilities are classified as sick, needing treatment or to be segregated and institutionalized. Because they are considered to require medical and professional care, they are subjected to a medical model which reinforces discriminatory and dehumanizing attitudes and practices.

Ironically, the medical model originally brought a change for the better, as new public policies for the mentally and physically impaired emerged between 1920 and 1960. Funds were committed, rehabilitation methods and programs were developed, living conditions for people with disabilities improved, and much more professional attention was paid to them. (It was, for example, during this period that the field of social work, which had its beginnings in the Progressive Era, as well as the mental health profession, fully came of age.) But, according to Robert Funk, director of the national legal arm of the disability rights movement, neither the status of people with disabilities nor public attitudes toward them changed.

> [T]he handicapped retained their caste status in the public mind as dependent, unhealthy deviants, who would, in the great majority, always require segregated care and protection. The charity, rehabilitation, and medical professionals ruled the day, providing better care and better services to a people who would, it appeared, retain their childlike dependent status in perpetuity.[10]

Almost three decades after the medical model took hold, the disabled continue to be oppressed by attitudes and images that perpetuate their caste status.[11] Alan Gartner and Tom Joe, in the introduction to their aptly titled edited collection *Images of the Disabled, Disabling Images*, in which Funk's article appears, state, "While the emergence of new views has tamed some of the extremes of the medical model, it still holds sway," especially in the training of the " 'helping professions.' "[12]

INHERENT DISABILITY

The medical model, because of its focus on the individual, reinforces the view that the impairment and its disabling consequences are lodged in the individual. In a study of the treatment of children with disabilities that probed parents' and pediatricians' attitudes, Darling and Darling describe a "clinical perspective" and a "curing model." Physicians do not consider the social context, having no "social system perspective," stressing rather the individual family's adjustment to the handicapped child.[13] By the same token, the person having a disability is expected to "adjust" to the world as given. Douglas Biklen, a director of special education programs, notes that the print media perpetuate an individualized approach, portraying the issue of treating seriously impaired newborns as an individual problem for parents, doctors, and disabled people themselves.[14] Darling and Darling have also found that the clinical perspective and the curing model actually "combine in many cases to produce negative attitudes toward congenitally handicapped children and their parents, especially when the parents refuse to accept either viewpoint."[15]

A clinical perspective appears as well in psychological approaches to disability. Comparing changes in practices and policies over a 40-year period from 1948 to 1988, social psychologist Lee Meyerson writes, "Our society has come a long way since the time when infants with disabilities were 'monsters' and adults with deviant physiques were 'freaks' . . . but we still have a long way to go." He expresses concern that clinical psychologists predominate in the new fields of health and community psychology. Noting that they receive different training and ask different questions than do social psychologists, he cautions, "If these clinical psychologists, like their medical counterparts, center their attention on defects, deformities, and disease whose origins and treatment are within the individual, the data that emerge are unlikely to support present trends." These "present trends" are embodied in the approach of health and community psychologists, who operate in a public health framework, oriented toward "person-environment interactions." These interactions can bring a "new and even more favorable Zeitgeist for people with disabilities."[16]

Us and Them: What Purposes Does Stigma Labeling Serve?

How do we explain why people with disabilities continue to be categorized and labeled? Why are they stigmatized? Why do such persons continue to be seen as biologically inferior, as sick and needing treatment, their whole lives colored, indeed dominated, by a particular functional limit? Why do we see disability as a "personal misfortune," the fault lying in the individual?

Goffman's classic study describes stigma as "an attribute that is deeply discrediting." A person with stigma possesses "an undesired differentness from what we had anticipated." "By definition," he continues, "we believe the person with a stigma is not quite human." And, on this assumption, the "normals" discriminate against and restrict the life chances of the stigmatized, constructing an ideology to explain their inferiority and account for the dangers they represent.[17]

Depth psychology theories find the sources of such attitudes in people's uncertainties about their own humanity. Just as I suggested in chapter three that "defectives" served a similar role for eugenicists, so John Gliedman and William Roth hold that people with disabilities are cast as "symbolic Other. In this role the disabled person becomes a kind of talisman, a visible incarnation of death, sexuality, and dependency, all of which arouse our deepest fears." Among the most fundamental is the fear "of the nonhuman and of becoming nonhuman ourselves." If one's humanity is achieved and proved through conflict and power over the Other, then the "handicapped person—by virtue of his disability—is the incarnation of our fear of failure, of losing out, of being mutilated and conquered by the Other." The "ultimate failure is death." In the mind of the able-bodied, "every handicapped person has . . . already died a little. . . . His lack—his blindness, or deafness, or paralysis—reminds us of the time when we shall all be blind, and deaf, and paralyzed." Making the psychoanalytic links between sex and death, this depth psychology theory argues that "the disabled person is a disturbing parody of a sexual object." So the retarded have been sterilized, and the sexual needs of the handicapped denied. "For what we fear in ourselves we deny to others."[18]

Relating the freak shows of the past to our continuing fascination with "freaks" and "abnormals"—as evidenced by the enormous success of the stage and film versions of *The Elephant Man*—literary and social critic Leslie Fiedler finds that "those wretched caricatures of our idealized body image . . . appear at first to represent the absolutely 'Other.'" But they are "really a revelation of what in our deepest psyches we recognize as the Secret Self. . . . in the depths of our unconscious . . . we seem forever freaks to ourselves."[19]

Harlan Hahn sums up the fears projected onto the disabled as "existential anxiety," the "perceived threat that a disability could interfere with functional capacities deemed necessary to the pursuit of a satisfactory life." Granting disability benefits therefore is preferred to attempting to increase capacities for those who have not met the expected levels of functional proficiency.

> The principal effects of existential anxiety have been to relegate disabled individuals to the role of helpless or dependent nonparticipants in community life, and to exacerbate nondisabled persons' worries about the potential loss of physical or behavioral capabilities that could result from a disability. In a society that appears to prize liberty more than equality, and that tends to equate freedom with personal autonomy rather than with the opportunity to exercise meaningful choice, the apprehensions aroused by functional restrictions resulting from a disability often seem overwhelming.[20]

Taking a societal view, Kaoru Yamamoto, a professor of education, has suggested that people who are physically and mentally "different" function to "preserve stability in society by embodying otherwise formless dangers." Thus non-deviates may perpetuate deviates' status because "society may indeed need the deviates as a symbol of evil, intangible dangers."[21]

Perhaps the most obvious examples of the ways the mentally or physically disabled represent danger, evil, and the other things people fear are in popular and literary culture. Among "the most persistent" of these representations, writes historian Paul Longmore, "is the association of disability with malevolence" and with criminality or villainy. "Deformity of body symbolizes deformity of soul."[22] Doctor No's and Doctor Strangelove's forearms are encased in black leather, " 'crippled' " as a result of their evil experiments; Doctor Strangelove is even " 'confined to a wheelchair.' " The TV adventure series *The Wild, Wild West* featured a "hunchbacked 'dwarf,' " a criminal genius who was also a doctor. Ronald Merrick, the "arrogant, deceitful, and viciously racist" British intelligence officer in the British-made TV series *The Jewel in the Crown,* has a disfigured face and a missing arm. Longmore points out that disability here is a punishment for evil; the disabled are seen as embittered people who resent and would even destroy the nondisabled.

"Closely related to the criminal characterization . . . is . . . the 'monster' " of horror films, and of horror classics such as *The Hunchback of Notre Dame* and *The Phantom of the Opera.* For both the criminal and the monster—even a sympathetic monster, such as the one in *Of Mice and Men* or *The Elephant Man*—the only solution is death. A genre of media images of the severely disabled that appeared in the 1970s and 1980s projected a similar outcome. For the quadriplegic in *Whose Life Is It Anyway?* the loss of function, and with it humanity, is so acute that death is "the only logical and humane solution." Suicide is chosen by the disabled character himself. The message is clear: "Better dead than disabled."[23] In the case of criminal characters, the "nondisabled audience is allowed to disown its fears and biases by 'blaming the victims,' making them responsible for their own ostracism and destruction." Through the sympathetic portrayals, the nondisabled preserve their own humanity, distancing themselves, avoiding having to deal with disability and its "problems" as social phenomena.

Leslie Fiedler links acts and expressions of pity and sympathy to deepseated terrors. When we would end the life of the crippled child (an archetype in literature) or of the severely disabled infant, to spare each a life of anguish, we may not do so out of "enlightened pity." Rather, our act "may in part be the product of the same primordial fear of difference and monstrosity that once prompted ritual infanticide." Pity, "the relevant literature seems to suggest, is only a disguised form of our aboriginal terror . . . leading us to evade rather than confront the problem of our relationship to the disabled by tempting us into weepy voyeurism and selfcongratulatory smugness." When we opt for quasi-miraculous cures, as in *The Secret Garden* and *Heidi,* we are expressing "a wish that there were no handicapped, that they would all finally go away."[24]

Robert Bogdan, on the other hand, faults socialization, rather than deep-seated fears. He argues that our responses to freak shows have been socially constructed by the way "our social institutions managed these people's identities." Covering the period from 1840 to 1940 when freak shows flourished, his *Freak Show: Presenting Human Oddities for Amusement and Profit* showed that while the persons on exhibit were exploited and degraded, they thought of themselves as "showmen," the experience earning them status and fame and fortune. " 'Freak' is not a quality that belongs to the person on display. It is something that we created: a perspective, a set of practices—a social construction." However, to the extent that freak shows still exist today, they are an affront to people with disabilities, projecting the message that they are freaks.[25]

Reviewing the popular media in the 1970s, Bogdan and Biklen found a pattern of social construction of "handicapism." Images associated physical ugliness with violence and crime; in horror films both physical and mental handicaps were linked with acts of violence and hate. Whether in children's stories, movies, or cartoons, the world of Disney reinforced stereotypes of mental impairment with frequent use of words such as "dumb," "moron," "crazy." News reports of murders often imputed the perpetrators' being alcoholic, incompetent psychotic, or mentally retarded as the cause of crime. In the media, the handicapped appeared generally as dependent and helpless.[26]

By the late 1970s portrayals had begun to change, increasing into the next decade. Longmore noted that TV commercials for hamburgers, jeans, and similar popular items started to show people in wheelchairs or with other disabilities in positive and active ways.[27] A weekly TV "family drama" in the late 1980s, *Life Goes On,* featured a teenager with Down syndrome who is "mainstreamed" into school and social life. He behaves as other teenagers do and is treated as they are.[28] Even as Down syndrome support groups have welcomed such changed portrayals as indications of a new trend, the effectiveness of their reach may be questioned. Longmore's 1987 analysis of literature and popular media suggests that old images, and the fears, anxieties, and behaviors they express, can exist alongside an emerging discourse of social awareness. In the same collection, Funk argues that denial of civil rights and equal opportunity is "rooted in the overriding influence of the persisting images of disabled people as deviant, incompetent, unhealthy objects of fear who are perpetually dependent upon the welfare and charity of others."[29]

Photographic images have come under scrutiny, for example by London-based photographer David Hevey, who is also disabled. Photographic representations are voyeuristic, manipulating the disabled person's image, he writes. Surveying photography collections, Hevey finds that the work of photographers such as Diane Arbus serves a purpose for the photographer, not for the disabled. "The use of disabled people is the anchor of the weird . . . the symbol of enfreakment or the surrealism of all society." In an article drawn from his book *The Creatures Time Forgot: Photography and Disability,* Hevey argues that, as the "site and symbol of all alienation . . . the 'contorted' body . . . does not function as the property of those disabled people observed. Its purpose was . . . as the voyeuristic property of the non-disabled gaze. . . . the impairment . . . became the mark, the target for a disavowal, a ridding, of the existential fears and fantasies of non-disabled people." He goes on to say that the newer work of the " 'post New Documentaries' " has made disabled people "an even more separate category. While the volume of representation is higher, the categorisation, control and manipulation have become deeper."[30]

In addition to "existential anxiety," Harlan Hahn has described an "aesthetic anxiety" experienced by those holding negative images of people with disabilities. The term "refers to the fears engendered by persons whose appearance deviates markedly from the usual human form or includes physical traits regarded as unappealing."[31] In Goffman's stigma typology such attributes are classed as "abominations of the body—the various physical deformities."[32] Held by some to be "experienced on sensory and visceral levels," feelings of "repulsion and discomfort" among the nondisabled are "triggered by the sight of a visibly disabled person." Such sights might include amputations, body deformities, cerebral palsy, or skin disorders.[33] Shunning and devaluing the physically unappealing and unattractive, the nondisabled may feel their own body image threatened. Their anxious preoccupation with appearance in turn reflects sociocultural norms. Writes Hahn, "[I]n a society that places extraordinary stress on beauty and attractiveness, aesthetic anxiety may be an important component of perceptions of disabled people."[34] Aesthetic aversion and anxiety presuppose social ideals not only of the "normal" but also of the perfect. As disabilities are measured against such norms, a hierarchy of standards for what is acceptable or unacceptable—aesthetically, physically, and mentally—can begin to emerge.

Setting Standards: A Hierarchy of Beauty and Brains

As Roth points out, "It seems hard for society to accept difference without somehow ranking it, thinking of it as inferior, deficient, dysfunctional."[35] Still, although people with disabilities are among the "different" who are labeled "inferior, deficient," and "dysfunctional," there are gradations of inferiority. Disabilities themselves are socially ranked. Sociologist Constantina Safilios-Rothschild points to seven interrelated factors—socioeconomic, political, and cultural—that influence the degree of prejudice directed toward the sick and disabled. Three are particularly relevant for studies that have measured social attitudes toward disability:

> (3) the prevailing notions about the etiology of illness and the degree of individual "responsibility" involved in falling ill and remaining disabled; (4) the cultural values or stigmata attached to different physical conditions or characteristics; (5) illness- or disability-connected factors, such as (a) the degree of visibility of the illness or disability, (b) whether or not the incapacitating illness is contagious, (c) the part of the body afflicted, (d) the nature of the illness (physical or mental) and the assumed "pervasiveness" of the disability, and (e) the severity of functional impairment and the degree of predictability of its course.[36]

In part because they are more readily measurable, attitudes toward physical impairments, that is, visible disabilities, have been studied more. One method to get at differences in and types of attitudes is picture-ranking. In a classic study from 1961, children aged 10 to 11, both normal and handicapped, were shown six pictures and asked to identify the boy or girl they "liked best." As each selected picture was removed, they were asked their "next best" choice, the process continuing until the last picture. Starting from "best," the children chose (1) a child with no handicap, (2) a child with crutches and a brace on the left leg, (3) a child in a wheelchair, a blanket covering both legs, (4) a child with the left hand missing, (5) a child facially disfigured on the left side of the mouth, and (6) an obese child.[37] Subsequent studies have revealed a surprising consistency of results, regardless of the race, physical handicap, socioeconomic status, urban-rural differences of the children questioned. Results for both sexes were constant as well, as were sex differences. Boys were more negative toward functional impairments, such as a child in a wheelchair or with missing limb, while girls looked less favorably on impairments with social consequences, that is, facial disfigurements and obesity. As they did for other findings, researchers ascribed these sex differences to cultural influences, including "stereotypes of physical beauty . . . identified with goodness and . . . physical ugliness . . . with evil."[38] A follow-up study showed similarly consistent preferences among children from grades 1 through 6 (ages 6 to 11), but some changes beginning to emerge among those in junior and senior high school. In the teen years, children's preferences began to approach those of the same-sex parent, the divergences along sex lines becoming stronger. Girls were more markedly prone to dislike cosmetically disfiguring impairments, boys to reject the functionally disabled. All, however, ranked obesity last.[39]

That younger children's preferences hold steady across many possible individual and social divides, and that children's preferences come closer to adults' as the children approach adulthood, indicate the extent to which these attitudes are learned, dependent on widely shared sociocultural values. Although these picture-ranking studies date mainly from the 1960s, reflecting the opinions prevalent then, and follow limited and perhaps simplistic methodologies,[40] the values and the practices they reflect persist. According to Funk, people with visible physical disabilities continue to be highly stigmatized, the intensity of discrimination depending on the severity and degree of disability.[41] The premium is on physical wholeness and attractiveness, as standards of health and beauty have become increasingly exacting.

The billion-dollar beauty, health, and fitness industries owe their success in promoting and selling their images in no small measure to tapping into the central role that physical attractiveness plays in our culture and in forming self-concepts.[42] The young, impossibly flawless specimens portrayed in the media are not just examples of perfect fitness and health. They represent unlimited material success and the good, the true, and the beautiful. As the physically flawed are associated with evil, so the physically attractive are linked with good. "What is beautiful is good," and "what is good is also beautiful."[43] And the "good" in our society is at one with success. Psychologist Rhoda Unger points out that physical attractiveness is associated with "perceptions of greater social influence, ability to succeed, competence, and likability," while "negative social judgments" are associated with people having "lower degrees of attractiveness." The less attractive are selected as more likely to show symptoms of psychopathology, even epilepsy; they are less desirable in high-status employment, and are more likely to be associated with social and political deviance.[44] While Unger's primary goal is to show how attractiveness stereotypes operate in the social control of women, her analysis applies equally to the way socially constructed norms of physical attractiveness can perpetuate negative assessments and reinforce social control of the physically disabled. Because of the beauty standards set for females, women with physical disabilities suffer a double burden, as Michelle Fine and Adrienne Asch, among others, have carefully pointed out.[45]

Within given cultures such standards are social and class-based. As Safilios-Rothschild writes,

> there are indications that the standards for physical integrity and perfection as well as for beauty are very strict in Anglo-Saxon countries (especially among the middle classes), and any deviation from the highly admired state of perfection is punished by social stigmatization. Not only physical deformities or chronic invalidating illnesses, but also obesity (or even overweight), pimples, oily hair, "bad" breath or sweating odors are considered intolerable and label the "afflicted" individuals as deviants. This labeling brings about devaluation, social isolation, and a more or less potent social stigma according to the nature and degree of the deviation.[46]

While physical health and attractiveness are important marks of success, in a highly industrialized culture intelligence is even more greatly prized.

> The higher the stage of industrialization and socioeconomic development in a country, the greater the tendency to value intelligence and all the qualities that are conducive to high achievement, productivity, competitiveness, and efficiency. Thus, stupidity is strongly stigmatized, since people with a low IQ have little chance of earning any kind of social status in societies in which one's personal ability and achievement determine his social standing practically to the exclusion of all other criteria.[47]

The increased value placed on intelligence translates into intolerance of mental illness or mental deviations of any kind. There is a growing tendency to discriminate against stupidity. Lewis Anthony Dexter noted that the Protestant ethic, with its "emphasis on achievement . . . as a justification of one's righteousness," and "Jacksonian democracy, with its emphasis on the rights and obligations of equality," interrelate to foster these attitudes. While the Protestant ethic "and its secular variants" have led people "to regard stupidity as a sin, rather than a common human failing," compulsory education, based on providing not only the opportunity but the obligation to be equal, has resulted in a "compulsory equality." Problems result for what Dexter terms "the high-grade retarded" (this was 1967) for themselves and for society.[48]

Bogdan and Taylor in the early 1980s questioned the validity of the term "mental retardation" itself, especially from the perspective of those so labeled. The term is "not just less than useful," but "seriously misleading." Its "scientific aura is deceptive in that it conceals subjective moral and cultural value judgments," mental retardation being "a demeaning concept which implies a deficiency in the humanity of those tagged." It is "a reification—a socially created category." It points to, not the state of mind "of the people who are alleged to have it, but the state of mind of those who use the concept in thinking about others." They conclude, "Mental retardation is a misnomer, a myth." Reviewing the dramatic rise in numbers of persons identified as retarded in the twentieth century, Bogdan and Taylor note how elaborate classification schemes were devised even as mental retardation continued to be thought of as an absolute condition. "[C]lassification of people as mentally retarded depends on organizational and societal values, beliefs, and processes." For those so labeled, the term "implies moral inferiority as well as intellectual deficiency," a comment that recalls the harsh moralisms of an earlier day. Moral judgment could well be added to intolerance of those who can't measure up in the "knowledge society."[49]

In current society, then, despite the fitness and body-building craze, brains are more important than brawn. Parents may hope for budding geniuses, but anything less than normal intelligence would be a disaster. And physical disabilities can at least be fixed. Even though images of beauty and health set exacting standards, medicine and technology are rising to the challenge. Plastic surgery can correct and even reconstruct "imperfect" body parts; prostheses and sophisticated mechanical and electronic devices are becoming available for the severely physically impaired. Masking the disability or making social participation easier, such measures could help to reduce social stigma of the physically impaired. But no comparable "fixes" (such as surgery to repair a "defective" brain) are in the immediate offing for the mentally impaired, unless we count mood- or behavior-altering drugs that may mask or temporarily reduce symptoms. Far less amenable to correction or technological fix, and of increasing importance to culturally dominant groups, mental disability is the least desirable attribute—at the bottom of the health hierarchy.

But, whether disability is mental or physical, past and current policy and practice have focused on making it disappear. Using whatever scientific, technological, social, or legal measures are available, the aim is to make disability just go away.

Social Policy and Practice: Then and Now

The prospect of eliminating "defectives" brings its own moral dilemmas. In the 1950s, evolutionary biologists posed the issue of "genetic load" (see chapter three). Because science and medicine were making it possible for more "bad genes" to survive and be transmitted to succeeding generations, natural selection no longer operated to prevent threatened deterioration of the human gene pool. Their patron saint, Charles Darwin, had raised this possibility almost a century earlier. For Darwin, the impetus to treat and protect the weak was moral, although also a product of evolution. Natural selection and the struggle for survival, he maintained, had produced not only physically and mentally superior human beings, but also a "higher morality." In civilized societies it was this developed moral sense that now worked to thwart natural selection and therefore to impede further race improvement. As he wrote in *The Descent of Man*, while among "savages, the weak in body and mind are soon eliminated,"

> We civilised men ... build asylums for the imbecile, the maimed, and the sick; we institute poor laws; and our medical men exert their utmost to save the life of every one to the last moment. . . . Thus the weak members of civilised societies propagate their kind. No one who has attended to the breeding of domestic animals will doubt that this must be highly injurious to the race of man.[50]

John Greene describes this as posing a dilemma for Darwin. Practicing a socially conscious morality would weaken and even eliminate the competitive struggle. Yet, much as he might have deplored the ethic of struggle in moral terms, Darwin found it necessary for both race survival and race progress. Could one "destroy the very basis of social progress" through practicing higher morality—itself a product of struggle—and still progress? For Greene, Darwin never dealt adequately with this contradiction.

Somehow Darwin believed that the "higher impulses" would win out, bringing humankind to moral perfection, a point at which struggle would presumably no longer be necessary.[51]

Evolutionary biologists and geneticists almost a century later expressed the conflict in terms of cultural and biological evolution. Science, as well as technology—with a little education and moral suasion added— would solve the problems of genetic deterioration that a scientific civilization had produced. They proposed artificial selection, the "new eugenics" variety. If voluntary artificial selection were instituted as societal practice, the genetic load would be sufficiently reduced so as to lessen the need to find and apply cures for genetic disorders. The practice of saving defectives would fall off, there being fewer to deal with. Genetic deterioration would stop, and the way opened for the human species to improve and progress. But what about measures in the interim, to save and care for the genetically unfortunate? As noted in chapter three, the geneticist Dobzhansky restated Darwin's dilemma in terms of twentieth-century technology. On the one hand he argued that we should accept an increasing dependence on technology to deal with genetic defects as part of modern life, even though using insulin, for example, might well increase the incidence of diabetes. "The remedy for our genetic dependence on technology," he wrote, "is more, not less, technology."[52] But Dobzhansky also favored using voluntary artificial selection to persuade the genetically defective not to procreate. The question then becomes, Would artificial selection succeed in decreasing the genetic load if technology continued to operate at cross-purposes? Today, the question is one of technology vs. technology. While prenatal screening carries out a type of artificial selection, even if unwittingly, medical technology enables increasing numbers of even the most severely disabled to survive.

As it was for Dobzhansky, for most of those involved in reproductive practice today, the "old eugenics" is unacceptable. Thus a form of Darwin's dilemma may still be with us. But perhaps the "dilemma" remains mainly as a rhetorical device to mask a mindset that supports eliminating the "defective," if socially acceptable means can be found. Harlan Hahn maintains that, if we look at people with disabilities as a minority group and not as individual cases, the attention paid to life-and-death decision controversies, telethons, and the "massive resources allocated to medical research" indicate that "the prevalent values of the nondisabled majority seem to denote a widespread belief that the principle [sic] solution to the problem of disability is to eradicate it."[53] The disabled, he points out, accounted for one million of the nine million human beings exterminated by the Nazis. Historically, the legal criteria for involuntary sterilization and for therapeutic abortion as they unfolded in the U.S. lend support to Hahn's harsh judgment, which could perhaps apply to reproductive practice today.

The eugenicists were the first to clearly link defectives to reproduction, justifying the connection "scientifically" and seeking to implement it legally and socially in the name of race survival and "betterment." Their technical solution was involuntary sterilization for the "unfit." As discussed in chapter two, the 1927 Supreme Court decision in *Buck v. Bell* that upheld the sterilization of a "feeble-minded" young woman in Virginia opened the way for the heyday of eugenic sterilizations in the U.S. Reaching a peak in the 1930s with over 2,000 a year, reported sterilizations were performed on more than 60,000 persons between 1907 and 1963.[54] Carefully crafted to meet court challenges, laws passed in the 1920s and '30s clearly rested on a eugenic rationale. For both criminals and the feeble-minded—the main objects of legislation—the purpose was to prevent their transmitting their defective genes to their offspring. In the beginning, both institutionalized males and females were sterilized. By the 1930s, "mentally defective" young women and girls had become the main targets.

Although the rate declined sharply in the 1940s as the courts began to chip away at the constitutionality of involuntary sterilization programs and the eugenic rationale became increasingly suspect and discredited, in 1975 twenty-four states still had eugenic sterilization laws. As late as 1981 such laws remained in 13 states.[55] After a brief rise in sterilizations in the 1950s, reported rates dropped off considerably, to below 500 a year after 1960. But it was not until the 1970s that reforms finally repudiated the eugenic theories on which the laws had rested. With reform came changes in the laws' rationale, arguments, and focus. As eugenic justification for sterilization was discredited and laws were increasingly challenged on the grounds of due process and the right to privacy, the focus shifted to the individual herself. The "state's compelling interest" in preventing procreation by the mentally retarded now became based on such issues as the individual's competency to care for a child as well as on social costs, and on "informed consent," not on the nature of the prospective child itself. But those labeled mentally retarded remained a suspect category, the wisdom of allowing persons so categorized to procreate still open to question by the law and mental health professionals alike.[56]

In a curious pattern of events, however, just as the onus shifted from defective offspring to defective adult and the eugenic rationale no longer served to support legal sterilization, the "defective fetus" was emerging as a legal justification for therapeutic abortion. Coincidentally, perhaps, abortion policy took over where sterilization left off to prevent the reproduction of so-called defectives. Abortions performed for fetal deformity actually predated mid-twentieth century attempts to legalize it as a criterion. By the late nineteenth century, mainly in response to the efforts of physicians, stringent state laws were in place to make abortion a crime except to save the life of the mother. Accepted practice had been to allow abortion until the point of "quickening," that is, until the woman felt movement. Acting less than out of moral concern, physicians sought to shut out competition and gain full control over reproductive medicine, including abortion. Medical practice, therefore, was not closely bound by the letter of the law. Between 1890 and 1950, physicians who performed abortions tacitly agreed to include among their criteria protection of the life and health of the mother, cases of rape or incest, and the possibility of "fetal deformity." Eugenic sympathies apparently played a role in the early period in supporting physicians' willingness to abort for possible fetal defects.[57] But medical criteria, especially dangers to the fetus from a woman's contracting rubella (German measles) or from being exposed to high levels of radiation from X-rays early in pregnancy, were more generally acknowledged and the case. In the post–World War II period, when most obstetrical care had moved into hospitals and medical records had become more readily obtainable, hospital surveys showed that approximately one in four abortions was performed for "fetal indications," with the highest proportion of these for rubella.[58]

In 1959, therefore, when the American Law Institute proposed reform of state abortion laws and offered a model statute, its provisions reflected what had been actual medical practice for more than half a century. Included among the special cases for approval were abortion to protect the life and health of the mother, cases of rape or incest, and "cases where there was a probability of congenital defects appearing in the embryo."[59] Greater public attention was building on the issue of possible fetal deformities, perhaps due in part to a number of rubella outbreaks. But it was the publicity surrounding the so-called Finkbine case in 1962 that served to heighten public awareness and provide a catalyst for legal reform. As Kristin Luker recounts, Sherri Finkbine's physician, learning that she had taken the sleeping pill Thalidomide, had recommended abortion. Reports had just begun to surface linking the drug to fetal malformations, including severe deformities of the limbs and hands. Just before the abortion was to take place, press stories (the original local story initiated by Finkbine herself to warn other women) made both the abortion and Finkbine a center of intense public controversy, and she was denied the abortion. Although Finkbine was able eventually to obtain an abortion in Sweden (afterward, the physician told her the fetus was so severely deformed it would not have survived), the debate on what had once been routine practice, though increasingly questioned by professionals, was now out in the open. Physicians who supported a broad interpretation of abortion indications—including psychiatric reasons—wanted legal protection for their practice. As the Finkbine case became a catalyst for professionally led efforts to reform abortion law, a fetal deformities provision was written into reform statutes enacted in the late 1960s and early '70s.[60]

The provision became highly controversial because, according to Luker, "strict" constructionists found it the most offensive criterion of all. It exposed the moral issue of the fetus as a person. When pregnancy endangered the life or health of the mother, or resulted from rape or incest, it could be argued that the fetus was being sacrificed for "some 'greater good.'" But the fetal indications provision meant that the fetus's existence could "be ended for its own good."[61] To those who held that the fetus was a "real" person, not merely a potential one, aborting a "damaged" embryo was totally unacceptable.

Although some medical professionals and later the "right-to-life" movement opposed making fetal indications a legal basis for abortion, they were in the minority among the public in the 1960s, and continue to be. Finkbine herself was not a crusader and suffered personally from becoming a symbol, but a Gallup poll at the time showed over half of those surveyed agreed with her position.[62] Support for the right to terminate a pregnancy for fetal abnormalities was to grow in the years that followed. Reviewing nine surveys of attitudes toward abortion sponsored by the National Opinion Research Center (NORC) of the University of Chicago over a 15-year period from 1965 to 1980, Donald and Beth Granberg found that the percentage of adults approving of legal abortion "if there is a strong chance of serious defect in the baby" rose from 57 percent in 1965 to 79 percent by 1972, and to 84 percent by 1973. Although it dipped slightly in the late 1970s, the figure was up to 83 percent in 1980.[63] In national surveys throughout most of the 1970s, more than four out of five adults surveyed approved of terminating a pregnancy for a defective fetus, a view that has held constant into the '80s and '90s.

In 1973, in *Roe v. Wade*, the Supreme Court ruled abortion to be a private right through the second trimester. Invalidating restrictive laws in the states, the legalization of abortion made controversy over a fetal indications provision moot. When prenatal diagnosis was developed in the 1970s and subsequently became accepted practice, it did so in this climate, in which abortion was legal up through the second trimester for any reason, and in which public thinking agreed that it was permissible, even desirable, to prevent the birth of a child *known* to be defective. Over the years since, abortion opponents' attempts to chip away at a woman's right to choose have succeeded in making it more difficult for some women—especially those younger or poorer—to obtain an abortion.[64] But, in pursuing their ultimate goal to outlaw all abortions, anti-choicers for the most part have not included attempts to restrict aborting for a fetal anomaly among their tactics.

At the sociocultural level, then, prenatal diagnosis seemingly takes over where sterilization leaves off. The nondisabled, write Gliedman and Roth, "deny the feelings evoked by disability by denying that the handicapped really are a problem." To soothe their consciences and handle their fears, the nondisabled readily turn to science and technology, invoking a technological fix.[65] Prenatal diagnosis, it could be argued, offers the supreme "technological fix." Enabling medicine to select out the defective and the disabled before they are born, reproductive science and technology offer the prospect of a future in which we will no longer have to deal with the effects of a gene or chromosome gone awry.

But with prenatal diagnosis came a shift in language and the stated medical objective. Sterilization policies and then therapeutic abortion policies singled out persons and their supposedly defective genes. Although an underlying rationale, especially for sterilizations, was to eliminate the defects and diseases that such persons carried and could perpetuate, the policies focused on the defective individuals. With prenatal diagnosis the stated objective of medical policy became the prevention of *disease*. In 1973, Michael Begab, president of the American Association on Mental Deficiency, saw in prenatal diagnosis a particularly effective means to "win the battle against mental retardation," once the procedure was "perfected." "In the right hands, diagnosis and abortion, coupled with an effective public education program to reach vulnerable women, is a powerful tool for the prevention of mental retardation."[66] The disorder itself was the scourge—whether CF, Down syndrome, spina bifida, or "mental retardation." Prevention became the key to making the problem of disability just go away.

Yet the means to do it still focus on the individual—in this case the potential individual: the fetus, or embryo. An interesting reversal has taken place. Just as the old medical model of disability, resting on biological inferiority, has begun to be seriously challenged, reproductive medicine, using the language of prevention, is serving to remedicalize and rebiologize disability. Prenatal diagnosis provides the means for reproductive medical professionals to renew medicine's claim to define disability and control its treatment. Professionals in reproductive medicine become the new arbiters of who and what is labeled and ranked as defective.

With the "geneticization" of disease,[67] the fault is again lodged in the individual, the bearer of flawed genes. But, unlike for the old model, there is reputable science to back it up. Genes take on renewed power to define and label the defective, to separate the imperfect from the perfect, and to justify eliminating the former. Under the new medical model, more tellingly than under the shaky rationale of the early eugenicists, the "defective" can once again be labeled biologically inferior. The model could make it easier to justify abstracting, dehumanizing, even eliminating people with disabilities.

The New Discourse of the Imperfect in Practice

When parents respond negatively to the diagnosis of a defect in their fetus, having opted for prenatal diagnosis in the first place, they reflect and reinforce the prevailing medicalized and biologized model of disability. This model of disability is the framework in which reproductive science and technology, medical professionals, and parents intersect within reproductive medical practice to produce a discourse of the imperfect, and perfect, child. Public acceptance of the disabled individual as a genetically defined, inferior deviant is strengthened as social-psychological, medical, and sociocultural approaches to disability converge. Gliedman and Roth point out that deviance analysis by social pathologists is only one approach of many used to study other disadvantaged groups, such as poor Blacks, alcoholics, or homosexuals, and therefore can be questioned. But for disability, the "expert" view of the pathologist is accepted as natural and thus prevails. "No professional needs to convince us that disability is a kind of deviance. Just as we see that handicaps are diseaselike conditions, it seems only natural that the handicapped role defines the legitimate needs of handicapped people." This is a "triumph of . . . therapeutic morality . . . without parallel in any other area of civil society."[68]

Reassigning a genetic basis to disability takes the deviance perspective one step further. Lost in the renewed obsession with genes and the precipitous rush to geneticize disability and disease is the critical fact that very few impairments have a genetic cause. Indeed, most disabling impairments are not due to inherited birth defects, nor are they congenital.[69] Nor are all prenatally diagnosable conditions genetic in origin. Of the approximately 3 percent of babies born in the U.S. with birth defects, the causes of 70 percent of them are unknown.[70] High on the list of causes are low birthweight babies, who are born disproportionately to very young mothers and others lacking proper prenatal care. Even as the Birth Defects Prevention Act of 1998 seeks to implement prevention through data collection, research, and education,[71] a genetic mindset persists. As the defect is re-lodged in the individual who harbors the malevolent gene, the distinction between an inborn, that is, "inherent," condition and one that is *inheritable,* that is, genetically transmittable, is lost. The type of prevention that captures the public relies on the miracle of medicine and technology to eradicate birth defects, rather than on less newsworthy preventive programs that try to improve prenatal care and efforts to extend adequate health care for all.

The medical and biological model of disability, with its genetic base, has been reborn just as a disability rights movement has come into its own. Advocates have sought to define their own needs and treatment, and, as will be discussed in chapter nine, have organized to change public policies as well as public images and attitudes. The reemergent disability model stands in direct opposition to these advocates' efforts. As Deborah Kaplan, a lawyer with the World Institute on Disability, writes, "Prenatal screening as a widespread social practice appears to be at odds with some of the goals of the disability rights movement. . . . many prominent disability leaders question its value and ethical basis."[72]

We now have a wheelchair-using Barbie doll, and more integrating of children with disabilities into regular school classrooms and programs.[73] But are these signs of new attitudes, or do the old ones persist as before? Four years after the 1990 Americans with Disabilities Act sought to outlaw employment discrimination, a *New York Times* article reported that the numbers of disabled people entering the workforce had not significantly increased, noting, "A well-intentioned law fails to erase prejudice and a lingering culture of dependency."[74] At a session on social attitudes and self-perceptions about disability at the 1996 meeting of the American Sociological Association, panelists and audience alike attested to the many ways people with disabilities still encountered stigma in almost every venue, and faced professionals whose attitudes still reflected the medical model.[75] In 1993, the National Center on Child Abuse and Neglect reported that children with a physical, mental, or emotional disability were twice as likely to be maltreated or abused as other children.[76]

In the 1970s ethicists raised questions about the effects of prenatal screening on the treatment of people with disabilities, only to see such concerns fade from mainstream discussion by the next decade (see chapter eight). In view of the persistence of negative attitudes and the availability of the technological fix to eliminate defects and the "defective," we need to ask more pointedly, What happens to those children with a condition whose birth could have been prevented? What happens to others living with the condition? Will people increasingly ask, Why should society be burdened by the presence and care of impaired individuals, since their condition and very existence were preventable?

A British psychologist, Theresa Marteau, extrapolating from a number of studies of attitudes toward genetic diseases, writes that "it is possible that attitudes towards those with genetic conditions for which screening is available will become more negative," given, first, that attribution for the causes will affect attitudes and second, that "attributions are influenced by the use of existing screening services."[77] Intolerance could be hardest on those with mental impairments, which have the highest incidence of all birth defects and are the most feared. Asked for an image of "serious genetic defects," respondents in a national sampling of adults in the U.S. in 1990 indicated "primarily that of Down's syndrome and other mental defects"; physical defects were mentioned much less frequently, though more often by the men than the women, bearing out earlier findings.[78] A study in Tel Aviv, Israel, found that the most frequently mentioned associations made about genetic disorders included the symptoms of mental retardation, pain, and visible malformations; self-directed emotions of fear, relief, and shame; and causes such as bad genes, heredity, and pregnancy complications.[79]

The major users of prenatal diagnosis continue to test and abort for mental impairments at a high rate. Given negative attitudes toward physical disabilities as well as toward mental ones, minor physical malformations such as a clubfoot, hip dislocation, or cleft lip, revealed through ultrasound, could also come to be less tolerated, even if they could be surgically corrected after birth. If the more privileged among users continue to select out the undesirable, and give birth to fewer children with mental and physical impairments, "unacceptable" children could become clustered increasingly in poorer and marginalized communities. A class- and culture-based hierarchy of birth criteria would then be built into the health care system. Among the consequences would be fewer social services for people with disabilities, greater gaps in opportunities between rich and poor, and diminished resources for research on causes, treatment, and cure of birth defects. Most disturbing, the eugenic claims linking mental and physical defects to the poor and selected racial and ethnic groups, once without empirical validity, could come closer to reality.[80]

The image of the desired child, the "perfect child," emerges White, privileged, and defect-free. Without blemish, it is the "perfectly beautiful" baby proclaimed by the March of Dimes, as their discourse conflates healthy, normal, and perfect. Discourses of the imperfect are no match for the image of perfectibility; they do not translate into pretty pictures so as to counter an emerging health-based birth hierarchy and the shaping of the ideal of the perfect child.

But just as anti-determinist scientists warn us against reducing genetic variety, so studying disability and exploring the dimensions of the imperfect remind us that the image and pursuit of the perfect child are exercises in essentializing the body, in denying differences. Writes Lennard Davis, we "can no longer essentialize [the body's] . . . differences, its eccentricities, its transgressions."[81] Counter-discourses to that of the perfect child, to include the voices of disability, along with those of pregnant women, medical professionals, ethicists, and feminists, are explored in part 3.

PART THREE

Counter-Discourses

Bioethics Discourse and
Reproductive Practice

Bioethics can be defined as the systematic study of value questions that arise in health care delivery and in biomedicine. Specific bioethical issues that have recently received national and international attention include euthanasia, assisted suicide, new reproductive technologies, human experimentation, genetic engineering, abortion, informed consent, acquired immunodeficiency syndrome (AIDS), organ donation and transplantation, and managed care and other concerns in the allocation of health care resources.[1]

Bioethics emerged as a distinct field in the late 1960s and early '70s. Responding to rapid changes in medical technologies and genetics research, bioethics became a growth industry. Yet, despite this growth, over the course of more than three decades bioethics discourse has remained marginal to reproductive medical and scientific practices. Even physician-initiated clinical ethics has had little impact on practice.

A largely closed circuit of bioethicists, grown more ideologically homogeneous and more media-driven over time, has set the tone. In the 1970s, bioethics discourse raised larger issues about eugenics, the meaning of normalcy, of disability, and of disease, as the uses of genetic research and the new technology of prenatal diagnosis were debated pro and con. By the 1980s, however, as a centrist mainstream emerged, the discourse narrowed, the larger issues relegated to the margins. As prenatal diagnosis came to be accepted practice, discussion shifted to such issues as assisted reproduction, as in IVF, with other reproductive subjects taking a back seat generally in bioethics discourse. The critical connections between the new genetics and prenatal diagnosis, central to the earlier discourse, were lost. In the '90s, discussions about germ-line gene therapy reforged these connections. But, for the most part, connections between reproductive practice and the new genetics did not occur.

Isolated, insulated, trapped in an individualistic, legalistic framework and the language of "rights," mainstream bioethics discourse fails to explore or affect the critical points of decision-making in medical practice. It fails to provide means and tools to probe issues about the relationship of prenatal diagnosis to the experiences of women and their families. Supporting and justifying the status quo, the discourse is an exercise in marginality, by default working to frame the discourse of the perfect child.

The Early Years

A distinctive feature of 1970s bioethics discourse was that it contained extreme positions about the new genetics and new reproductive technologies, and the ways they intersect, within the prevailing discourse. Genetic engineering and eugenics were central to the debates. Champions of genetic manipulation and brave-new-world alarmists alike met in bioethics forums and in the pages of medical journals and texts. They, together with moderate centrists, put broad philosophical and social issues on the table.

Epitomizing the pro–genetic engineering and eugenics position, and perhaps its most uncompromising advocate, was the Reverend Joseph Fletcher. An ordained Episcopal minister—although no longer practicing by the 1960s—Dr. Fletcher was atypical of the clergy, who often were outspoken critics. Wrote Fletcher in an early article, "The right to conceive and bear children has to stop short of knowingly making crippled children —and genetics gives us that knowledge." Stating that what is rational and willed is human, and what is random is not, Fletcher argued that "engineering" procreation is "more human" than the so-called "natural"

method, precisely because it gives us rational control! Appearing originally in the *New England Journal of Medicine* in 1971, this article continued to be quoted from and reprinted into the '90s.[2] Two decades earlier,
in the 1950s, Fletcher had advocated sterilization for those unfit to be
parents. By the late 1980s, Fletcher was to hail the possibilities of "ortho-
genic genetic control" through germ-line gene therapy. Instead of denying
the "genetically unfortunate" the chance to have children, as under the old
eugenics, we would now be able to "improve their germ-line" so their
children would not suffer "genetic problems."[3]

Although critics of such views soon faded from bioethics discourse,
supporters of genetic engineering have continued to have a voice and
command some respect within the bioethics mainstream, albeit with
views more tempered and less stridently expressed. Some of this was
generational, especially among scientists. Born in 1906, the same year as
Fletcher, biologist Bentley Glass was a former student of geneticist H. J.
Muller, one of the generation of scientists advocating eugenics who came
of age in the early decades of the twentieth century (see chapter three).
Addressing the first annual meeting of the Society for Health and Human
Values in 1972, Glass spoke to the old issue of degeneration of the gene
pool. He argued that curbing natural selection through negative eugenics
—such as preventing people from marrying—would not be enough to
counter the effects of medical advances that enable people with serious
defects to survive and procreate. But there was no Darwin dilemma for Dr.
Glass. He advocated positive eugenics or "genetic engineering." Acknowledging that not all desirable characteristics were genetic in origin, he
nevertheless proposed a list of favored intellectual, moral, artistic, and
physical capacities, including the behavioral.[4] Looking ahead, he favored
"engineering" at the reproductive cell stage, that is, before fertilization,
since procreation required some form of human gestation, or "foster
mother." Glass questioned whether the "right" to reproduce declared by
the United Nations

> is indeed to remain unrestricted. Is it not equally a right of every person
> to be born physically and mentally sound, capable of developing fully
> into a mature individual? Has society . . . no right at all to protect itself
> from the increasing [genetic] misfortune? Should not the abortion of a
> seriously defective fetus be obligatory?[5]

In a slightly revised version of this 1972 talk reprinted in a collection of his
essays in 1985, Glass had not changed these positions.[6] Throughout the
1970s and 1980s, Glass continued to be a respected member of the scien-

tific community, his expertise called for in symposia, conferences, and publications on genetic issues.

At a symposium in 1971, molecular biologist Robert Sinsheimer supported designed genetic change. This symposium, held at the National Institutes of Health (NIH), reflected the pro and con positions of the time as well as the beginnings of the moderate middle, as participants explored the ethical implications of the new genetics. Entitled "Ethical Issues in Human Genetics: Genetic Counseling and the Use of Genetic Knowledge,"[7] the symposium placed eugenics and genetic engineering on the agenda. Cautioning that we were still "grossly ignorant of the genetic factors that underlie intelligence or emotion or conscience" and that much more genetic research was necessary, Sinsheimer nevertheless endorsed using "all the wisdom we can develop" to "find the way to a higher state." By "higher state" he meant a "higher form of intellectual and moral existence," a state he thought possible for human beings, as the "highest" species and "potentially immortal." Sounding much like the evolutionary scientists at the Darwin Centennial a dozen years earlier who sought to control evolutionary progress, Sinsheimer concluded, "The next step for evolution is ours."[8] He tempered this stance somewhat a few years later,[9] yet apparently granted permission for a much earlier article of his, in which he unequivocally supported the "new genetics" for the "genetic improvement of man," to appear in a 1987 collection.[10]

Dr. James Neel, a prominent medical geneticist who was involved in early genetic counseling, took issue with Sinsheimer's advocacy of genetic engineering to improve "genetic man," pointing out our as yet limited knowledge of the potentialities of the human genotype. Yet among his priorities and objectives for using genetic knowledge were not only reducing the proportion of persons with genetic disease, but also "the improvement of the expression of existing genotypes" including "cultural engineering," "the creation of genetically superior individuals by artificial insemination" (invoking Muller's "germinal choice"), and "protection of the present gene pool by a world population policy."[11] Here, clearly, was a eugenic agenda, despite his criticism of Sinsheimer.

Among the sharpest critics of such a eugenic agenda at the symposium were members of the clergy, along with some scientists and medical professionals. Topics that included the meaning of genetic disease, the "problem of the right to life," privacy rights, "potential problems for the future," and especially the "control and applications of genetic knowledge"[12] enabled the imposing array of medical geneticists, research scientists, theologians, philosophers, lawyers, physicians, and NIH representatives to range widely about attitudes toward "defectives," concepts of the "abnormal," or what constitutes the "normal" or "perfect."

Clearly opposed to use of the new genetic knowledge was theologian and ethicist Paul Ramsey. Linking abortion to attitudes toward and concepts of normality and abnormality, he wondered if society would become so intolerant of "abnormals" that women would be denied the choice to continue such a pregnancy. He envisioned demands even to do away with a Down syndrome baby once born. With "intrauterine screening," the "concept of 'normality' . . . is bound to be 'upgraded,' and the acceptance of 'abnormality' and care for abnormals is bound to be degraded." Ramsey foresaw abnormals as outcasts through imposition of a "standard of 'normality' which every individual must meet to have a life deemed by others to be worth living."[13]

Physician and biochemist Leon Kass advanced the "slippery slope" argument. Once the principle is accepted that " 'Defectives should not be born,' " the bases for elimination will not stop at the cytological or biochemical, but will extend to the sociopsychological or economic. " 'What price the perfect baby?' " asked Kass. An opponent of abortion in almost all instances, he found no justification for "genetic abortion."[14] Kass also voiced concern about the second-class status of "living defectives" if affected fetuses were aborted. Named chairman of the President's Council on Bioethics by President Bush in 2002, Dr. Kass has not changed his opposition to any sort of genetic intervention in the intervening thirty years.[15]

One of the few practicing physicians at the symposium made a similar point about status. Speaking to concerns of physicians and patients about genetic counseling, Dr. Judith Hall, a pediatrician from Johns Hopkins, asked, "Will we make second-class or less privileged citizens by our concern for quality? Will we deny mentally retarded or handicapped individuals the right to procreate?" Predicting that "[p]rocreation will inevitably become more and more a laboratory science in order to obtain normal babies," she wondered whether we were willing to pay the price.[16] One of only eight women participating in the symposium, Dr. Hall also foresaw laws to promote population control and mandate genetic screening.

An even more outspoken critic, who explicitly connected prenatal diagnosis and eugenics, was Jerome Lejeune, the French physician and geneticist who had discovered that a tripling of chromosome 21 caused Down syndrome. When medicine treats and cures, said Lejeune at the symposium, it works against natural selection. But when prenatal diagnosis and selective abortion work to reinforce natural selection, that is eugenics.[17] In a later discussion of how to view the abnormal or defective, Lejeune stated, "as medical men we have to hate the diseases but love the disabled."[18] There was no doubt as to how he resolved the Darwin dilemma. Although he continued his genetic research and medical practice until his death in 1994, he also continued to oppose prenatal diagnosis and abortion, and their eugenic implications.

Sociopolitical arguments were also advanced against eugenic uses of genetic research, especially by the few African Americans at the symposium. Dr. Robert Murray of Howard University Medical School, and a practicing physician, sharply criticized the cultural imperialism implied by the eugenic social policies advocated by Sinsheimer and Neel.[19] Such population control measures, he pointed out, would reduce the number of minorities; he questioned whether acquisitive Western man should be the prototype. Dr. Murray also remarked on the elitism of the symposium. Challenging the pervading "myth" of individualism, Reverend David Eaton of the All Souls Unitarian Church in Washington took the assembly to task directly for ignoring issues of race and poverty.[20] He reminded participants that in the "non-white" community neither abortion nor genetic counseling were the issues, while such concerns as malnutrition and prenatal health care were. Eaton laid such problems squarely at the door of institutionalized racism and White racism. The Black community did not want counselors to "tell us," but rather to have them work within the community, with community members.[21] In the 1980s, genetic counselors, speaking to the cultural and class differences between counselors and their clientele, would voice similar criticisms.

Scientists at other venues also weighed in with a sociopolitical critique of the new genetics in the 1970s. At a conference at the New York Academy of Sciences in 1975 that focused on the role and responsibility of the scientist in relation to new developments in molecular genetics,[22] Jon Beckwith of Harvard Medical School specifically cited and reacted to views of scientists such as Sinsheimer and Glass. A microbiologist and molecular geneticist, and a continuing critic of genetic determinism, Beckwith stated that the social and political climate was ripe for a new eugenics movement. In an analysis that could equally serve as a critique of *The Bell Curve*, written by Harvard colleagues 20 years later, Beckwith argued that unrest over civil rights, equal opportunity, poverty, and crime underwrote people's willingness to accept claims that differences in IQ were genetic, or that an extra Y chromosome signified criminality. A then much publicized decision of a woman to abort an XYY male fetus, based on the prognosis that she could be carrying a future criminal, was, said

Beckwith, "heavily influenced by the social and political context" in which it was made.[23] Scientists will promote these genetic studies instead of examining the social and political roots of violence and inequality, while doctors who accept scientists' interpretation do so because it "fits comfortably with their own biases." The parents "live in a society where most of the prevailing social values are heavily influenced by a dominant class determined to protect its privileges."[24]

But this kind of social analysis of genetic research was rarely linked directly to reproductive medical issues. Reproduction was barely on the agenda at the 1975 New York Academy of Sciences conference.[25] Although other critics in the '70s did consider the negative effects of the new genetics on reproduction, commentary tended to be philosophical and abstract, rather than sociopolitical.

This was generally the case at the 1971 NIH symposium. Assessing future images of disease, disability, and perfection, Rev. Ramsey spoke of "society's repulsion to disease" and the possible consequences of a "lack of biological perfection."[26] Ethicist Daniel Callahan supposed that "behind the human horror at genetic defectiveness lurks . . . an image of the perfect human being." The "very language of 'defect,' 'abnormality,' 'disease,' and 'risk' presupposes such an image, a kind of prototype of perfection." Although he claimed that the "monistic" vision of a "perfect human being" had given way to a respect for pluralism and "human diversity," Callahan noted that with "advances in the detection and cure of genetic disease—the ghost of the perfect human being, once sensibly laid to rest, is putting in his appearance again." He feared that social pressures would mount on parents not to bear children "deviating from the norm of perfection," even denying them the right to bring such children into the world.[27]

These ethicists, theologians, and research scientists, although linking issues about "normals" and "defectives" and perfect humans to reproduction, did not connect further to reproductive practice. Except for those few, such as Ramsey and Kass, who would ban all testing and screening, ethicists steered clear of explicitly linking cultural beliefs to actual practices.[28] Callahan expressed concern that prenatal diagnosis threatened to revive people's "horror" at "genetic defectiveness" and "our ancestors'" view of the "defective child as a curse." Yet he did not carry this to the point of opposing further testing and screening. A co-founder and president of the Institute of Society, Ethics and the Life Sciences, a co-sponsor of the symposium, Callahan was in effect staking out a moderate position. His was the liberal option of support with cautions. Endorsing "further development and refinement of genetic knowledge," he wanted us to "manage both to live humanely with genetic disease and yet to conquer it at the same time."[29] By the end of the '70s, this position would be codified in the moderate ethical mainstream. The institute Callahan headed, which was renamed the Hastings Center in the 1980s, came to epitomize this mainstream.

Although the 1971 symposium was able to encompass strongly pro and anti views of uses of the new genetics and those who advocated them, it also represented the coming together of the distinct group who would constitute the closed mainstream bioethics community that would function in the succeeding decades. Even allowing for natural attrition and the addition of newly minted experts, the philosophers or "ethicists," joined by lawyers, theologians, and social and natural scientists who make up this self-described "our crowd," has exhibited a remarkable continuity. Operating outside the clinical setting, this core includes few medical professionals, who are more often invited experts than central members. Although omissions of other key participants have been less glaring in recent years, largely missing from the 1971 symposium were the perspectives of women professionals, patients, and racial and socioeconomic under-classes.[30] White males from a limited set of professions have continued to be the major accredited bioethics spokespersons at forums, in the literature, and in the popular media.

The 1971 symposium was to play a key role in shaping mainstream bioethics discourse in the following decades. Focusing on prospects and possibilities for human genetics, the symposium underscored a growing consensus on the promised benefits of genetic research, especially by lifting the "burden" of disease. With the exception of those opposed to "genetic abortion," even participants leery about the possible effects of amniocentesis did not question the value of prenatal diagnosis itself. Nor did they question continued research into genetics and reproductive medical technologies. Instead, they cautioned about assuring "safety," "thoughtful application," and exercise of "individual choice" to guard against misuse. Their philosophic, abstracted discussions about "defectives," and about eugenics, were just that: abstracted and removed from practice, such topics to become more marginalized in subsequent ethical discourse. In thus avoiding practical and critical issues about reproductive technologies, which amounted to giving them a cautionary blessing, the symposium laid the groundwork for a negative eugenics consensus that developed during the 1970s, as prenatal diagnosis gained momentum and came to be accepted as routine in medical practice. An ethical discourse that could link the issues of genetic research and genetic engineering to prenatal diagnosis would be further precluded.

The 1980s: The Bioethics Mainstream

By the end of the 1970s, bioethics discourse on genetics and reproductive medicine had decisively shifted. It now increasingly accepted research into, and wider use of, prenatal diagnosis, with little or no critique of the research or the procedures. Adopting the language of medical culture, mainstream bioethics discourse joined the social consensus that prenatal screening was of value to eliminate the "burden" of genetic disease, reinforcing the negative attitudes toward "defectives" implicit in that view. Specific topics, such as testing safeguards, took over, the scope of ethical issues narrowing as a consequence. Discussion of societal implications or philosophical meanings of disease and what is "normal" or "perfect" shifted to the margins, as did extreme positions. The prevailing concepts and language of mainstream discourse became those of individual choice, patient autonomy, privacy, and of "rights" and the law, putting a premium on individual cases and minimizing social contexts and consequences.

Underpinning mainstream discourse was a liberal gestalt that had begun to be articulated by leading ethicists in the 1970s. At a wide-ranging symposium entitled "Genetics, Man, and Society" at the annual meeting of the American Association for the Advancement of Science (AAAS) in 1972,[31] John Fletcher—not to be confused with Joseph Fletcher, as their views were poles apart—did not agree with certain radical critics at the meeting that eugenic manipulation or evolutionary controls were real threats. Rather, for Fletcher, Western culture's commitment to voluntarism would effectively counter the "possibility of mounting a widespread program of mandatory positive eugenics." Nor did he find anything "in the promise of the application of genetic knowledge which will automat ically raise us to a higher state of development in the history of evolution." He continued, "Mankind will not be saved from destruction by genetic knowledge, but neither will we be dehumanized by its careful and restrained use."[32] Sociologist James Sorenson had similarly expressed faith in wise individual choice as a safeguard against a socially engineered eugenics. "[F]inal decisions," he had noted at the 1971 NIH symposium, "are largely left to the family, with the doctor, the technical expert, assisting" with information "for an informed decision."[33] This belief—that somehow those involved can be trusted to do the "right thing"—remains a bedrock of mainstream bioethics discourse.

The report of a 1983 presidential commission on ethical problems in medicine and biomedical and behavioral research typified the circumscribed approach of bioethics in the 1980s. Although framed by ethical caveats, the report, *Screening and Counseling for Genetic Conditions*, did not question the meaning and purpose of prenatal diagnosis and genetic screening.[34] Policy recommendations were narrowly construed, confined to the specific subject matter. Drawing on the expert testimony of geneticists, other medical personnel, lawyers, and ethicists, plus representatives of cystic fibrosis organizations for a case study of cystic fibrosis, the report limited itself to ethical issues of autonomy, choice, and confidentiality, focusing on the individual and the immediate family. Nor did the ethical and procedural policy recommendations for professionals and for government provide for policy follow-up.

In a foretaste of the marginalization and isolation of ethics that would come to characterize the discourse in the '80s, a collection published by the March of Dimes in its Birth Defects series in 1979, *Genetic Counseling: Facts, Values and Norms,* organized the topics in such a way as to separate practical concerns from ethics. In part 1 were grouped philosophical articles about the relation of human genetics to health and disease. Parts 2 and 3, on the other hand, focused on the immediate and practical, with articles specifically oriented toward psychological, social, moral, and legal issues of genetic counseling.[35] This pattern of separation would continue in subsequent collections, including those prepared by physicians. Further, the amount of space allocated to philosophical issues would shrink, marginalizing them further.

The law's relation to reproductive issues formed a distinct genre within the discourse. Special symposia entitled "Genetics and the Law," started in the 1970s, were followed by further symposia, books, and law journal articles on genetics and related topics. Several volumes in a "Genetics and the Law" series, co-edited by medical geneticist Aubrey Milunsky and lawyer George Annas, were published.[36] Yet here, too, although criticisms accompanied the technical material, the content of these volumes supported research and technology and did not probe deeply; the topics and debate were limited and narrowly structured. Reviewing a book co-authored by obstetrician-gynecologist Dr. Sherman Elias and George Annas, *Reproductive Genetics and the Law,*[37] together with the 1987 volume in the Milunsky and Annas series, John Fletcher pointed out that Elias and Annas were long on explaining and synthesizing scientific, medical, and legal information, but short on discussing societal impacts and serious socio-moral problems.[38] John Robertson, another frequent contributor to bioethics and the law discussions and who favors the liberal, individualistic approach, has generally supported much of the new reproductive research and its applications in the name of "reproductive freedom."[39]

Philosophical discussions of the time also did not connect the ethics of genetic engineering and reproduction. At the nineteenth Nobel Conference, in Minnesota in 1983, participating scientists and theologians explored such broad issues of genetic engineering as the long-term risks of bio-engineering, what it means to be human, and the anxieties created by the god- and Satan-like powers of humans to manipulate life. But with no medical practitioners present at the conference, such ethical issues remained unrelated to practice. When Karen Lebacqz, a professor of Christian ethics at the Pacific School of Religion, questioned the usefulness of relying on the paradigm of logic and rationality to explore fears about genetic manipulation and asked for new approaches, she was misinterpreted by her male colleagues as someone who opposed the technologies. Instead of asking about "playing God," Lebacqz was saying that we need to be suspicious about the ways we think about the issues of knowledge and control of these technologies and to seek new paradigms.[40] Hers was a lonely voice.

Perhaps in part reflecting the political quiescence of the Reagan years of the '80s and postmodernism's attempts to divorce intellectual discourse from the real world, ethical discussions of genetic research, including gene therapy, remained muted. On the reproductive front, alternative reproductive strategies such as IVF and "surrogate" motherhood, not prenatal diagnosis, took center stage. On the genetics front, at least, the emphasis would in part change in the 1990s.

The Nineties: Re-enter Genetics—A Discourse Shift?

Accelerating research in molecular genetics in the '90s renewed a focus on genes, the consequences for medicine, and possibilities for altering the human condition. Two particular developments captured the ethical debates: the launching of the international effort to map and sequence the human genome,[41] and the prospects for germ-line gene therapy. Germ-line therapy discussions reconnected genetics and reproduction, but most ethical evaluations of the human genome project did not.

GERM-LINE GENE THERAPY

As explained in chapter four, germ-line gene therapy is far more controversial than somatic. While somatic cell therapy alters the genetic makeup only of the treated individual and can be performed prenatally or on living humans, germ-line therapy affects the reproductive cells, producing permanent genetic change that can be passed on to offspring. It must take place in the very early embryo or even before conception, in the reproductive cells of the parents. "While somatic cell gene therapy raises no new ethical problems," wrote two Dartmouth professors in the *Journal of Medicine and Philosophy* in 1991, "gene therapy of gametes, fertilized eggs or early embryos does raise several novel concerns."[42] The entire issue in which this article appeared was on the topic of human germ-line engineering.

In the 1980s, when the prospect of germ-line therapy still seemed remote, ethicists separated the ethics of genetic intervention from the ethics of reproductive technologies. John Fletcher traced "two streams of evolving ethical issues in medical genetics." The "older and wider stream" included "moral problems in genetic screening and prenatal diagnosis." A "newer stream" then "emerged with moral concern about creating new knowledge and new life forms by molecular biologists in recombinant DNA research." He continued, "the use of human DNA itself in prenatal diagnosis, screening, and now perhaps for treatment, links the two streams."[43] But in 1985, Fletcher did not go on to develop an ethical discourse that could link gene therapy, prenatal diagnosis, and DNA research. The ethical consensus reached went only so far as to oppose therapy for "eugenic enhancement,"[44] while approving corrective therapy with "suitable safeguards."[45]

By the 1990s, as germ-line therapy moved closer to the possible, the old distinctions between "somatic" and "germ-line" in the ethical dialogue had begun to break down. Some ethicists backed the research, suggesting that germ-line therapy might not be such a bad thing after all. Was "eugenics" necessarily a dirty word? At a symposium in Los Angeles in 1998 entitled "Engineering the Human Germ Line," John Fletcher pointed out to a panel of "high-level scientists and other experts" that the symposium tended to dispute the premise "virtually enshrined in public policy" that germ line is "a Rubicon not to be crossed, and [one] as being 'sanctified.' "[46]

A new distinction, between "prevention" and "enhancement," underlay a developing qualified support for germ-line therapy. It could be both medically and ethically justified if it was used to prevent or fight disease. But using it to enhance the individual remained problematic. In an article in the 1991 issue of the *Journal of Medicine and Philosophy* mentioned above, Burke K. Zimmerman made what became the classic, oft-cited case for the development and use of germ-line therapy. He argued that

> it is the moral obligation of the medical profession to make available to the public any technology that can cure or prevent pathology leading to death and disability, in both the present and future generations. . . . Because prenatal screening and even early embryo screening and selection can prevent only a subset of known genetic disorders, direct genetic intervention is the *only* way in which certain couples can exercise their rights to reproductive health.[47] (emphasis in original)

Zimmerman proposed directly modifying the DNA of early-stage embryos, created through IVF, in such cases. Among his stringent criteria for "[d]irect manipulation of the pre-embryo" were that the procedure will be highly likely to succeed in correcting the defective gene and that no genetic errors or genetic material would be introduced that could have unpredictable effects on future generations.[48]

Thus an ethical consensus grew that germ-line therapy can be morally and ethically justifiable if it is necessary to benefit the individual as the only means to permanently prevent the transmission of disease genes. Participants at the 1998 Los Angeles symposium were reported to have agreed that germ-line therapy's potential for curing disease was too great for it not to be implemented, whatever ethical problems might ensue. In 1997 ethicist Arthur Caplan wrote that if it were possible to "eliminate diseases such as Tay-Sachs, thalassemia, or Hurler's syndrome . . . from the human population by germ-line alterations, is there any convincing moral reason why this should not be done?"[49]

Genetic enhancement when it is not medically necessary, however, elicits considerable and varying caveats. There are the theorists and the realists, the optimists and the cynics, and the noncommittal.[50] Along with others, Zimmerman left the door open, cautioning about the need to know a lot more before attempting to modify complex characteristics, and the profound social implications. Marc Lappé, in the same issue of the *Journal of Medicine and Philosophy*, spoke to the problem that somatic alteration might inadvertently affect the germ line. If modification occurred as an indirect or secondary effect of somatic cell therapy it would be morally acceptable; if intentional, it would not be. "Germ line engineering as a directed attempt to change the genotype of future generations cannot ethically be justified."[51]

The "slippery slope" argument—that using germ-line therapy for preventive and medical reasons could lead to enhancement—has lost ground. Professors Edward Berger and Bernard Gert offer the criterion of *malady* as a way to distinguish between negative and positive eugenics. Thus hemophilia, Tay-Sachs disease, Lesch-Nyhan syndrome, cystic fibrosis, and sickle cell anemia, for example, are maladies, as are cancer and tuberculosis, and so can be classified as candidates for germ-line gene therapy. While they see "no theoretical reason for not using germ-line therapy," they find that "real world considerations" dictate severe limits on its use. "[W]e do not believe that all researchers are sufficiently responsible to limit their use of this exciting new technology in the appropriate way." Given that such "technologies tend to get over used," the potential "for causing great harm to very many" cannot justify this technology's use "in order to provide benefits, even great benefits, for a very few."[52]

Inevitability becomes the strongest argument supporting germ-line therapy's use for enhancement. David Resnik, believing that we will move down the slippery slope from prevention to enhancement, argues there is no point in banning germ-line. Rather, we should accept the possibilities, insuring that use "is conducted in a safe, just, and proper way, not [following] a policy that tries to close Pandora's box." But he is not making "an unabashed endorsement of genetic enhancement," since the "main reason for conducting human germ-line therapy is to prevent genetic diseases."[53]

William Gardner, in law and psychiatry research at the University of Pittsburgh School of Medicine goes much farther. Germ-line enhancement is inevitable because parents will demand it. Seeking to have offspring who can compete successfully in an increasingly competitive world, parents will out of rational choice, elect to enhance their children's abilities. He argues further that such choices will be self-reinforcing. As safety and efficiency of the procedure grow, as greater global competition will require enhanced skills, and as the unenhanced fall further and further behind, the pressures would grow for even those opposed to sign on. The actions of "pioneering parents" would be persuasive for others to adopt enhancement. Though its use might not become universal in the short run—objectors might organize successfully and social changes might limit its spread—his model suggests that "for a considerable time humanity will be divided into populations that either do or do not use enhancement."[54] He further argues that nations will come to adopt enhancement out of economic necessity.

His is a wake-up call. His purpose is to alert those ethicists who would prohibit genetic enhancement to the enormous difficulties of enforcing such a ban, especially in view of the threat that stringent regulations would pose to liberal societies' principles of freedom and privacy. He concludes,

> Most discussions of the bioethical control of human genetic enhancement liken it to the professional regulation of an innovative medical treatment. However, if the argument presented here is correct, then prohibiting genetic enhancement would be similar to, but perhaps even more challenging than the (so-called) control of nuclear weapons.[55]

But increasingly, mainstream bioethicists talk less about prohibition and exhibit less alarm about its possible use for enhancement. For John Fletcher and physician co-author Gerd Richter, somatic cell therapy for the fetus, along with preimplantation genetic diagnosis, is deemed "morally praiseworthy" because they offer another option to women who face the trauma of aborting a much-wanted child. The use of such therapy will be "very limited," however, taking only a "modest place in the nation's biomedical research goals." Keeping to the distinction between prevention and enhancement, they see no danger of a " 'slippery slope,' " holding that "a moral line ought to be drawn between somatic cell gene therapy and enhancement of culturally desirable traits in individuals who do not have diseases that carry severe morbidity or mortality."[56]

Yet the moral line is distinctly wavering. For some mainstream ethicists, the eugenics line is redrawn between individual acts and social policy. Arthur Caplan sees the danger coming from population eugenics imposed by government, not from choices by individuals. "Insofar as coercion and force are absent and *individual choice* is allowed to hold sway, then," he writes, "*presuming fairness* in access to the means of enhancing our offspring, it is hard to see what is wrong with trying to create better babies."[57] The emphases are mine, not Dr. Caplan's. I have used italics to contrast Dr. Caplan's view to that of the realists, such as Gardner, and Berger and Gert, who predict very different consequences from the aggregate of individuals' rational and apparently well-intentioned choices. Mainstream bioethics' construction of a just society of rational, liberal-minded individuals fails to see that faith in liberal individualism is part of the problem, not the solution—a point I will discuss further in the final section of this chapter.

THE HUMAN GENOME PROJECT

The stepped-up pace of the Human Genome Project (HGP) in the late 1990s, the publishing of the "working draft" of the genome's sequencing in 2001, and the announcement of the completion of sequencing in 2003 have had an important effect on ethical discourse surrounding the project.[58] Though specific topics related to policy have remained salient, conceptual and social issues and the linkage of genetics and reproduction have gained new emphasis, mainly through the Ethical, Legal and Social Implications (ELSI) program of the National Center for Human Genome Research. When the HGP was set up in 1990, under the joint auspices of the National Institutes of Health (NIH) and the Office of Biological and Environmental Research (OBER) at the Department of Energy (DOE), 5 percent of the initial $100 million budget for the newly constituted National Center for Human Genome Research (NCHGR) was earmarked for ELSI.[59] Doing this at the outset was

> unique in the history of science. This support gives us the opportunity to "worry in advance" about the implications and impacts of the mapping and sequencing of the human genome, including several thousand human disease genes, *before* wide-scale genetic diagnosis, testing and screening comes into practice, rather than *after* the problems have presented themselves in full relief.[60] (emphasis in original)

Setting out to identify the most urgent issues and key research areas, ELSI sponsored symposia and workshops which drew on professionals from the sciences, the humanities and social sciences, medicine, ethics, and the law. A 1991 NIH workshop defined four "high-priority areas" which guided social policy research throughout the decade. They were "(1) the use and interpretation of genetic information, (2) clinical integration of genetic technologies, (3) issues surrounding genetics research, and (4) public and professional education and training about these issues."[61]

Since its mission was to produce policy recommendations for the HGP, ELSI tended to focus on concrete and specific, rather than conceptual or abstract, topics in each area. Concerns over privacy and confidentiality of genetic information, over its misuse, for example, in discrimination by employers and insurers, became key research subjects under area one, the use and interpretation of genetic information. Topics for area three, genetics research, were informed consent, safety, and quality. The NIH workshop which generated these research priorities, however, did pose conceptual questions. As discussed in the published volume based on the workshop, priority number four had originally asked, "How might the Human Genome Project affect our concepts of 'disease,' 'normalcy,' and 'humanness'?"[62] Editors George Annas and Sherman Elias commented further, "Related to concepts of health and disease are concepts of reductionism and determinism . . . [and] related to all these notions is the overriding issue of eugenics." Finally they pointed out, "Perhaps the most important social policy issue of all—should the Human Genome Project proceed at this time?—received no priority rating." However, neither of these issues was carried further.[63]

ELSI reflected its policy priorities in research grants, workshops, conferences, and task forces. Of 172 research grants awarded from 1990 to 1998, only a few focused on broadly ethical questions, these mostly in the first few years.[64] Reproductive issues received little attention; grants under priority number two, on integrating new genetic screening technologies into clinical practice, focused on carrier screening and predictive testing of living, often adult, persons. Only six grants (including one to me) were related specifically to prenatal testing and/or screening. Another early exception was a conference at NIH in November 1991, "Reproduction and Genetic Testing: Impact on Women," in which a fairly wide range of researchers and practitioners, mainly women, participated. A conference book was published as a supplement to the journal *Fetal Diagnosis and Therapy*, but there was no further sponsored follow-up.[65]

ELSI's Task Force on Genetic Screening, a major project organized with the DOE from 1995 to 1997, illustrated ELSI's focus. With the goal of making "recommendations that will assure the public that genetic tests will be safe and effective but will not stifle progress in this exciting field," the project focused mainly on predictive testing, that is, on the genetic testing of individuals to predict future onset of disease, as for Huntington's disease or breast cancer. Its recommendations covered the clinical setting, the laboratory, and education of both providers and the public. Discussion of prenatal testing was limited mainly to issues of informed consent, patient autonomy, quality of personnel, and safety of test results.[66] In both its charge and its work, the task force reflected ELSI's research and policy priorities for genetic testing. The lack of attention to prenatal testing issues also perhaps reflected the fact that, after two decades of expanding use, prenatal diagnosis was so fully absorbed into reproductive practice that it did not present itself as a problem under ELSI's priority area number two, clinical integration of new genetic technologies. Using the language of patient autonomy, voluntarism, privacy, and informed consent, ELSI remained within the bioethics mainstream that held prenatal testing decisions to be an individual family, not a social, matter.

Responding in part to the speed with which genome sequencing was progressing, in the mid-1990s ELSI launched a process of self-evaluation and a series of planning and program reviews.[67] The final report of ELSI's Research, Planning and Evaluation Group (ERPEG), published in 2000,[68] articulated five goals for the five-year period 1998–2003 that had already been set forth in earlier reports. These goals, which in turn were reflected in adjustments in ELSI's four program areas,[69] emphasized greater attention to cultural, social, and conceptual issues recommended in the 2000 report.

Goal four, for example, which is to "[e]xplore ways in which new genetic knowledge may interact with a variety of philosophical, theological, and ethical perspectives," reintroduces the kinds of conceptual questions raised at the outset of the ELSI program, but then for the most part not pursued, and includes calls for more broadly cross-disciplinary, "worldview" research. Goal number five, to "[e]xplore how socioeconomic factors and concepts of race and ethnicity influence the use, understanding, and interpretation of genetic information, the utilization of genetic services, and the development of policy," speaks to the perceived need for ELSI-funded research to increase attention to social concerns.[70]

Although the ERPEG report of 2000—as well as the HGP report of 1998—charted the ELSI program's success in influencing policy in a number of areas, it also clearly spelled out content weaknesses in the four program areas. While grants since 1998 do deal with the "emerging issues" of genetic enhancement, behavioral genetics, and preimplantation genetic diagnosis, ERPEG noted that "'empirical' and 'applied' studies" that use standard methodologies need to be supplemented with "more studies that use 'theoretical' or 'analytical' approaches . . . [so as] to examine these same issues in broader contexts," and that members of other disciplines and "of minority racial or ethnic communities" need to be better represented among principal investigators.[71] ELSI's grant portfolio has reflected such emphases. One-third of the grants since 1998 (up through 2001) cover social and conceptual areas such as race and ethnicity, disability and quality of life, public health, and equity and access. A number of the grants were long range, extending to 2003 and 2004.

ELSI's relatively little attention to reproductive topics, especially prenatal diagnosis, in the earlier research portfolio has begun to be addressed in more recent sponsored research. At a conference in January 2001 at NIH, entitled "A Decade of ELSI Research," the second of the three days was devoted to genetic testing, with two of the sessions focused on prenatal testing. The day's final session was on genetic enhancement.

Clinical Ethics

Physicians have had a mixed and sometimes rocky relationship with ethics discourse and with ethicists,[72] given the underlying tensions between the practicing physician and the "ivory tower" philosopher. In the 1970s physicians appeared at bioethicists' forums mainly as invited experts; by the '80s, physicians were calling on bioethicists to lend their expertise to medical professionals' forums and publications. In the '90s, clinical ethics became a distinct field, physicians taking it upon themselves to focus on ethics in clinical practice, founding the *Journal of Clinical Ethics* in 1990, and establishing physician-headed programs and departments of medical ethics, whose numbers increased markedly within schools of medicine.

Physicians have paid more attention to the ethics of reproductive medicine, and especially prenatal diagnosis, than have bioethicists. In 1971, Dr. Theodore Friedmann, referring to prenatal diagnosis, wrote in *Scientific American,* "it is not difficult to imagine the emergence of pressures to set standards for desirability in genetically determined characteristics."[73] Dr. Judith Hall, at the 1971 NIH ethics symposium, wondered whether we were willing to pay the price of making procreation a laboratory science in order to have normal babies. By the end of the '70s, however, even as bioethics discourse grew narrower and more specific, physicians raised fewer ethical questions of this kind.

As physicians in the '80s sought ethicists, legal experts, and social commentators on medical issues for their own symposia, ethical issues were compartmentalized. Often appearing at the beginning and/or end of a volume on clinical practice and the state of the art in reproductive medicine, the chapters on ethical, social, and legal issues seemed tacked on. Thus book-ended, the main clinical information was undisturbed, unconnected to the ethical analysis presented.

A 1989 volume on fetal diagnosis and therapy with four co-editors from different fields broke this format by interspersing technical and scientific chapters with ethical, legal, and sociopolitical discussions.[74] In this format perfectibility issues in relation to prenatal diagnosis were raised. In part 1, for example, ethicist John Fletcher deplored the "trend toward perfectionism."[75] Dorothy Wertz and James Sorenson, in the closing section, explored the sociological implications of the desire for a "perfect child." They predicted several outcomes stemming from prevailing beliefs in the "right" to become parents and to have " 'perfect' children," the commitment to patient autonomy, and an "implicit two-class system for fetuses: the wanted, for whom no expense should be spared, and the unwanted, which can be aborted with impunity." Among their predicted outcomes were that prenatal diagnosis for all pregnancies and abortion of defective fetuses would become routine; that the medical profession would gain even greater control over pregnancy and birth; that to parents' existing right to choose the number, spacing, and quality of their children would be added the right to choose their sex; and that, given the inequalities of health care and the lavish outlay of resources for specialized procedures, most of the new technologies would benefit the few, not the many, and others not at all.[76]

Yet further dialogue, that could extend discussion in this vein and perhaps bring changes in practice, did not occur in the clinical literature. A symposium on the implications of the "new reproductive genetics" on women and their physicians appearing in *Clinical Obstetrics and Gynecology* in 1993 and guest-edited by Dr. Mark Evans returned to the separated format. Articles on legal and social issues were grouped at the end, including one on the impact of prenatal screening on people with disabilities, with apparently no interchange with clinical materials in the rest of the volume.[77]

The issue of abortion as virtually the only "treatment" for a diagnosed defect continues to be ethically troubling for physicians. As pointed out in chapter five, the emergence of the fetus as a patient can compound the dilemma, the solution a further example of compartmentalization. The autonomy of the living patient, the pregnant woman, becomes overriding, as she is the one who must decide, and thus take responsibility for, what happens to her fetus, otherwise defined as the "other patient." Dr. Michael

Kaback has termed diagnosis and abortion a *"secondary form of prevention"* (emphasis in original) of genetic disease, since "conception of affected individuals is not prevented." But he offers only the hope of finding "effective therapies or even cures. . . . [which] would obviate greatly the use of abortion as a means of disease control."[78] Even as preventing conception or correcting the defect begin to seem possible through preimplantation diagnosis and germ-line therapy, "secondary prevention" prevails, and with it continuing debates over therapy vs. abortion.[79]

During the 1980s, medical professionals did raise other conceptual questions about undesirable fetuses and the "perfect baby," treading into territory often avoided by physicians and ethicists alike. Dr. Theodore Friedmann, in a report on a 1983 conference on gene therapy, commented on the possible manipulation of genes.

> In general, any programs designed to promote ideals or a specific good should be suspect. Not all rational people can agree on what is "good," and attempts to promote or enhance nonuniversally held goals may lead to placing social stamps of approval or disapproval onto genetic traits and to using social and political institutions for unacceptable eugenic purposes. Arguments for the design of a "better" human genome, or for the elimination of "defective" genes, would also seem to fall into this category at the moment—at least until we know much more than we do now.[80]

Noting the troubled history of sterilization, marriage, and immigration policies in the U.S., and the Nazi experience, Friedmann's parting concern was over the use of gene therapy to do "good" for eugenic purposes. In 1989, he would suggest that we withhold judgment and not close the door to germ-line gene therapy, despite many technical and ethical uncertainties.[81]

In the late 1970s, Drs. Edmond Murphy, Gary Chase, and Alejandro Rodriguez pointed out that the statement "every person 'has the right to be born healthy'" could be interpreted to mean "only healthy persons have a right to be born." If so, then the choice concerning an affected fetus is not between a healthy and non-healthy existence, but between a non-healthy existence or none at all.[82] In the early 1980s Dr. Kaback also addressed the issue of quality and choice.

> Does our technology provide us with sufficient information to judge a pregnancy as not being of sufficient "quality" to go to completion? Who has the right to make such a decision? Does our increasing technical capability to evaluate lesser and lesser imperfections in the fetus lead into a state of growing intolerance for any imperfection?

What would be the implications of such a notion on a societywide scale? . . . Others have raised the question of whether individuals afflicted with disorders that could have been prevented through prenatal diagnosis and selective abortion will come to be considered as less than equal members of society. Would prejudices occur against [them] . . . and what might be the social implications of such attitudes?[83]

Dr. Perri Klass, the Boston pediatrician whose article "The Perfect Baby?" in the *New York Times Magazine* was referred to in chapter five, noted the difficulty of even defining what is "perfect." Addressing lay readers, she explained that prenatally diagnosable abnormalities cover a "wide spectrum," from usually fatal trisomies (such as having three copies of chromosome 13 or 18) to non-lethal conditions such as sex chromosome anomalies or Down syndrome. Each diagnosis compounds the moral dilemmas posed by testing. As have other physicians and genetic counselors, she cautioned that testing is no guarantee of certainty. "Can, or should, we seek a perfect child?"[84]

Yet most physicians at the time did not pay the attention to broader moral and social questions that Drs. Klass, Kaback, Friedmann, and Murphy and his colleagues did.[85] Speculation was left to the ethicists, while the gap between physicians and ethicists persisted. Attempting to bridge that gap, in the late 1970s William Ruddick, a philosophy professor at New York University, developed a four-year project at NYU and Montefiore hospitals which sought to promote dialogue and interchange between the physician, geared to the concrete immediate situation, and the philosopher working at the abstract level to formulate principles as guides to action.[86] Although participating physicians supported the project,[87] others have questioned the professional ethicist's relevance to medicine. Dr. Edward Hill, the obstetrician quoted in chapter five, noted in 1986 that the over 200 medical ethics articles published monthly are irrelevant to medical practice.[88] In 1979 Dr. Mark Siegler, from the Pritzker School of Medicine in Chicago, set up a "Clinical Ethics" editorial department in the *Archives of Internal Medicine* as a forum in which physicians could discuss issues relevant to their daily interactions with patients. Siegler, highly critical of the field of bioethics, saw no place for the professional ethicist in the clinical setting.[89]

Dr. Siegler in some ways anticipated the direct involvement of physicians in clinical ethics that came about in the 1990s. The *Journal of Clinical Ethics,* which was established in 1990, sought to fill the need for a journal about applying medical ethics that was directed primarily to care providers, that is, physicians, nurses, and others who interact directly with patients.[90] The number of books and journal articles devoted to clinical ethics and written by physicians has markedly increased. Advances in research genetics and the Human Genome Project have spurred ethical responses to their effects on prenatal diagnosis and germ-line therapy.

In 1994 the American Medical Association stated its position on genetic selection:

> In general, it would be ethically permissible to participate in genetic selection (abortion or embryo discard) or genetic manipulation to prevent, cure, or treat genetic disease. It would not be ethical to engage in selection on the basis of benign characteristics. Genetic manipulation of benign traits, though generally unacceptable, may be permissible under exceptional circumstances.

As published in the *Archives of Family Medicine,* the summary of the AMA report continued:

> At a minimum, three criteria [for genetic manipulation] would have to be satisfied: there would have to be clear and meaningful benefit to the child, there could be no trade-off with other characteristics or traits, and all citizens would have to have equal access to the genetic technology, irrespective of income or other socioeconomic characteristics.[91]

Though the technology of modifying the human genome was still in "rudimentary stages" and future developments uncertain, the report sought to clarify such issues as parental choice, abortion, therapeutic goals to eliminate and cure disease, discriminatory practices, and eugenics as new applications of technology emerge.

Among medical professionals examining these issues in the medical and scientific journals, ob/gyn Eugene Pergament and Morris Fiddler considered the clinical applications of prenatal gene therapy. Writing in *Prenatal Diagnosis,* they weighed its pros and cons, medical rationale, the technical aspects—their concerns including safety and efficacy and responsibilities toward the embryo and fetus and future generations.[92] Two medical geneticists, Drs. Kenneth Garver and Bettylee Garver, urged ELSI to take up eugenics as an issue. Arguing in the *American Journal of Human Genetics* that "a eugenic mentality has existed in the United States during the entire 20th century," the Garvers stated, "Prenatal diagnosis, a new form of negative eugenics, is becoming a routine part of prenatal care. It is vital that the growing desire to have 'normal' babies does not erode our acceptance and care of those who have disabilities, otherwise the advances made through the Americans with Disabilities Act will be nullified."[93]

Dr. Allan Jacobs of the Department of Obstetrics and Gynecology at Beth Israel Medical Center in New York, concerned that an unchecked use of genetic selection in a free market will result in class inequities—liberty trumping equality—has urged the medical profession to inform society of the impact of genetic selection techniques. Criticizing contemporary clinical ethics, Dr. Jacobs states that the beneficence-based and autonomy-based paradigms which motivate medical decisions do not provide "sufficient ethical guidance to resolve public policy questions regarding management of genetic technology."[94]

The 1990s were characterized by this increased physician involvement in ethical issues. An editorial in a special section of the *American Journal of Human Genetics* on genetics education addressed "our added responsibilities" concerning the new genetic technologies.[95] Lisa Parker, a professor of human genetics at the University of Pittsburgh, in a featured article suggested adapting bioethics reasoning, especially ELSI's "preventive ethics," to the teaching of ethics. In contrast to medicine's criticisms of bioethicists a decade earlier, Parker held that the "evolution, literature, and methods of the American bioethics movement" can "have a beneficial effect on the relationship between these professionals [clinicians and researchers] and the public they serve and on the acceptance and efficacy of new genetic technology."[96]

Yet this level of critique in the '90s was the exception and not the rule. Following the legacy of the '80s, ethical focus has tended to be narrow and specific, concentrating on such subjects as risks, safety, quality control, and informed consent. Even when broader questions are raised, especially about the impact of genetic research, the technologies are generally accepted and not questioned in any fundamental way. The *Journal of Clinical Ethics* reported on surveys that showed a consensus among clinicians in support of prenatal testing and the use of abortion for a diagnosed birth defect, and wide support among both physicians and the lay public for abortion if the woman's health is endangered or there is a strong chance of a serious defect in the baby.[97] Clinicians' continuing concern is that cure will keep lagging well behind the growing ability to test and diagnose, with moral discussions continuing to center on abortion. And, despite more attention to reproductive issues than in mainstream bioethics, clinical ethics as a whole devotes relatively little space to the subject of reproduction, and even less to prenatal testing. Ethics texts for clinicians and medical students, even as they focus on the clinical uses of genetics, pay relatively little attention to prenatal testing and diagnosis issues.[98]

Among the medical journals, the *Journal of Clinical Ethics* makes the most concerted attempt to deal with ethical issues directly affecting prac-

ticing physicians. While not devoting much space to the subject of reproduction, especially in its early years, it has recognized a role for feminist
perspectives on bioethics and the ethic of care. The Spring 1992 issue
offered a discussion of the ethic of care, pro and con, and Spring 1994
featured a comprehensive review of three important books by feminists on
feminist approaches to medical ethics.[99] In 1996 the journal published a
four-part series entitled "Feminist Approaches to Bioethics," guest-edited
by feminist ethicist Rosemary Tong.[100] Yet, among the variety of issues and
subjects contributed by many feminist thinkers there was little on reproduction and no article dealt with prenatal diagnosis. The articles in the
series also conform to the individualistic, legalistic model of mainstream
bioethics which is limited as an approach to challenge the status quo.
Edmund Howe, the journal's editor in chief, in his introduction to the
series made clear his interest in the contributions of feminist perspectives,
as he did in his article on IVF in the Winter 1999 issue, "The Need for
Original Ethical Analysis for Women."[101] Thus, more recent issues have
shown a trend to more attention to testing and reproductive issues.[102]

The Limits of Bioethics Discourse

ISSUES AND INDEPENDENCE

Bioethics discourse should attempt to raise significant issues in biomedicine, generate meaningful dialogue, and so have an impact on practice.
Over the past three decades and more, genetic research and reproductive
medical practice have become increasingly intertwined. Yet mainstream
bioethics has by and large failed to explore critically relevant issues about
this relationship and to promote a two-way conversation both with the
medical community and with the wider public. It has remained marginal to
professional medical practice. Even when ethical critique originates within
the medical profession itself, at times asking penetrating questions relating
to reproduction, there is virtually no influence on reproductive medical
practice. Medical ethics commentaries are mostly specific and contained,
and not about to rock the medical boat.

One of the impediments to raising meaningful issues is the question
of the degree to which funded research can remain independent, free from
the hand that feeds it. Noting its location within the Human Genome
Project, which was federally sponsored and housed within the federal
government, ELSI acknowledged the problem, asking whether it could
assure "an independent, critical assessment of the ethical, legal, and social
implications" of the HGP's work. The response in ELSI's 1996 report was

that the committee's recommendations were "intended to assure so far as possible that there is an open and unfettered review of genetic research and the social consequences of that research."[103]

Daniel Callahan, founder and president of the Hastings Center, was less sparing, however. Addressing a symposium upon his retirement, he commented it "is hardly likely" that the NIH's Human Genome Project would have set aside 5 percent of its annual budget for ELSI "if there had been even the faintest likelihood it would turn into a source of trouble and opposition; and it indeed hasn't." But his sharpest barbs were reserved for his fellow ethicists. Excoriating what he called "our crowd" for having been coopted, Callahan declared bioethics had become an "accommodating handmaiden" to the "biomedical establishment." We became "insiders by default."

> [In the] early days of bioethics . . . there was an interesting debate between the views of Joseph Fletcher—who never said no—and those of Paul Ramsey—who usually said no. . . . It appears that Fletcher won the day. . . . While bioethics creates problems now and then for mainstream, right-thinking trends, it mainly serves to legitimate them, adding the imprimatur of ethical expertise to what somebody or other wants to do.[104]

In his talk, "Bioethics, Our Crowd, and Ideology," which opened the symposium to assess the state of bioethics as a discipline, "our crowd" referred to the core group, mainly ethicists, plus lawyers and medical professionals, many of whom were present. For Callahan, the shared ideology of the bioethics mainstream and biomedicine meant support of the status quo.

DISTANCING

Bioethics discourse is distanced and detached from clinical practice, which is so even for that of medical personnel themselves. The difference between the ethicist outside and ethics within medicine is in method of analysis. The bioethics professional employs methods that promote distancing and abstraction. Chief among these is the "situational" or "consequentialist" approach to determining moral obligation. Asking what the consequences of an action may be, the ethicist follows the utilitarian principle of choosing what will do the least harm. Ethicists develop hypothetical situations that pose a variety of ethical dilemmas, such as whether to test or abort solely to select for sex. Even though the situation may be based on an actual case, discussion of actors' options and consequences of their choices takes place in a detached setting of ethical experts. "Case studies" become little more than academic exercises.[105] Ethicists also can apply the deontological theory of moral obligation. Here moral action is based on the concept of rights and respect for persons without reference to the consequences of actions.[106] Abstraction rules, since there is no attempt to refer to actual people.

Whether bioethics professionals use a situational or deontological method, they take the atomized individual as their reference point, using the legalistic terminology of rights of Western liberalism. The language of "patient autonomy" and "informed consent" rests on the concept of the right of the individual patient to choose and to be informed, and the right of the physician to give or withhold information. While individual rights may be seen to be in tension with public or social goods, the discourse of rights keeps the ethicist's focus on the individual as an abstract entity who is detached from the social setting or social consequences.

By contrast, the practicing physician must deal with real persons; the situations are not hypothetical. Yet the physician, too, is committed to the language and practice of individualism, to "patient autonomy," and to the privatized setting of patient care. The focus on the fetus, which places fetal rights in opposition to the woman's rights, locates the physician squarely in an atomized rights framework.[107] Objectifying the patient is another aspect of distancing.

IDEOLOGICAL SYMBIOSIS

A commitment to a common terminology and the language of rights is a further example of the ideological symbiosis of physician and ethicist that Daniel Callahan remarked on. Despite continuing differences and tensions, the gatekeepers of reproductive medicine and ethicists of the bioethics mainstream have much in common. As professional elites, they are "experts," set apart from the "public" they would benefit. In reproductive science and technology, they generally accept as givens, and often as goods, prenatal diagnosis, carrier screening, fetal therapeutic measures with appropriate safeguards, and continuing research in medical genetics. Bioethicists' rationale is the same as that of the medical practitioner: to eliminate disease, and to relieve suffering. The credo is the same: above all, to do no harm, and to confer benefit. Ethicist and physician alike view advances in molecular genetics and prenatal diagnosis as ways to lift the "burden" of disease. Even though ethicists, and some physicians as well, voice growing concern about testing and aborting for "trivial" purposes or for conditions that are untreatable, they belong to a mainstream that perpetuates negative attitudes toward "defectives." Dissenters from and critics of such thinking, such as the late Paul Ramsey, remain minor voices, and are almost unheard today. Prevailing cultural attitudes die hard, as people with disabilities can poignantly attest. When ethicists and medical professionals settle for cautioning against improper use of genetics and technologies, relying on individual choice as moral guardian, they underwrite the status quo.

Mainstream bioethics ends up supporting the power of the gatekeepers of reproductive medicine to set the norms for reproductive practice. These norms exert influence on those who must make decisions, on those most intimately involved: women and their families. Although White middle- to upper-middle-class clientele for sophisticated prenatal technologies often share many of these cultural values, they vary considerably in their attitudes toward disability and the value of prenatal diagnosis itself. But prevailing norms remain powerful, given their supports by the mainstream.

LIMITED OUTREACH

The clientele for prenatal diagnosis by and large is not part of bioethics conversations, even though bioethicists have called for public discussion and educating the public on important issues. Bioethics discourse is virtually a closed circle. Conversations usually take place at specialized institutions which have proliferated over the past three decades, the Kennedy Institute of Ethics at Georgetown University in Washington, established in 1971, one of the earliest and now perhaps one of the most extensive. Several dozen centers in the U.S., including independent centers such as Hastings, think tanks, scientific academies, and government agencies, join with centers in Australia, New Zealand, Canada, France, Germany, Sweden, and elsewhere to form an international network supporting research and discussion. Access to the symposia, conferences, and forums they sponsor is generally limited to experts, counting consumers of medical care among the missing. Their reports and proceedings appear in journals, books, and other formats, which are aimed at specialized professional audiences. Although the Internet has made the work of bioethics organizations and centers much more readily available—most centers have Web sites—these resources serve mainly scholars, students, and professionals in health or related fields, not laypersons.[108] Bioethics texts—which unfortunately are perfunctory and limited on reproductive issues—are for academic teaching and reference, not general public consumption.

Unlike most other bioethics institutions, the HGP's ELSI program sought from the outset to reach out beyond the circumscribed ethical community, including calling for education in genetics and genetic issues for the public and professionals alike. Its revamped goals reemphasize these commitments for its grants policies, taking a more inclusive world-view of the impact of genetic research, as well as revisiting the intersections of genetics and reproductive practice.[109] These policies may signal a continuing departure from the confining practices of mainstream bio-ethics.

A troubling lack of outreach of bioethics discourse is the failure to bring balance to public perceptions of the findings and uses of genetic research, resulting in a field day for genetic reductionism. Throughout the '80s, articles appeared in respected law journals and books favoring eugenics and genetic engineering, and apparently accepting genetic reductionist claims at face value. Citing Harvard professors Eysenck, Jensen, and Herrnstein, among others with genetic determinist views, a "Notes" article in the *Harvard Law Review*, "Eugenic Artificial Insemination: A Cure for Mediocrity?" endorsed the Nobel Sperm Bank and the use of sperm from intellectually superior donors to "produce intellectually superior off-spring."[110] George P. Smith, a law professor at the Catholic University of America, wrote in the *Southern Illinois University Law Journal* that the law must be ready for "public acceptance" of "[c]ontrolled breeding through genetic manipulation."[111] In his *The New Biology*, he favored using the law to promote "[g]enetic integrity, eugenic advancement, and a strong genetic pool designed to eliminate illness and suffering."[112] Legal critique within the bioethics mainstream—which is not wittingly pro-eugenics or genetic reductionism—apparently has had little effect in countering an uncritical belief in the deterministic power of genes among a highly educated segment of the public outside medicine and science.

For the wider public, the message in the popular media is a sensationalized genetic determinism. Heralding each new "discovery" of a gene, whether for homosexuality, alcoholism, or schizophrenia, the popular media celebrate the power of genes and the triumphs of genetic science and reproductive technologies. Blatantly supporting genetic determinism are such books as *The Bell Curve*, published in 1994, which, in equating IQ tests with intelligence and measuring differences by race and class, has called up the specter of the old eugenics.[113] Five years later IQ genes were alive and well as *Time* magazine hailed scientists' genetic enhancement of memory in a strain of mice with a cover story headlined "The IQ Gene?"[114] As discussed in chapter five, Dr. Aubrey Milunsky at Boston University has since the 1970s consistently provided a medical imprimatur for genetic determinism in books aimed at the layperson.

In contrast to the celebrations are the dire warnings, which in their way also attest to the power of genes. Starting in the '70s, "playing God" has outrun "brave new worlds" for the singularly unimaginative titles of a spate of books alerting us to the dangers lurking in a bio-engineered genetic future.[115] Although those published in the '90s are more tempered and less fanciful than the earlier books—compare, for example, Jeremy Rifkin's *The Biotech Century* (1998) to his *Who Should Play God?* (1977, with Ted Howard) and *Algeny* (1984, with Nicanor Perlas)[116]—they are short or misleading on facts and frame the issues superficially. The 1997 film *Gattaca* painted a scary future of children made to order. *Twilight of the Golds,* a 1993 play, dramatized the plight of a family having to decide whether to abort a fetus prenatally diagnosed as homosexual, even though such diagnosis was not possible.[117]

Cautionary tales by science writers and scientists in the '90s are better grounded scientifically. Bryan Appleyard, a columnist for the London *Sunday Times,* sees the elimination of undesirable fetuses as a "form of privatized eugenics in which millions of individual decisions will change society." His solution is to resist through a "spiritual search."[118] Journalist Gina Maranto's *Quest for Perfection,* in which she traces medical and technological attempts to create perfect humans back to Plato, sees IVF combining with genetic manipulation to produce eugenics.[119] Lee Silver, on the other hand, a professor of biology at Princeton but writing in a popular vein in *Remaking Eden,* asks for a reality check about eugenics, criticizing Maranto and others who condemn eugenics out of hand. Outlining how "reprogenetics"—the joining of genetics with current technologies in reproductive biology—will enhance children and "turn science fiction into reality,"[120] he ends the book with scenarios of gross future inequalities: in two centuries a "GenRich" class is ranged against the "Naturals"; in thirty centuries' time the two groups have become different species, unable to reproduce with each other. His book is both a wake-up call and an argument for a rational, clearheaded look at the whole issue of genetic enhancement.[121] Philosopher-ethicists Allen Buchanan, Dan Brock, Norman Daniels, and Daniel Wickler, in their *From Chance to Choice,* express concern over the "benevolent parental impulse" to do what's best for children as "the capability for genetic intervention increases." Distinguishing "between permissible and obligatory genetic enhancements," and examining the "social implications of some of the enhancements that parents might consider undertaking," they "argue that . . . the child's right to an open future places significant limitations on what it is permissible for parents to do in this regard."[122]

Genetic reductionism has also met substantial criticism. *The Bell Curve,* for example, elicited well-aimed, cutting responses in the popular and scholarly press.[123] The journal *Science for the People* and the Committee for Responsible Genetics have continued to be important voices among the critics of determinism.[124] Books in the '90s have joined Richard Lewontin, Steven Rose, and Leon J. Kamin's *Not in Our Genes,* published in 1984,[125] in measured attempts to cut through the misinformation and claims of a reductionist science, exposing the race, ethnic, class, and sex biases barely disguised under the veneer of scientific "fact." Ruth Hubbard and Elijah Wald's *Exploding the Gene Myth* (1993) and Philip Kitcher's *The Lives to Come* (1996) are especially well-argued examples of such critiques.[126] In her *Genetic Maps and Human Imaginations,* published in 1998, Barbara Katz Rothman writes, "What genetic thinking—what all reductionist thinking—lacks is an imagination, the leap of the mind that takes us beyond the pieces to see the whole."[127]

ON THE MARGINS

Yet, even though aimed at a general audience and accessible in paperback, these works on the dimensions of genetic futures are, like the bioethics mainstream in this respect, removed from reproductive practice. Penetrating criticisms of the status quo find their audience among those who share such views in the first place: like-minded scientists, ethicists, or interested others, such as myself.[128] Public debate remains elusive, and practice and perfectibility discourse remain unaffected.

For its part, the mainstream of professional bioethics has become increasingly media-driven. Responding to each new "hot" topic, whether test-tube baby Louise Brown in the '70s, Baby M and surrogate motherhood in the '80s, Dolly the cloned sheep in the '90s, or cloned human embryos in '04, the mainstream is reactive. Increasingly, it fails to take the lead in defining the critical questions. With the exception of some recent discussions about germ-line gene therapy, mainstream bioethics skirts the issues that arise at the point where DNA research and reproductive technologies intersect: at the point of medical practice. Ignored are the ways technologies and science combine to operate as disciplining technologies. In failing to explore the process by which reproductive medical decisions are made, mainstream bioethics avoids examining the process through which criteria emerge that mark the imperfect child, and begin to define the qualities for the child that would be perfect.

The price of avoidance can be high. As prenatal diagnosis expands to reach ever-widening groups of pregnant women and moves back to the preimplantation and even pre-conception stages, and as genetic science and technology expand the detecting of diagnosable conditions, the imperfect and perfect become more carefully defined. To ignore the aggregate effects of individual actions at the critical point of decision-making in medical practice is to ignore the social effects of those decisions. The result is mainstream bioethics' implicit support for negative eugenics. It is a eugenics by default, not by grand design. Accepting genetic research and the "promise" of new diagnostic technologies, ethicists buy into prevailing values about "defectives," submerging old doubts and how to define *normalcy, health,* and the *perfect.* Abdicating critical stance and remaining outside practice, mainstream bioethicists are marginalized "experts" who support the status quo.

N I N E

Sites of Resistance

Mainstream bioethics discourse is ineffective and marginalized partly because it is situated outside the practice of reproductive medicine. Effective opposition to a dominant discourse, according to Foucault, comes from within. Arising from within the networks of power, dissenting voices constitute what he terms "sites of resistance." Such voices inside or directly focused on the practice of reproductive medicine contrast with the abstracted rhetoric of mainstream bioethics. Although disparate and often deflected and submerged, voices of medical professionals, pregnant women, and people with disabilities and their advocates are such sites. Potentially, they contribute to framing counter-discourses to the perfectibility discourse of reproductive medicine.

Medical Professionals

Technology itself is a target of some medical professionals, who challenge or at least question its uncritical acceptance by colleagues and public alike. In his critique of the rhetoric of medical ethics, Dr. Edward Hill is among those expressing concern over the way the public is lulled into thinking that technology is the great panacea. Dr. David Grimes, an ob/gyn at San Francisco General Hospital, directly attacked technology and medical practice. In the provocatively titled "Technology Follies: The Uncritical Acceptance of Medical Innovation," published in the *Journal of the American Medical Association,* he asked, what "procedures or practices . . . will rank with bloodletting as a folly of our time?" Because "women's health issues have traditionally received less attention than those of other groups," he wrote, "unproved technologies have been especially problematic in reproductive health." His examples include a former practice of testing pregnant women's urine for estriol (a form of estrogen) to monitor the fetus—a test which was subsequently found worthless—and today's electronic fetal monitoring and certain infertility tests, which have yet to be proved of real value. Among underlying reasons for these "follies," noted Grimes, are the " 'false idol of technology,' " the inability of medicine and medical education to let "sleeping dogmas lie," and the role of the market in promoting and perpetuating medical technologies of questionable value and efficacy. He called for better use of scientific method, including the practice of "randomized controlled trials," which were not practiced by his catalog of "technology follies."[1] A study subsequently reported in the *New England Journal of Medicine* substantiated Grimes on fetal monitoring, which is routinely practiced in hospital delivery rooms. When over 150,000 babies in California were tested to show whether fetal monitoring was effective in preventing brain damage during childbirth, researchers found that 99.8 percent of the signs of injury detected were false.[2]

Within reproductive medicine, queries about prenatal screening have similarly focused on effectiveness, but less on the technology itself. Testing procedures are evaluated particularly according to risks and benefits, skill of the operator, and cost-benefits. In France, prenatal screening did come under attack in the 1980s when Dr. Jacques Testart refused to continue doing IVF, which he foresaw rapidly developing into a vehicle to promote genetic testing and selective abortion, and thus to foster eugenics.[3] Although U.S. medical professionals do not generally echo his concern, U.S. reproductive medicine has produced critiques of particular prenatal diagnosis procedures, including the triple screen and ultrasound, and also of the meanings of "choice."

The triple screen, which, as described in chapter four, tests for levels of three substances in a pregnant woman's blood, was advanced for use in the early '90s particularly for detecting Down syndrome. At the time, some physicians argued that it would be cost-effective to apply the screen not just to women over 35 or at high risk for other reasons, but to all pregnant women regardless of age, since more Down syndrome births occur among younger women, who have more children. In an article in *Clinical Obstetrics and Gynecology* in 1993, ob/gyn Thomas Elkins and medical geneticist Douglas Brown from Louisiana State Medical School challenged this argument on two sets of grounds: "simple" economic, and "complex" human and social.[4] Their analysis of "simple" economic costs was straightforward, refuting the claims made for the screen's savings in dollars and cents terms. Out of 2,067 pregnancies of teenagers, 19 and younger, the testing process, which moved from triple screen to ultrasound to amniocentesis to winnow down the group at risk, yielded only one fetus with Down syndrome. The total cost of this one diagnosis was approximately $106,980. The similar progressive screening of 8,431 patients under 35, which included the 2,067 teenagers, yielded four fetuses with Down syndrome, again at a cost of about $100,000 per fetus detected. Combining data from other centers, Elkins and Brown projected costs in the "millions" to extend the triple screen to all women. "By what standard is this screening cost effective?" they asked.

Their analysis of "complex" costs went further, however, to raise disability and societal issues, linking them to loss of "choice," for which the price was "too high." Encouraging the use of the triple screen for Down syndrome demands analysis of much more than "brief economic concerns." The "validity of using such a dehumanizing approach toward a population group also must be questioned," wrote Elkins and Brown. In singling out people with Down syndrome, such screening proposals foster and perpetuate negative assumptions and biases. Taking issue with classifying Down syndrome as a "serious anomaly," like the lethal trisomies 13 and 18, Elkins and Brown state that while the "true prognosis for a fetus with Down syndrome is not known . . . the vast majority will do well medically (with routine, equivalent care), will be highly functional mentally, and will be integrated socially into today's world."[5] The two authors spare no one for sharing and contributing to false assumptions about Down syndrome, from the marketers of the tests to ob/gyns and genetic counselors, and including the medical literature, which emphasizes burdens against benefits, with accent on the burdens. Rather, materials showing the "positive side of Down syndrome" should be made available to medical professionals and prospective parents. Citing evidence of coercive counseling by medical professionals, the authors express concern for the integrity of the medical profession. Drs. Elkins and Brown ask finally what "attaching a price tag to persons with Down syndrome" says about our moral and social character. They suggest a "value analysis" for screening procedures and use that would bring together a range of perspectives and viewpoints.

That the triple screen has since become routinely offered to women in categories usually recommended for prenatal testing, with use becoming even more widespread as serum screening is extended to new populations, indicates how far critical reevaluations of prenatal testing need to go to have impact, especially concerning disability perspectives. In the introduction to the third edition of the *Catalog of Prenatally Diagnosed Conditions,* published in 1999, Dr. David Weaver notes that the triple screen, listed as a major procedure, has come under criticism for its very high false positive rate.[6] As the study cited by Elkins and Brown illustrates, among 2,067 pregnancies, the triple screen showed 150 to be at "high risk"; ultrasound reduced this number to 53 who were recommended for amniocentesis; of the 31 pregnancies tested, only one fetus had Down syndrome.

When doctors expect women to test and to abort for a diagnosed anomaly and are dismayed when women don't, and when doctors and genetic counselors present only negative aspects of Down syndrome, Elkins and Brown argue they are limiting, not expanding, women's choices. "One of the greatest costs of the triple screen for Down syndrome, as it is now being discussed, is the loss of choice that occurs."[7] Elkins and Brown cite Barbara Katz Rothman on the "illusion of choice" offered by prenatal diagnosis, which, because of inherent pressures, actually narrows choices.

Other medical professionals reflect similar concerns of social scientists that pressures to test skew and structure choice for pregnant women. At two schools of nursing in California, a qualitative, descriptive study revealed the ways "choice" was problematic for women whose fetus was diagnosed with an anomaly. Whether they chose to terminate or to continue the pregnancy, they needed to construct " 'healing fictions' " in order to be comfortable with that choice. But the women and their partners also suggested they were often " 'backed into' " prenatal testing in the first place, "as opposed to having actively chosen or refused" it.[8] Miriam Kuppermann and her colleagues at the University of California, San Francisco, questioning the rationales for offering prenatal diagnosis, conclude that women's preferences rather than criteria such as availability of resources (which are now adequate) and women's age, should be paramount. Although the authors' recommendations could result in extending use of prenatal diagnosis, through widening and equalizing access, their aim is to develop "sophisticated decision-assisting tools" so that "pregnant women and their partners make choices that reflect both their own values and the best available scientific information regarding whether to undergo prenatal diagnosis and which tests to use."[9]

Evaluations of the routine use of ultrasound, which are confined to effectiveness and cost-benefit criteria, are more typical of the internal critiques of prenatal testing in U.S. reproductive medicine. The RADIUS study, reported in 1993 and based on randomized controlled trials involving over 15,000 pregnant women, found that use of ultrasound had no effect on pregnancy outcomes among low-risk women. Even though more fetal defects appeared in the women screened than in the control group, both groups had the same rate of fetal loss or other adverse outcomes.[10] Based on findings on effectiveness of the procedure itself to affect pregnancy outcomes, the study recommended that physicians use ultrasound more selectively. An editorial by Dr. Richard Berkowitz in the same journal issue reporting the study recommended against advocating a nationwide policy of routine use of ultrasound because it would not be cost-effective.[11] In shifting the criterion to cost-effectiveness, Dr. Berkowitz was suggesting that lack of resources was the reason not to advocate more widespread use, not usefulness of the procedure itself. This seems to contradict the study's findings: that use of ultrasound was unable to change fetal loss and thus affect pregnancy outcome.

The results of the RADIUS study were subsequently questioned by the Eurofetus project, a much larger study based in Europe, which faulted Radius on assessing the accuracy of success in detecting fetal anomalies. A two-thirds accuracy rate for Eurofetus was contrasted to one-third accuracy for Radius, thus implying that ultrasound was more effective than Radius suggested. At a 1997 meeting of the New York Academy of Sciences entitled "Ultrasound Screening for Fetal Anomalies: Is It Worth It?" there was apparently some agreement among medical professionals attending that all women should be offered an ultrasound scan whether there was a problem or not, the procedure's benefits outweighing risks. A report of the meeting published in the *New York Times* noted, however, that "there were dissenters and caveators aplenty." Among the concerns expressed were false negatives, which could fail to detect an anomaly, especially a serious one.[12]

Despite inconsistencies and lack of clear lines of critique, such studies and discussion by medical professionals signal that a process of self-criticism and evaluation of prenatal diagnosis issues is taking place within reproductive medicine. These studies were well publicized in professional journals and in the mainstream press.

Among other strands of critique from within medicine are those of Dr. Neil Holtzman of the Johns Hopkins School of Medicine, who has worked closely with ELSI and the Human Genome Project. Dr. Holtzman has warned repeatedly about the trend toward increasing commercialization in reproductive medicine. In his book *Proceed with Caution,* published in 1989, he described the growth of commercialized laboratory testing, its problems and pitfalls, as well as those of unregulated genetic testing and research.[13] Dr. Holtzman has also called on physicians to speak out against genetic determinism.[14]

Contrary to a widely held view that medicine wants hands-off from government, the 1980s and early '90s found medical geneticists and genetic counselors deploring the policies of the Reagan and Bush administrations which precluded government involvement in genetic and reproductive research. Such policies meant not only lack of funding for much needed medical research, but also lack of public dialogue to frame proper rules and research guidelines. The use of embryos for research on stem cells and fetal tissue has been continually buffeted by the politics of abortion, alternatively banned and reapproved under succeeding U.S. presidents since the '80s; the controversy reignited in early 2004 with the cloning of human embryos. Because of its critical role in finding causes of and cures for a range of diseases, such research has support among medical and other science professionals, as well as many advocacy groups. Loss of federal supports and funding for scientific and medical research not only hampers major fields of research, but also can allow privately funded research to go ahead without proper oversight and increase the prospects for commercialization.

Within the practice of medical genetics there have been calls urging more dialogue between the medical profession and the public, and for greater feedback and communication among medical professionals themselves. Dr. Jessica Davis, then a medical geneticist at North Shore University Hospital on Long Island, New York, and subsequently director of genetic services at Weill Cornell Medical Center, made the case for public involvement at a conference on medical ethics in the 1970s. Dr. Davis pointed out that it was not until public demands forced the issue that the medical profession accepted controls over medical experimentation involving human beings. The "lesson to the experimental scientist is a practical one in which he may not recognize the presence of any ethical imperatives," she argued. Dr. Davis urged an "ongoing dialogue" between biological scientists and the rest of the scientific community, especially the medical community, and between with the general public. One of the few conference participants to particularize, Dr. Davis spoke "on behalf of my patients," their questions and needs, to emphasize the "importance of sharing information about new technologies and techniques as well as involving a concerned and interested public."[15]

[193]

The adequacy of genetic counseling, the biases found in it, and the status, class, and cultural gaps between medical professionals and their clientele have come under continuing scrutiny within reproductive medicine. In 1998, a study in the Department of Pediatrics at Johns Hopkins, which looked at the context of discussions between pregnant women and obstetricians and nurse-midwives, found that information about genetic testing provided at the first prenatal visit was inadequate to ensure "informed and autonomous decision-making." The study concluded that guidelines to address the content of these discussions should be developed with input from obstetricians, nurse-midwives, genetic counselors, and pregnant women.[16]

In 1992 Seymour Kessler discussed five "process issues" that should be considered in genetic counseling: language and communication of risks, discordant agendas of counselors and counselees, emphasis on facts but little on psychosocial factors, the influence of counselor's gender on the outcome, and cases of directiveness in counseling.[17] Genetic counseling has been exploring some of these issues in the patient-provider relationship at least since the mid-1980s. Along with their colleagues in reproductive medicine, genetic counselors generally support prenatal testing. But within that framework, some genetic counselors have sought to raise questions about the whole process of communication with their clients.

Among the first to note problems and gaps were counselors whose clientele were other than middle- and upper-class Whites. At the education conference of the National Society of Genetic Counselors in 1985, therapist Maria Vargas took aim at the individualized model in therapy and genetic counseling. The model reflects "dominant trends in this country" and seeks to have people conform "to this modality."[18] Juliet Yuen, an Asian-American genetic counselor at the University of Hawaii, pointed to the prevailing Euro-American counseling norms on the U.S. mainland. The "majority group genetic counselor is the product of a middle-class Euro-American culture."[19] Culture influences counseling through the counselor's culture, the client's culture, and the culture of the environment in which counseling takes place. Yuen argued that counselors had to have this level of cultural awareness in order to treat the whole person. Rodger Lum, of the Asian Community Mental Health Services in Oakland, California, noted that research has "amply demonstrated that counseling outcome is strongly influenced by social class."[20] Age, sex, and counselor and client expectations are further important influences on the counseling process and its outcome.

The Division of Medical Genetics at Beth Israel Medical Center in New York, emphasizing that genetic counseling services need to be responsive to the social and cultural backgrounds of patients, developed a program particularly to serve its population of Chinese ancestry in Lower Manhattan. The program took into account the various barriers to access and use of services—including communication, language, culture, economics, and education—reporting a marked increase in use of genetic services by Chinese patients.[21]

Although medical geneticists, who are more often male, do some counseling, most professional genetic counselors in the U.S. are female. What effect, if any, does sex have on the counseling process and on attitudes, given that the patient too is female? Studies comparing women and men counselors across a number of countries show men more directive than women. Pregnant women in the U.S. do request obstetricians who are female and have reported being more satisfied with female obstetricians than with male.[22] Some research shows female physicians in various fields to be more caring toward patients than are male physicians.[23] Calls to bridge culture and class gaps, to improve communication, and to be more sensitive to patients' needs have come particularly from the mostly female genetic counselors. Perhaps a shared experience of pregnancy also contributes to the apparent rapport of female providers with their patients.

But when it comes to attitudes, it is questionable whether female providers are specially affected by concerns and fears about testing that may be expressed by their patients. There is no evidence that female obstetricians, or female doctors in family practice who care for pregnant women, are critical of testing procedures or are any less or more supportive of the extension and use of prenatal diagnosis than are their male counterparts. Nor do we find such critique among genetic counselors. Professional roles and position in the medical hierarchy may be more important.

The genetic counselor, through her professional role as a communicator of information in an intimate setting, is well situated to be an agent of change, such as concerning the subject of disability. Here, the counselor's sex—as it is related to her position in the medical structure of power—is relevant since it can limit her ability to make significant impact on reproductive practices. Chapter five pointed out that genetic counselors have the least status (based on claimed expertise, professional degree, and sex) of the trio of physicians, medical geneticists, and genetic counselor serving the prenatal patient. Presumably, then, genetic counselors have the least power among these professionals to effect changes. They are also restricted by the individualized, privatized setting of medical practice in which they operate, which confines them to the prevailing tools of method and style to improve communication with an increasingly diverse clientele. The one-on-one setting, focused on the immediate situation, operates to exclude materials whose content depends on broadening the social and cultural context in which testing decisions can be made.

To the extent that some genetic counselors seek to bridge class and culture gaps, yet are limited in the ways they might pursue such ends and effect change, they embody Foucault's "subjugated knowledges." Such knowledges, although arising within the power configurations of the dominant discourse, do not fundamentally change that discourse. But counselors are also a link to those pregnant women whose voices, too, are subjugated, in that they deviate from the norm of support for prenatal testing.

Pregnant Women

The majority of women recommended to test do so. Some, however, refuse or have serious reservations. Even though both partners may well be involved in decisions and men may have considerable influence, most studies of responses to prenatal diagnosis, and my own interviews, focus on women. The following discussion, therefore, will reflect mainly what women have reported. It will also reflect, for the most part, decisions about amniocentesis, which is the most studied procedure, plus some reactions to ultrasound and to maternal serum alpha-fetoprotein (MSAFP) screens.

Women opt out of prenatal screening for a variety of reasons. A major one is opposition to abortion, whether for themselves or generally. Being opposed or unwilling to abort can cut across class, race, or cultural background, though religion is often a contributing factor for those who hold this view.[24] For these women, there is no point to testing if it will not change the outcome of their pregnancy. Where this reason overrules all others, prenatal testing is not problematic, and so I will not include this group of refusers in my discussion.[25]

Another set of responses to testing comes from women who have given birth to an affected child, or who have one or more family members with the condition in question. Although they may choose to test, most do not abort if the diagnosis is positive. These women's preferences, discussed in chapter six, coincide most closely with the views of disability rights advocates, whose attitudes I discuss in the next section.

Personal perceptions, contexts, and specific situations play a part among women's other varied reasons for refusing prenatal testing. The refusers come mainly from those who are "routinely" offered prenatal screens because of age or because screening is mandated to be offered, as is the case for MSAFP screening in California. These women fall into two groups. One is those who are from the majority still recommended for testing: largely White, middle- and upper-middle-class, age 35 and over, and the original testing recipients. The other group is of women often labeled "minorities" because of class, race, or ethnicity, to whom testing has been more recently and more widely extended. The reasons offered by both groups for refusing overlap, but there are sufficient differences to warrant considering the groups separately. A key difference is the proportionately higher rate of refusal for the second group.

"You mean you're not being tested?" "You have a right to say no?" "Didn't they make you take the test?" "What will you do if your baby has Down's?" For women in the first group, it is expected that they will test, indeed that they will seek testing as a matter of course. If they don't, they meet with incredulity, even hostility. When Anna Quindlen wrote in her *New York Times* column that, at age 35 and pregnant with her third child, she would not have amniocentesis, reader response was heavy and mainly critical.[26] My conversations with pregnant or recently pregnant women, and interviews by others, tell the same story: surprise, disbelief, often disapproval, and even blame if the woman does give birth to an affected child.[27] Social and peer pressures can make matters even more difficult for a woman already conflicted about a usually difficult decision. Instead of finding sympathetic listeners and supports as she goes against the experts and conventional wisdom, she may be judged, and feel isolated.

Why do women of "advanced maternal age" refuse prenatal tests, despite the pressures, the statistically documented risks of fetal defects, and the irreversible consequences of their decisions? For some women, the reason is that they will not abort *this* pregnancy. If their position is tied to religious or other ethical or moral beliefs, then they overlap with anti-abortion women. But women in this group tend to be pro-choice. Their unwillingness to abort is highly specific to this pregnancy. They are determined to have *this* child, no matter what. A woman of 38, four months pregnant with her second child, told me just that. What if the child has Down syndrome, I asked? "It would devastate our lives," she answered, adding, "My husband and I try not to think about it." Both were working professionals.

This same woman also referred to her family history and her own health as positive factors, which were mentioned also by others. These factors included late and successful pregnancies of their mothers and/or other women relatives, and no family incidence of birth defects or major physical or mental disease. Since birth disorders such as Down syndrome occur randomly, this sort of reasoning amounted to faith, or gut feeling that they were not "high risk." Yet, at the same time, it gave rational support to statistical evidence that high risk is particularly associated with family incidence of a condition. Some women linked family history and health factors to their views of established medicine and health care. A 40-year-old woman having her first child, although choosing a hospital delivery because of her age, told me she had had no prenatal tests or screens at all, not even "routine" ultrasound, and was attended by midwives throughout her pregnancy. By no means totally rejecting conventional medicine (her child, born healthy, sees a pediatrician regularly), she reflects thinking and practices characteristic of the women's health movement in the late '60s and the 1970s. Feminists' continuing critique of patriarchal medicine, especially as it has dealt with pregnancy and childbirth and high-tech procedures, has encouraged combining traditional and modern medical approaches so as to consider the whole person and the body's natural healing processes.

Among other reasons for refusing testing are concerns about risks from the procedures themselves. Women fear miscarriage, damage to the fetus, pain, or even the need to repeat the test because of errors or other complications.[28] Women here may draw on their own experiences or those of friends. Even though she is presented with statistical evidence that benefits outweigh risks, her own perceptions of risk can be stronger. Once again, the abstracted rationality of the medical argument clashes with what a woman experiences and feels. The medico-scientific rationale does not allow a patient's perceptions to be factored in. When researchers in California compared women who accepted MSAFP screening with those who refused it, they found that differences hinged on how the women interpreted and applied biomedical concepts of "risk," and not on rejection of or resistance to the offerings of science and technology.[29]

Attitudes toward disability also influence decisions. Nancy Adler and her colleagues who looked at psychological issues found that "[w]omen who view genetic defects more negatively are more likely to undergo amniocentesis than are those who are less distressed by the possibility of having an affected child."[30] A woman who does not share prevailing negative views of disability may be willing to cope with raising such a child (and indeed, may not see it as "coping" at all). One woman told me that she did not want a world in which there was no room for those who were different. She recognized, however, that she might find it hard to sustain this level of moral commitment if she were faced with the prospect of a disabled child. A study in California by Nancy Press, Carole Browner, and others of pregnant women's views of disability revealed a similar inconsistency: women who expressed upbeat and positive views of children with disabilities became negative and fearful when asked about the possible implications of a disability in a child of their own.[31]

What happens if the testing decision involves a second child rather than the first? A woman pregnant for the second time and who had decided not to test smiled when I asked if she would do so if it were her first. "When my son was born" (before she was 35), she answered, "I thought I would have control over what he would be like and how he would develop." This she found not to be the case at all. Her boy was now six. She saw no compelling logic to try to control the outcome before birth. Another woman who refused testing the first time around—and had a healthy child—told me the decision not to test in her second pregnancy was far easier, even though she was now past 40 and therefore statistically at "higher risk." Other conversations indicate that the decision about testing for a first pregnancy can produce an anxiety level that is not matched for subsequent ones.

Male partners' attitudes and influences on prenatal testing decisions—to the extent they are studied—reveal pressures, usually to test and to abort if the result is positive. Especially among White middle- and upper-middle-class parents, as discussed in chapter six, men's self-image as successful males appears to be bound up with the quality of their offspring. A "damaged" child is a blow to their self-esteem, even though they may blame their wives for "bad genes."

Poorer and ethnically and racially "minority" women who refuse testing often give reasons similar to those of more affluent Whites. Class and/or cultural differences produce differences in emphasis, such as reasons for not aborting or the kinds of fears expressed about medical procedures. But there are also contrasts. While women in poorer and more ethnically diverse communities into which programs have been extended are accepting testing, they still refuse at a higher rate than do middle-class White women. Opposition to abortion is more widespread, and there is greater willingness to accept disabled children. Suspicion and fear of medical science and technology are often more marked; yet here, too, views are diverse.

In 1979, New York City initiated a program funded by Medicaid and the Department of Health to offer genetic services to an inner-city population. Studies conducted in the 1980s showed substantial increase in use of these services by the population served.[32] In the mid-1980s anthropologist Rayna Rapp undertook intensive research among pregnant women participating in this subsidized program.[33] She spent an initial four years doing in-depth interviews and participant observation at the Prenatal

Diagnosis Laboratory (PDL), the major genetic services laboratory in the program. She later supplemented her work with research at the Division of Medical Genetics at Beth Israel Hospital, where she could study a greater proportion of White middle-class women for comparison. The inner-city population served by the PDL was approximately one-third Hispanic, one-third African American, and one-third White. Rapp's findings from the first two years of her research prefigured the diversity and contrasts she would continue to find, such as the importance of the meaning and interpretation of language.[34] African American women, for example, "were far less likely [than White middle-class women] to either accept, or to be transformed by, the medical discourse of prenatal diagnosis."[35] Among the reasons both Hispanics and African Americans (including Caribbean Blacks) rejected amniocentesis were "anti-abortion attitudes often (but not always) articulated in religious terms; fear of losing the baby after medical invasion; anger and mistrust of the medical system; and fear of needles." The last reason was especially strong among Hispanic women.[36] By contrast, middle-class women, who were "disproportionately white," tended to accept amniocentesis, even though they might be ambivalent. Rapp quoted one woman: "I always knew I'd have amnio. Science is there to make life better, so why not use its power? Bill and I really want a child, but we don't want a baby with Down's, if we can avoid it."[37]

Attitudes toward science and technology revealed class and cultural contrasts among those who accepted testing. While White middle-class women expressed a positive view and saw technology transforming their choices on a personal level, a Hispanic immigrant woman wanted the test because the miraculous powers of science could reveal what God had in store. Rapp likened her view to that of the native-born professional woman who felt that in providing amniotic fluid for research she would contribute to the progress of science. Both women were in awe of science, but their reverence was grounded quite differently. A 1988 report on genetic services at the PDL found that patients were suspicious "of the 'test with the needle,' which has been imbued by street lore with great pain and frequent miscarriage."[38]

In California, a 1986 law that mandated MSAFP screening be offered to all pregnant women drew new constituencies into the world of prenatal diagnosis. Although mostly accepting MSAFP, which was presented as a routine and simple blood test, the newly served ethnically diverse working- and lower-class women found themselves unprepared for the prospect of amniocentesis should the MSAFP reading be positive. Unlike the earlier middle-class clients for prenatal diagnosis, this new group of women had not previously sought genetic services, in part because they tended to complete their childbearing earlier. Research in California since the mid-1980s, especially by Carole Browner and Mabel Preloran at UCLA, has confirmed findings from elsewhere that women from these constituencies, with the exception of certain Asian groups,[39] refuse amniocentesis at significantly higher rates than do others.

Studies conducted at three public hospitals in southern California explored this refusal among newly emigrated Mexican women, asking why they were more than twice as likely as European American women to refuse amniocentesis. As in New York, ethnicity and culture mattered up to a point. But "deep-rooted cultural givens—such as religion, *machismo*,[40] or opposition to abortion. . . . [were] far from being the deciding factors in their amniocentesis decisions." Rather, the most important factors included the "women's understanding of the risks of amniocentesis, their fear of birth defects, their faith in medicine, and their relationships with their doctors."[41] Their two main reasons for declining amniocentesis were a continuing belief "that the pregnancy was normal despite the positive screening test result" and fear that "the procedure could harm the fetus."[42] Displaying some skepticism of medical accuracy and authority, they chose to trust their own knowledge, derived from experience, while at the same time not rejecting other aspects of prenatal care, such as monthly check-ups, which would enhance the well-being of their fetus. Here we see similarities that cross class, race, and ethnicity, as refusers among middle-class women also express distrust of the medical establishment, relying rather on their own feelings and experience. They too struggle to choose the course that will best ensure the health of their fetus.

Ultrasound, which is offered more and more routinely, is accepted by women in part to help them toward such reassurance. While medical professionals have expressed concerns about false negatives, when the screening fails to detect an anomaly, false positives have brought some women anxiety, indeed agony. A *New York Times* science reporter, Natalie Angier, recounted the ordeal she underwent with ultrasound while she was pregnant with her daughter. Ultrasound seemed to show the child had a clubfoot, but it was not so—which Angier discovered only when her daughter was born.[43] Her anger is shared by women who have had similar experiences. The situation can be particularly difficult when ultrasound reveals a suspected genetic or chromosomal disorder when it is too late to have amniocentesis. Among reader responses to Angier were women who echoed her experience of a false positive; others told of the pain of false negatives from ultrasound, and from amniocentesis, which had failed to detect even a devastatingly abnormal fetus.[44] Then there are ultrasound indicators so ambiguous that no determination can be made between a diagnosis of massive abnormality or one of apparent fetal health.[45]

As suggested above, attitudes toward people with disabilities can figure into middle-class women's decisions about prenatal diagnosis. Many of the poor and working-class women Rayna Rapp interviewed identified with disabled children they knew, whether their own or those of relatives and friends, and with children with disabilities they saw in TV telethons (which were popular fund-raisers at the time). These women described positive relationships with children who were "slow" and talked about how physically or mentally disabled children needed love and caring. By contrast, White middle-class women separated themselves from mothers of Down syndrome children whom they encountered. While they admired the self-sacrifice of women caring for disabled children, most drew the line at such sacrifice for themselves, arguing the need for their own self-actualization and fulfillment. Although Rapp describes a "running battle on the question of selfishness and self-actualization" on the part of White middle-class women as they sought to justify their decisions to test and to abort, they more often came down on the side of their own needs. They—or their husbands—sometimes inverted the selfishness issue to argue that it was selfish to bring a disabled child into the world.[46]

Class and cultural differences in attitudes toward disabled children surface in perceptions of who is disabled and what disability is. Screening for the sickle cell anemia trait, which is found mainly among African Americans, has a painful history in the U.S. Sickle cell anemia is a recessive blood disease, which means that a person must inherit the trait, or allele, from both parents in order for it to be expressed. Characterized by persistent anemia, impaired growth and development, and susceptibility to infection, it is still less severely disabling than a number of other diagnosable conditions. Mass screening programs for African Americans of marriageable age legislated in the 1970s were charged as racist and even genocidal, and subsequently abandoned. Whether or not the earlier experience is remembered, African Americans regardless of class continue to be ambivalent about sickle cell screening, which began to be resumed in selected centers as genetic services expanded. Rejection of tests is common, even as ambiguous attitudes toward the disease persist. Researchers have found that persons diagnosed with the trait felt stigmatized, even though they did not have the disorder. Non-carriers had an even more negative view of the disease.[47] Yet a (White) medical geneticist, commenting on the high rate of refusal of testing, remarked to me, "Sickle cell is not viewed as a problem in the Black community" (a view that is not necessarily shared in the dominant White culture).

Those who refuse prenatal testing remain a relatively small percentage of pregnant women, most of whom continue to accept amniocentesis when their age or prior screening results indicate a possible problem. But this high rate of acceptance seemed to be lessening in the late 1990s. Comparing two groups of patients who were referred to genetic counseling because of advanced maternal age, abnormal serum screening results, or ultrasound abnormalities, a study at the New Jersey–Robert Wood Johnson Medical School found differences between the 1995 and 1998 groups. Fewer patients at risk for Down syndrome desired amniocentesis in 1998 than did those in 1995, both before and after the two groups had received genetic counseling and ultrasound. The authors of the study cite these results among "changing trends" in patient decisions.[48] If the numbers of refusals are growing, perhaps the increasingly articulate voices of people with disabilities have played a role.

People with Disabilities

Potentially the strongest voices among counter-discourses are those from people with disabilities. Until recently, however, spokespersons and advocates, with a few exceptions, have shied away from the sensitive issue of prenatal testing and selective abortion—for understandable reasons. Disability advocates focused on improving the lives and prospects of persons with disabilities and on promoting public awareness through research, support services, legislation, and education. By the '90s, however, a strong, politically active disability rights movement had developed. Drawing on feminist analysis as well, a disability rights critique of prenatal testing emerged—articulate enough for a lagging mainstream bioethics to take notice.

Among the results of a Hastings Center two-year project in the mid-1990s was *Prenatal Testing and Disability Rights* (2000), the first book devoted to such a critique. The critique argues that testing and selective abortion are morally problematic and are based on misinformation. Edited by Adrienne Asch of Wellesley College and Erik Parens of the Hastings Center, the book presents varied perceptions of disability rights advocates, ethicists, medical professionals, and social scientists.[49] While participants in the project failed to reach a consensus about drawing lines on prenatal testing, they did agree on the critical need to correct misperceptions about disability among medical practitioners and parents and to change the public climate.

The development of the disability rights critique represents an important phase in efforts to call attention to disability issues. Making the clear linkage to prenatal testing, the critique has served to considerably extend the existing aims and work of disability advocates up to this point. For over three decades, genetic support groups and organizations for particular conditions, in serving their own clientele and raising public awareness, have helped to shape the background for disability-based counter-discourses.

These support groups, usually organized at national and local levels, have grown dramatically in size and scope. Two of the oldest and largest are the National Down Syndrome Society (NDSS) and the Spina Bifida Association of America (SBAA). The NDSS, founded in 1979, now "represents more than 100,000 individuals including persons with Down syndrome, parents, educators, health care professionals and interested community members."[50] The SBAA was founded in 1973, and serves the 70,000 adults and children with spina bifida through a network of almost 60 chapters, i.e., Group Members, in more than 125 communities throughout the country.[51] The words "Education. Research. Advocacy," which appear under the NDSS logo on its Web site, could well characterize the work and goals of similar organizations. Engaging in both support and advocacy for affected persons and families, these groups maintain Web sites, offer information and referral services, publish newsletters and other materials, promote relevant medical and genetic research, sponsor conferences and scientific symposia, and conduct public information campaigns.

In 1986 the Alliance of Genetic Support Groups was formed to give these lay advocacy organizations—who make up about 70 percent of the Alliance membership—a stronger voice. Self-described as a coalition of "support groups, consumers, and professionals," the Genetic Alliance, as it is now known, has grown to include 300 consumer groups, health coalitions, professional organizations, genetics clinics, hospitals, and biotech companies, plus approximately 250 individual consumers and professionals among its members.[52] At the "heart" of the Alliance is building "communication between genetics professionals and consumers," as well as engaging in "educational programs . . . and advocacy for health care policies." The "goal of both endeavors is the assurance of universal access to high quality and culturally sensitive genetic services."[53]

My queries about prenatal testing policy drew these responses. In an interview in June 1990, Alliance founder and executive director Joan Weiss told me it is a matter of individual choice. If consumers are educated and informed, then testing decisions will be made responsibly and ethically, and not for "trivial" reasons. Ten years later, the Alliance put it this way:

The mission of the Genetic Alliance on this topic has always been to provide information and resources in a nondirective way and this has not changed. Our focus regarding prenatal diagnosis remains to try to provide support and to help people find all the available information so that they can make the best decisions for themselves and for their families.[54]

Reflecting the growing importance of genetics and genetic testing issues in the '90s, the Alliance maintains a liaison with the National Human Genome Research Institute (NHGRI) and its ethics arm ELSI, and was previously so associated with the Council of Regional Networks for Genetic Services (CORN).

Organizations representing particular genetic conditions usually do not take positions on prenatal testing. In answer to my query, the Spina Bifida Association of America replied, "Prenatal testing issues are not on our advocacy agenda."[55] The National Down Syndrome Society, however, issued a position statement on prenatal testing in April 2004,[56] and a booklet on the topic that was in preparation is now available as *Prenatal Testing and Down Syndrome.* The SBAA, for its part, actively promotes the use of folic acid in foods and supplements early in and prior to pregnancy to prevent neural tube defects. But encouraging health measures to prevent a condition from occurring is one thing; preventing through testing and possibly aborting an affected fetus is another. Avoidance of advocacy positions on prenatal testing is consistent with these organizations' wish to avoid conflict with their primary aim, which is to serve individuals and families affected by the condition, and at the same time not to endanger wider goals to inform and educate so as bring public understanding and attitude change.

While these organizations and the Alliance lobby for changes in public policies, especially concerning research and services, their advocacy is not overtly political in the sense that the disability rights perspective is. Disability rights activist Marsha Saxton locates the beginnings of the growing disability rights movement in the mid-1970s.[57] A measure of the movement's political success was the passage of the 1990 Americans with Disabilities Act (ADA), which went into effect in 1992.[58] Its major provisions cover four areas: public accommodations, employment, public transportation, and telecommunications. The law mandates making properties which are open to the public accessible to disabled people; prohibits discrimination in hiring, advancement, compensation, and training; requires that buses, trains, subway cars, and rail stations be accessible; and requires ready access to telephone and telecommunications services for hearing- or voice-impaired persons.[59] Geared to physical disabilities, the legislation focuses on ensuring equal access, treatment, and opportunity: for example, employers may not discriminate against "qualified" disabled individuals, that is, those who are "mentally able" to do the job even if physically impaired.

By the end of the decade, effects of the law were starting to be measured. In a Harris survey taken in 1998, people with disabilities, while acknowledging some improvements, reported continuing areas of discrimination and social stigma. Fewer than half (only 45 percent) of the respondents felt they were treated equally when people learned of their disability.[60] Gauging public reactions as people with disabilities gain greater visibility can continue to be elusive. Does awareness of "difference" make people more positive, or does intolerance increase when, for instance, harried commuters have to wait for a passenger in a wheelchair to board a city bus? Businesses that had lobbied against the legislation as too costly could now face image problems in addition to being cited or sued if they do not comply with the law.

The view that prenatal testing fosters discriminatory attitudes is central to the disability rights critique. As articulated in the Parens and Asch book, the critique is explicitly directed at prenatal testing and selective abortion. Faulting programs for separating the consequences of testing from testing itself, Parens and Asch directly link the two.

> [T]he motivation for the disability critique is the reality of using prenatal testing and selective abortion to avoid bringing to term fetuses that carry disabling traits.

Their argument makes "two broad claims: that prenatal testing followed by selective abortion is morally problematic, and that it is driven by misinformation." Central to the first claim is what is called the "expressivist" argument. Testing prenatally to select against disabling traits "expresses a hurtful attitude and sends a hurtful message to people who live with those same traits." It disparages their lives and the lives of disabled people in the future.[61] Extending the argument, Nancy Press asks, what does the very offering of prenatal testing say about our society and our attitudes toward people with disabilities? If we look at the social context in which testing is offered, she writes, we discover the real message is that some lives are less worthy than others, a message confirmed by the fact that most women do abort for a positive diagnosis.[62]

Like other contributors in *Prenatal Testing and Disability Rights,* and as Asch and others have argued elsewhere, Press addresses the second claim, that such attitudes and actions are based on misinformation about disability, and that this situation needs to change. The heart of such proposals is information to counter widely held assumptions that the lives of people with disabilities are unrewarding and indeed not worth living, that the burdens to themselves and their families are insurmountable. A chapter by education researchers in *Prenatal Testing and Disability Rights* says otherwise. Reviewing several bodies of research, the authors show that, contrary to popular views, families with and without children with disabilities have similar patterns of adjustment and well-being, even as "family responses to disability are immensely variable."[63] Press has proposed working with genetic counselors specifically, as they are the medical professionals in closest contact with women and families contemplating testing. Barbara Bowles Biesecker and Lori Hamby from the Genetic Counseling Graduate Program at Johns Hopkins, pointing out that counselors are inadequately prepared to discuss disability, call for more education and exposure for them to "difference" and disability experiences.[64] Though counseling's watchword is to be "nondirective," as I noted previously no one is neutral and prevailing societal attitudes are powerful.

The point emphasized by Press, by Asch, and by others explicitly taking feminist perspectives, is that information about disability must be introduced at the point of practice. Writing in the *American Journal of Public Health,* Asch calls for revamping the education of "obstetricians, midwives, nurses, and genetics professionals." Until this happens, they "cannot properly counsel prospective parents." Asch details the kinds of information that should be made available to parents by "responsible practice . . . concerned with genuine informed decision making" at each stage of the process: from prior to testing to disclosure of a disabling trait in the fetus. Such information would include "a detailed description of the biological, cognitive, or psychological impairments associated with specific disabilities," discussion about functioning, support services, and financial assistance, and the direct experiences of members of families with disabled children and of disabled persons themselves. Addressing her journal audience directly, Asch admonishes public health professionals to "do more than they have been doing to change the climate in which prenatal tests are offered." She further calls on practitioners and policy-makers to adapt programs to accommodate all children, so programs will "fit the people who exist in the world," rather than claiming "that some people should not exist because society is not prepared for them."[65]

More than a decade earlier Asch and Michelle Fine, in their co-edited book on women with disabilities, had proposed taking disability issues into the doctor's and genetic counselor's office so as to make a far greater range of information available to the pregnant woman. In a jointly authored essay, they argued that while a woman carrying a fetus diagnosed with Down syndrome has the right to make her decision "in whatever way she needs," if genetic counselors, physicians, and others involved would provide information, often not "customarily available," about "how disabled children and adults live, many women might not choose to abort."[66] Asch's argument has become stronger since then. As she had argued in the American Journal of Public Health, in a separate article in Prenatal Testing and Disability Rights she strongly repeats her call to change the social climate and the practice of medical and health professionals: the "message" about disability in the professional literature must be changed.[67]

The bolstering of Asch's arguments, the initiation of the Hastings project, and publication of Parens and Asch's co-edited book all indicate that changes prefigured as early as the late 1980s remain a long way off. A sense of urgency marks the newer work. A complicating issue for many disability rights advocates is their pro-choice position. They cannot see themselves asking women not to have an abortion for a disabling trait. To propose banning or stringently curtailing testing is also untenable, since this would also deny women choice. Yet if no limits are placed on testing and women retain the absolute right to choose, disabled people's rights are critically compromised. The tensions between women's rights and disability rights create an acute dilemma for feminist disability advocates.

In Women with Disabilities, Asch and Fine tackle the dilemma this way. First they distinguish between a fetus residing within the body of a woman and a live newborn. They then argue: while newborns with disabilities have every right to medical treatment—even over parents' wishes—women have every right to abortion for whatever reason they choose. Asch and Fine's perspective rests on connecting rights to "personhood." Based on a woman's right to control her body, a woman must have absolute right over the fetus inside her. "On the basis of women's rights alone, abortion must be safe, legal, and funded." But, once the child is born, it is a person with its own rights to be protected. "As a society, our constitution accepts personhood as starting at birth. We cannot simply decide that 'defective' persons are not really persons and not entitled to all the care and protection we grant other citizens." In pressing for medical treatment for all newborns, regardless of prognosis, Asch and Fine criticize the selectivity that is practiced. Costly treatments are supported when "procedures result in a perfect, 'normal' child." But they are questioned if "no amount of medical treatment" will prevent that infant from remaining "throughout its life as a person with some level of disability."[68]

Asch and Fine are also critical of feminist reproductive rights advocates who link abortion rights and disability. Assuming that women would automatically abort for a disabling trait, activists exploit the "defective" fetus as the "good or compelling reason" to guard women's right and access to abortion. For Asch and Fine abortion must be an unequivocal right, available on "the basis of women's rights alone . . . not to rid our society of some of its 'defective' members."[69]

By the end of the '90s, pro-choice was less of an issue as such for disability rights advocates as they developed the prenatal testing and selective abortion critique. In the Parens and Asch book pro-choice is assumed, but is not expressed in an explicitly feminist context. Reproductive choice becomes part of broader discussions of rights and freedoms, specifically as to how efforts to ban or restrict testing might legally and ethically impinge on rights guarantees. The lack of consensus on how to resolve conflicts over rights and thus to decide to draw lines for prenatal testing illustrates the limits of the bioethics approach for the disability critique. Advocates like Marsha Saxton and Adrienne Asch herself take strong issue with testing. But they represent one pole within a critique which settles for taking a stance only on the critique's second claim, that of misinformation. In recommending only that more information be provided to practitioners and parents, and that greater efforts be made to change societal views about disability, the Hastings project skirted the critique's first and central claim, namely that prenatal testing and selective abortion are morally problematic. While moral issues were discussed from the perspective of rights and the expressivity argument, the project took no stance.

As I argued in chapter eight, and will do so further in the following chapter, the legalistic and ethical framework of individual rights at the core of mainstream bioethics impedes taking a critical or controversial stance that can translate into policy. Feminist advocates of disability rights often, too, have little choice but to use the limiting language of individual rights. When Asch and Fine, for example, defend equally a woman's right to choose and a disabled newborn's right to treatment, they apply the concepts of individual rights and personhood to separate points in time so as to avoid the trap of pitting the woman against her fetus. But the rights language limits discourse to the individual level—and to a universalized abstract—which precludes placing disability and prenatal testing in the social contexts that Asch and Fine and other feminists call for elsewhere.

That disability rights advocates, however, have taken on the difficult issue of prenatal testing marks a significant step toward creating a disability counter-discourse. Critically important is their recognition of the need to reach professionals and parents with their message at the point of reproductive practice, a course originally promoted by feminist advocates. A continuing obstacle here is the privatized and individualized setting in which testing decisions take place. Given limited time for counseling and information dense with statistics and probabilities, the setting is not conducive to receiving alternative messages about disability and placing them in social context. Efforts to change practice must thus be accompanied by parallel efforts to transform the social climate. When genetic support groups and the Genetic Alliance seek to increase communication between professionals and consumers and to educate and inform the public so as to change negative attitudes, they contribute to building a more favorable climate for people with disabilities. In this way their work complements that of disability rights advocates.

But the politically activist stance of disability rights advocates and their willingness to at least discuss the prenatal testing issue—even if consensus is elusive—is different from that of genetic support groups. Focusing on improved education, research, and services, genetic support groups seek to promote public information and achieve ameliorative reforms within existing scientific and political systems. While not rejecting this liberal pragmatist approach to policy change, disability rights advocates go further to scrutinize prevailing medical practices and social and scientific mindsets. Such differences in approach among spokespersons for people with disabilities can hinder framing a disability-based counter-discourse. Yet their common efforts to change the social climate, though separately pursued and differing in method and intensity, may work positively toward changing the atmosphere in which the pregnant woman confronts prenatal testing and selective abortion decisions.

Creating Networks and Connections

To what extent do these three sites—medical professionals, pregnant women, and people with disabilities—present a challenge to the dominant perfectibility discourse? Foucault argues that changes in discourse are effected by forces within the networks of power, as they connect to articulate changes in the practice in which the forces are rooted. The discourse of the perfect child is an ideology framed, not through elite conspiracy, but through decisions made and actions taken within reproductive medical practice. A critical link among the three sites, is that, in contrast to mainstream bioethics, they speak from within reproductive practice or from advocacy positions for changes to that practice. The three sites are also concerned about communication, exposing and seeking to repair knowledge gaps between practitioner and patient, and between people with disabilities, medical professionals, and pregnant women. The sites confront common dilemmas and explore the meanings of language. These links surface in a number of ways.

Among medical professionals, a critical discourse on genetic testing and attitudes toward disability has been slow in coming. Chapter eight noted that some physicians early on expressed concerns about possible stigmatizing effects of testing and selective abortion. In 1978 Dr. Edmond Murphy and his colleagues called for developing principles to guide choices. It is not just a matter of cost influencing choice, they pointed out, but that a person with a genetic disease is thought to be "inherently undesirable." Stereotypes about various defects influence those who are making the prenatal decisions.[70] Fifteen years later, Drs. Elkins and Brown spoke pointedly to the misinformation and biases about Down syndrome among medical professionals and the damage done to a specific group by singling out its members as targets for the triple screen. As noted above, Elkins and Brown were highly critical of the biases and coercion evident in professional attitudes and counseling and the limits imposed on pregnant women's choices.

More recently, Dr. Steven J. Ralston, a perinatologist and obstetrician invited to participate in the Hastings project on testing and disability, spoke of persisting negative views. Medical professionals had little exposure to the viewpoints and lived experiences of people with disabilities. His medical training taught that "disability—no matter what its form—is a bad thing and to be avoided at all costs." The Hastings meetings caused Dr. Ralston to question these assumptions, prompting him, as a doctor specializing in high-risk pregnancies, to seek to resolve the conflict he found now between "my belief that society would be better if it were more tolerant and accepting of those with different abilities and needs, and my belief that insofar as the world is not yet ideal, the decision to terminate a pregnancy with an abnormal fetus is reasonable."[71] Acknowledging the complexity of decision-making, and taking into account his own experience as a CF carrier, he affirmed his pro-choice position. He found a new sensitivity to language and to the kinds of information that should be made available to doctors and patients alike.

Dr. Allan Jacobs of the Department of Obstetrics and Gynecology at Beth Israel Medical Center in New York, whose criticism of clinical ethics was discussed in chapter eight, has taken the issue of choice to the level of genetic enhancement and its wider social consequences. He is concerned about the increased social inequality that will result if genetic choice is freely pursued. Framing the conflict as one between liberty and equality, Dr. Jacobs warns that the "potential impact of genetic selection for the purpose of enhancing normal traits to improve the economic and social status of individuals" will be immense. We cannot suppress the technology of genetic selection even if we would want to. Yet we are loath to exercise social controls over the freedom to choose. He calls on the medical profession to act in the wider social arena so that the "potential effects of genetic science, including . . . genetic selection," can be "in the forefront of consideration by the public and its governments."[72]

Genetic counselors are a further locus for linking medical professionals and disability concerns. Situated at the point of decision-making in reproductive practice, counselors, whose own awareness of their difficult role has evolved, become a point of entry for disability rights advocates, who can, through the counselors, link to pregnant women and their partners. As counselors become more sensitive to the issues and values involved in the decision-making process, they can be better prepared to meet the varied responses of women to testing, including refusal. Genetic counselors in turn can connect with other medical professionals within reproductive practice who are raising cautionary signs about the uncritical acceptance, widening use, and social and ethical implications of prenatal diagnosis technology. These medical professionals and disability rights advocates alike support increased training and information about disability issues.

Genetic support groups and the Genetic Alliance seek to open dialogue between experts and consumers, to educate the public, and to foster and facilitate more input into medical and policy issues by the publics involved. Medical professionals, too, have supported such public input. Medical geneticist Dr. Jessica Davis, who had served on the Alliance board and on the health issues sector of a commission set up by the government for the year 2000, had early on pointed to the public's important role in calling attention to ethical issues in medicine, and so influencing changes in practice and public policy.[73]

Although pregnant women who refuse testing differ in their reasons why, they also share attitudes which will cross racial, ethnic, and class divides. They are often wary of the promises of established medicine and its technologies. They would rather place more trust in their own feelings, in a sense of self, in what feels right for "me." For the well-educated, more affluent woman, her reliance on self reflects the individualism of the dominant culture to which she belongs, even as she rejects equally strong cultural attitudes toward disease, health, and social status, and social pressures to conform. The poorer or "minority" woman who also calls on her own resources in resisting the medical experts may, by contrast, find supports in her cultural milieu for her stance. Some women who refuse prenatal testing, as well as those who choose not to abort for a diagnosed disabling trait, may also share a willingness, for whatever reasons, to accept an "imperfect" child. Here there are links with the views of disability rights advocates and even with cautionary medical professionals.

The question remains as to whether overlapping concerns of dissenters and questioners could serve to link their several discourses into a counter-discourse to that of the perfect child. Are there means to fashion these sites into networks of resistance? Perhaps the answer is a postmodern one: not to try to unify, but to recognize and support the role of multiple counter-discourses to strengthen and keep dissent alive; yet at the same time to address the possibilities of language to provide bases for coherent counter-voices to emerge.

"No longer do words like 'risk,' 'abnormality,' or 'problem' seem innocent of judgment and bias," wrote Dr. Ralston in Parens and Asch. "I am much more cognizant and wary—if not worried—about the impact and power of the language I use when counseling patients."[74] So, too, have other medical professionals such as genetic counselors found it necessary to rethink the language they use to communicate with a varied clientele about issues surrounding prenatal testing. Disability rights advocates' conscious attempts to change the terms used about disability are critical to their efforts to change attitudes. Although new language does not necessarily transform the ways people think, at the least it raises consciousness, while it continues subtly to persuade. When, in the opening chapter, Parens and Asch reconfigure diagnosing a "defective fetus" into discovering a "disabling trait" in the fetus, they set guidelines for a new discourse to explore the ways disability rights and prenatal testing intersect.

Medical discourse profoundly affects women in reproductive health care. Women candidates for prenatal testing find themselves distanced from the abstracted language of scientific probability. These feelings can be particularly strong for women who refuse testing, who look to their own sensibilities to guide their choices. A medically and statistically oriented discourse has little relevance for decisions they are making and the dilemmas they face. Needed is language which can speak to the unique experiences of pregnant women, while at the same time be relevant for others involved in the process.

Feminist critique, drawing on feminist ethics and women's multiple experiences, offers a different conceptual language for reproductive medical discourse. It may serve as a possible framework for counter-voices, to create alternatives to the dominant discourse.

TEN

Transforming the Dream of
the Perfect Child

As *healthy* and *perfect* are conflated in reproductive medical practice, the discourse of the perfect child distorts the pregnant woman's hopes and plays on her fears. At the heart of the discourse is the way in which prenatal testing further alienates her from the pregnancy experience. As the defective fetus becomes the focus of medical attention, the pregnant woman is eclipsed as primary patient. She becomes almost an observer to what is happening. Masked is the degree to which the discourse disempowers her, robs her of agency, reducing her claim as active, embodied subject with control over her pregnancy.

How then to reclaim agency? How to enable women to participate in framing a discourse that counters the illusion of the perfect child, yet preserves the goals that the illusion masks? How can a reproductive medical discourse and practice emerge that will transform the dream?

Feminist perspectives have long focused on women's experiences to understand the dimensions of women's power, in concept and in practice. In the second wave of feminism, feminists of varying approaches and persuasions have brought intense attention to women's relationship to their bodies and to their reproductive lives. For radical feminists, organizing as FINRRAGE (Feminist International Network of Resistance to Reproductive and Genetic Engineering) internationally in the mid-1980s, this meant strong opposition to almost all "reproductive and genetic engineering," casting women as victims of a male medical profession and technology. Although their extensive research called attention to very real abuses, their position was criticized for not differentiating among women's varied needs and lost saliency over time.[1] For liberal feminists, this focus has meant being in the forefront of struggles for reproductive rights and equal rights, actions which have brought important gains for women before the law. Liberal feminists' commitment to women's autonomy and freedom to choose, however, operating as it does within the individual rights framework of the U.S. legal system and democratic beliefs, does not sufficiently critique the ideology and contexts of practices, such as that of reproductive medicine, when they operate as oppressive discourses for women.

Among feminist responses that can speak directly to women's empowerment and transforming the discourse of the perfect child is the work of feminist philosophers. Feminist philosophers are engaged in an ongoing dialogue on the female subject in social context. Starting from the concept that the female subject is a relational being, they explore what this means for feminist ethics, the ethic of care, and postmodernism, resituating subjectivity and identity in a feminist postmodernist framework. As their work deconstructs traditional ontologies and substitutes concepts of being grounded in women's experiences, it suggests ways to change the discourse of reproductive medical practice and so counter the dominant discourse of the perfect child.

A Feminist Relational Concept of Being and the Ethic of Care

Feminist philosophers have taken sharp exception to traditional moral and ethical theory and what this means for the female subject. In the introduction to their edited collection on feminist perspectives on philosophical methods and morals, Lorraine Code, Sheila Mullett, and Christine Overall write,

> the moral universe as it is construed in the philosophical tradition is not one in which women can live. It is a universe that denies value to the fundamental experience of caring for other human beings, and erects standards of moral maturity according to which female moral responses are accorded minimal esteem.[2]

[215]

In her influential 1982 study *In a Different Voice,* psychologist Carol Gilligan offered a counter to Lawrence Kohlberg's reigning model that moral decisions are made in a hierarchical, step by step order. She found that her female subjects made moral decisions in a relational and contextual framework, not in a hierarchical one. Although Gilligan's work has been criticized for appearing to universalize women's moral behavior on the basis of a narrow sampling of subjects,[3] it has been important in the development of feminist ethical theory, which looks to women's experiences to critique existing theory and to develop alternatives.[4]

Feminist ethics has been defined by feminist philosophers in this way:

> Most generally we mean by ethics the normative analysis of issues and concepts concerning right action, the human and non-human good, and social justice. Feminist ethics criticizes the gender blindness and biases in much traditional ethical theory, and develops new theories and concepts that are more gender sensitive. Feminist ethics also works to conceptualize issues of right action, social justice, and the human good from out of the specifically gendered experience of diverse groups of women.[5]

Among the concepts feminist ethics questions is the basis of the theory of moral rights that underlies traditional ethics. "According to the rights view of ethics," writes Caroline Whitbeck, "the concept of a moral right is the fundamental moral notion. . . . People are viewed as social and moral atoms, armed with rights and reason, and actually or potentially in conflict with one another."[6] Whitbeck criticizes this quintessentially masculine rights view of ethics as rooted in a "self-other *opposition* that underlies much of so-called 'Western thought.' "[7] Following the legacy of Hobbes and Locke, political organization, formed by contract among potentially warring individuals, bequeaths a law and moral theory that rest on the opposition of self and other.[8]

Conforming to this pattern of atomized, adversarial discourse, traditional bioethics is distant, removed, non-contextual, based on conflicting claims of "rights." Its moral and ethical situations fail to be relevant for women making critical decisions about reproductive technologies. By contrast, a feminist concept of being and the ethic it proposes look to women's experiences and to the social embeddedness of those experiences. In the introduction to her *Making the Connections,* Beverly Wildung Harrison writes that her essays "illustrate the significance to ethics of starting with reflection on real women's real experiences, however different those experiences are, before moving inductively to a definition of the moral situation and claims about what we ought to do."[9]

The pregnancy experience directly contradicts antagonistic self-other dualisms. Noting that women are usually erased in discussions of reproductive ethics, Christine Overall points out, "on the rare occasions on which women are discussed within the context of abortion or birth, the fetus-woman relationship is most often seen as one of competition and antagonism rather than interaction and support."[10] In the abortion literature, writes Whitbeck, "being pregnant is represented on the one hand as similar to having a tumor, or on the other as being hooked up to an adult stranger who is dependent on that hookup for survival, or more remote yet, as occupying a house with another person whose presence constitutes more or less of a threat to one's life."[11] As Whitbeck and others are quick to point out, the absurdity of these characterizations, along with the adversarial model, fly in the face of the complexity and highly subjective nature of what women experience while pregnant.

Applying a phenomenological approach to her own pregnancy, Iris Young offers a distinct alternative to the oppositional model.[12] Starting from existential phenomenology that locates consciousness and subjectivity in the body itself, Young explores her experience of the "lived pregnant body," drawing on Julia Kristeva's and Adrienne Rich's ideas of pregnancy as a split subjectivity. Young describes the "doubling" experience of pregnancy as a "body subjectivity that is de-centered, myself in the mode of not being myself." As the first movements of the fetus produce the sense of splitting subject, "I experience my insides as the space of another, yet my own body." Even as the outside boundaries of the pregnant body are in flux, it is still her body, allowing her—however differently—to accomplish her aims. Indeed, the weight and materiality of pregnancy "often produce a sense of power, solidity and validity." Pregnancy is a dynamic process of movement, growth, and change. "The pregnant subject is not simply a splitting in which the two halves lie open and still, but a dialectic. The pregnant woman experiences herself as a source and participant in a creative process. . . . she is this process, this change."[13] Young adds that the encounter with obstetrical medicine works to undermine this subjectivity and to alienate the woman from the experience of pregnancy and birthing.

The caring ethic also counters atomized perspectives. For Sheila Mullett, the caring ethic relies on a feminist "double consciousness," for "part of caring is the ability to apprehend the world through the eyes of the other." The "double perspective of feminism" has "the ability to see and feel the limitations of the present while imagining alternatives to it. It also involves relinquishing the perspective of a solitary moral agent operating alone and contributing to the construction of a consensual perspective by a process of sharing experiences and seeking to articulate and explain these experiences so as to generate new categories of interpretation." Al though the caring ethic has been criticized for reinforcing the idea that stereotypical female roles are "natural," Mullett argues that double consciousness enables women to be aware of such distortions as they use the caring experience to imagine possible moral paradigms. The feminist perspective then becomes "an experimental consciousness, a method of paying attention to suffering, a toleration of ambiguities."[14] Gilligan, carefully defining a *feminist* ethic of care, as distinct from a *feminine* ethic of care, states a "feminist ethic of care begins with connection, theorized as primary and fundamental in human life."[15]

The experiences of both pregnancy and mothering help to develop a relational view of human interaction, which would begin, writes Overall, "by rejecting the alienated view of the self and its connection with others." Drawing on Whitbeck, Overall notes that pregnancy's "simultaneous relationship to what both is and is not oneself" continues through the early stages after birth, when "the well-being of mother and child are inextricably linked." "[F]or the woman involved, all of these interactions constitute immediate lived experience that she is not unique, not a solipsistic self in an indifferent universe inhabited by programmed robots. As Whitbeck expresses it, 'bringing another person into full social being requires continual renegotiation of the self-other boundaries.'"[16]

Whitbeck develops this relational concept of being into a relation-based feminist ethic. Taking human interrelatedness as the fundamental factor of human development, she holds that an individual "acquires the moral status of a person in and through relationships with other people."[17] She proposes a "'responsibilities view of ethics'" to replace the "rights view of ethics." Instead of an ethic based on moral rights of atomized individuals, her ethic has "moral responsibility arising out of relationships as the fundamental moral notion."[18] Our necessary interdependence as human beings thus becomes a central underlying condition for making moral decisions. Moral decisions do not occur in isolation. "Rights" exist, according to Whitbeck, not as claims against each other, but as claims made on society, and are translated into moral obligations. Under a feminist relational ethic, then, moral decisions occur in the social realm. Writes Overall, even though moral choices are individual choices, they "are not and cannot be made independently of their social context."[19] For decisions about reproductive technologies, context extends from the families involved to the wider medical, socioeconomic, and cultural frameworks in which they are situated.[20]

This feminist relational ethic challenges the prevailing abstracted and disembodied character of the atomized, adversarial ethical model, which erases women. As ethicists debate the moral and metaphysical status of the fetus, writes Overall, there is "relatively little discussion of the woman who is the co-creator and sole sustainer of the embryo/fetus, except insofar as she is treated as a container or 'environment' for it."[21] Denied are women's bodily integrity and personhood.[22] The abstracted rights model denies the critical factor of bodily experience, that human beings are embodied beings, and further, that embodied beings are gendered. Iris Young points out that even existential phenomenologists, whose "lived body" theories seek to overcome Cartesian dualism, fail the gender test, since they cannot explain the uniquely female bodily experiences of pregnancy and birth. For them the body remains an impediment, something alien, outside; body is again the inferior Other.

Female Embodiment and Female Subjectivity

As they have sought to reclaim the female body, reembodying women as subjects who engage the world as intentional agents, feminist theorists have adopted feminist interpretations of postmodernism. If we start from the feminist phenomenological view that locates the sense of self, one's subjectivity, in bodily experience, the question arises as to what happens to the sense of self, to one's consciousness of identity, during the split-body experience of pregnancy Young describes. Does identity split too? Postmodernism posits a fragmented and fractured identity. Does fragmentation preclude the possibility of female embodiment? Or, on the contrary, does it provide a way to deal with the disembodied and estranged experiences of women that reproductive technologies intensify?

Donna Haraway has used the image of the cyborg to capture the fractured identity of postmodernism for feminism. The cyborg—who, like women, is culturally and biologically constructed—represents the fragmentation of both body and identity that occurs under a postmodern technological "informatics of domination." Because feminist theory sees female identity as multi-dimensional, with feminists struggling for "new couplings, new coalitions," Haraway finds in the cyborg an apt metaphor. The cyborg is "a kind of disassembled and reassembled, postmodern collective and personal self . . . the self feminists must code."[23] Mapping the identity of woman onto the cyborg, Haraway offers the possibility of endlessly changing shape and form, of multiple identities, of an end to antagonistic dualisms, and of the chance to transcend gender.

Susan Bordo, acknowledging the undeniable appeal of Haraway's archetypes of fluid, sexually ambiguous shape-changers, of multiple, changing identities, faults them as deconstructionist images: they "refuse to assume a shape for which they must take responsibility."

> To deny the unity and stability of identity is one thing. The epistemologi-
> cal fantasy of becoming multiplicity—the dream of limitless multiple
> embodiments, allowing one to dance from place to place and self to
> self—is another. What sort of body is it that is free to change its shape
> and location at will, that can become anyone and travel anywhere? If the
> body is a metaphor for our locatedness in space and time and thus for
> the finitude of human perception and knowledge, then the postmodern
> body is no body at all.[24]

For Bordo, the body must be "somewhere." Held up to a deconstructionist
analysis, Haraway's cyborg image threatens disembodiment. Bordo argues
for the "locatedness" of the body, and the gendered nature of that locatedness. For Bordo, gendered embodiment is central to feminist analysis.

Suzanne Damarin finds the cyborg world is gendered. In cyberpunk
science fiction, cyborg reproduction "is clearly postheterosexual and . . .
postsex," but the cyborg is not "constructing itself as postgender." Instead,
she points out that the way that "traditional gender identities and practices . . . appear to be defining the subjectivities of individual cyborgs"
indicates that the cyborg is "a return to the prefeminist era."[25] As she looks
at how new technologies of the postmodern act to socially reconstruct
women individually and collectively, Damarin warns that woman as subject could disappear under the "informatics of domination." Yet, despite
implicitly criticizing Haraway, Damarin also finds a postmodern subjectivity to be a way out and means of resistance for women, calling on
women to participate in shaping evolving technological visions.

Postmodernism, says Damarin, frees women from the subjectivity of
modernity that has essentialized women in a failed attempt to represent all
women. Instead of representation, a postmodern subjectivity offers a
many-faceted simulation. This subjectivity "cannot represent but simu-
lates woman/women/womyn as ever changing, always becoming, responding to and/or resisting the inputs, outputs, and programs of domination." It "removes experience from the constraints of the linearity of time
. . . and the materiality of 'legitimate' experience." It "is never complete, and
neither true nor false nor falsifiable, but invites continual revisits and
revisions." Its "ever changing boundaries and surfaces. . . . provide opportunity for interpretation(s) of the changing functions and positions of the
minds and bodies of women in response to the inputs of postmodern
reproductive and artificial intelligence technologies."[26] Damarin, like
Bordo and other feminist theorists, believes that a transformed female
subjectivity that overcomes both dualisms and an essentialized, fixed female identity is critically necessary. Without some sort of subjectivity,
women will be unable to develop "sites of resistance" to a technical ra-

tionality that converts patriarchal technological visions into experiences ultimately destructive of women's minds and bodies. Damarin seeks this subjectivity in the very postmodernism that could threaten a disembodied future for women.

The view of female subjectivity as changing and yet embodied complements feminist ethic's relational concept of being to provide a conceptual basis for a woman's active participation in her pregnancy experience, as technologies impinge upon and distort that experience. Overcoming self-other dualism, the feminist relational concept does not separate body and mind, but integrates them. Physical self and identity can be reconciled. While the body may change shape or form—as it does dramatically in pregnancy—it still has locatedness as a physical self. So, too, with consciousness, sense of self. The pregnant woman, like anyone else, has a variety of changing experiences, apprehended through the body, as she engages the world and interacts with other human beings. Consciousness reflects the many dimensions of experiences for a kind of multiple consciousness, or multiple identity in that sense. Yet we remain embodied beings.[27]

Connecting: A Feminist Ethical Framework

Perhaps the most critical insight of feminist ethics is that the relational model, not the oppositional, atomized model, describes human interaction and the development of social and moral identity—for all sexes. "Persons *are* relational and interdependent," writes Virginia Held. "We can and should value autonomy," she continues, "but it must be sustained and developed within a framework of relations of trust."[28] Humans exist mainly as social beings, making decisions, not as abstract entities, but as real persons in human contexts. They decide about medical and reproductive technologies not as moral and social atoms, but in relation to those most concerned and affected: women, parents, families.[29]

Seeking to explore further how autonomy and the relational model interrelate, feminist ethicists have proposed *relational autonomy,* which is the title of an edited collection of essays on the subject. Applying her analysis specifically to medical decision-making and the health care professional–patient relationship, Anne Donchin proposes a "*strong relational autonomy*" as the model to be followed. "Autonomy in the strong relational sense is both reciprocal and collaborative," she writes. "It is reciprocal in that it is not solely an individual enterprise but involves a dynamic balance among interdependent people tied to overlapping projects. Moreover, the self-determining self is continually remaking itself in response to relationships that are seldom static."[30] The feminist relational ethic rests squarely on this concept of human interdependence as the defining quality of the human condition. It rests, as Gilligan and others point out, on connectedness, unlike the patriarchal model, which is based on disconnection. Disconnections, writes Gilligan, are "at the root of violence, violation and oppression, or the unjust use of unequal power." Contrasting the two modes, Gilligan speaks to the question I ask: how can we frame a discourse that rests on the relational model? Citing her earlier work, she points out that the "tension between a relational psychology and a patriarchal social order is caught by a paradox: living within the structures of patriarchy, women find themselves giving up relationship in order to have relationships. . . . *A feminist ethic of care became the voice of the resistance*"[31] (emphasis added).

This ethic of relation and connection is based on a conceptual language different from that of the prevailing reproductive discourse. It can offer a framework to articulate and link resistances into alternative discourses. When Foucault describes power as a series of "relationships of force" which are sustained by confrontations among unequal groups and forces within the social body, he shows that not only dominant forces but also resistances play pivotal roles. Located everywhere within the power network, the "multiplicity of points of resistance" are diverse in character and distributed in irregular fashion. The "strategic codification of these points of resistance . . . makes a revolution possible."[32]

Adapting Foucault for feminist praxis, Jana Sawicki applies his view of power and its incorporation of multiple resistances to deconstruct the seemingly hegemonic power of reproductive technologies. Using "a bottom-up [Foucauldian] analysis" to trace the origins of the present situation, she finds it "the outcome of a myriad of micro-practices, struggles, tactics and counter-tactics" among the various non-feminist, anti-feminist, and feminist forces. Thus she includes not only dominant discourses and practices, but also the "moments of resistance" that have transformed these practices over the years. Writes Sawicki,

> Although it is crucial to continue to identify the ways in which new reproductive technologies threaten to erode women's power over their reproductive lives, it is also important to locate the potential for resistance in the current social field, that is, what Foucault refers to as "subjugated knowledges"—forms of experience and knowledge that "have been disqualified as inadequate . . . or insufficiently elaborated."[33]

Women's use of and support for reproductive technologies have built-in undersides of resistance. So, too, do the myriad experiences of others in reproductive medical practices generate resistances. Because the decisions that people make about prenatal diagnosis exhibit "context, experience, and particularity,"[34] they do not fit the reigning abstract, isolating model of decision-making. Yet women and others involved are forced into that model, leaving the complexities and difficulties of their compromises not understood, and their voices often unheard and ignored. The feminist relational model and ethic can provide a framework in which to explore and link resistances not only among women who reject or are ambiguous about prenatal testing, but also extending to others who question, including medical personnel and disability advocates, so that shared concerns and values can be aired and articulated.

A common concern of questioners and dissenters, though they do not necessarily agree on specifics, is that important elements are left out of the decision-making process. High on the list is lack of attention to social contingencies and consequences of choices. What does it mean to raise a child with a disability, and what are the arguments for and against? What about social supports? What are possible effects of a disability on the child? on the particular family? on other families and particular social groups? For many, a critical issue is that the pregnant woman is increasingly ignored, that her needs are subsumed as the fetus takes center stage and she declines as participating subject. While questioners and dissenters will vary as to attitudes about prenatal testing itself, they voice concerns about its effectiveness, about its proper use, under what circumstances, and for whom.

As to changes proposed, questioners and dissenters often agree on placing greater emphasis on prenatal health care, on pursuing research for treatment and cures, on developing medical priorities that are not necessarily geared to a commodified product. They will suggest listening more carefully to those involved in prenatal testing, from parents to families to those with a stake in the process whose voices may have been muted. Some may share a concern that research and prenatal care priorities are not necessarily delivering the trouble-free pregnancies and healthier babies hoped for, indeed that the promise itself may be flawed.

These concerns suggest, implicitly if not explicitly, a different set of values from those that underlie the discourse of the perfect child. They are values that run counter to the medical and biological ranking of human beings, with its built-in biases of class, race, ethnicity, and gender that are furthered under current practices.[35] The feminist ethical framework offers an alternative set of values that put the relational model of human interaction at its core and the striving for connectedness as a prime guide for action. Feminist values prompt questions about practice that seek to change practice, further prompting reappraisal of values as they operate and are informed in practice.

How would this work for reproductive medical practice? Going beyond and redirecting the traditional goal of medical ethics—to do no harm and to confer benefit—a feminist ethic asks, "Who benefits?" More significant than asking whether new reproductive technologies are good or bad, write Judith Rodin and Aila Collins, are "questions related to for whom they are good, in what instances, and for whom they should be made accessible."[36] Feminist ethics reassert focus on woman and fetus as a unit. Evaluations and treatment are to flow from that premise and not from the fractured and contentious model. Medicine can then refocus to ask, How can medical research and new technologies improve the health and enhance quality of care of both woman and fetus? From here decisions about prenatal care and the possible use of technologies can widen to include the complex of relationships and communications among families and others who want to be involved in the process,[37] especially those born with genetic "defects." Pressures can build to take up such issues as social supports and to redirect research priorities to treatment and cure of particular conditions.

Shifts in reproductive practice would mean working within a set of health care norms other than those prevailing, and locating prenatal diagnosis within this different set of norms. Instead of the individualized model, we have a "health model." Sheryl Ruzek has called for a "broad, socially based health model" for reproductive health issues, one that "includes all aspects of life conditions as well as services that promote or impede health."[38] Well-being becomes the focus, not just absence of infirmity. When health is a "core issue," it "shapes what we view as the important social and ethical issues in birth." These include equitable delivery of services to all pregnant women and scrutiny of our research priorities, especially for their effects on clinical practice. While "we elevate research to an exalted status," writes Ruzek, we "simultaneously ignore its implications for clinical practice when it contradicts other 'system needs.'"

> The social and economic consequences of supporting unjustifiable medical tinkering and failing to provide a "floor of equity" for birth are so enormous that the pattern must be changed. A first step is reconceptualizing the nature of health for pregnant women and their families in a manner that promotes community and social stability rather than purely self-interest.

Ruzek notes that a social health model reflects the World Health Organization's definition of health as "'a state of complete physical, mental, and social well-being and not merely the absence of infirmity.'"[39]

The social health model counters prevailing notions of health as they are reflected in the discourse of the perfect child. Instead of concentrating narrowly on disease or "defects" lodged in the individual, health practices would shift their focus to a more broadly conceived state of well-being for the future child, as well as for its mother. The dimensions of that well-being can then be framed through a social process that brings in parents, medical personnel, health workers, as well as state-of-the-art science and technology that is relevant. Reflecting a variety of social and cultural experiences, the process suggests shifting and fluid, rather than absolute, health criteria. Procreative health, for mother and child, is a continuously evolving state of well-being, rather than a search for the "perfect child."

A medical practice pointed in this direction would reframe the discourse of reproductive technologies, now one of disease and the "imperfect," into one of health, access, and quality of prenatal care. The focus becomes: What constitutes health, for whom, and by whom defined? A discourse turned away from the imperfect or perfectible individual reins in genetic determinism. Genes and genetic heritage are now cut down to size as only one set of factors contributing to procreative health, and to the decisions made about that health. Being "imperfect," no longer a matter of individual genetic fault, is revealed for what it is, a social construct used to label the socially unacceptable.

Perfectibility Revisited: A Different Dream

From its birth as a secular ideology in the Enlightenment, newly wedded to science, medicine, and the Idea of Progress, perfectibility discourse over the next two centuries took on the language and ideology of the positivists, evolutionary biologists, and the eugenicists, to emerge today as the discourse of the perfect child. In today's wedding of technology, science, and ideology, the dream of human perfectibility is no longer a matter of misapplied science and science fiction fantasy. Incorporated into reproductive medical practice, the explosive changes in science, medicine, and technologies of the past half century inscribe the dream on the human fetus. Replacing the eugenicists' crude attempts to mark the bodies of the unfit as Other—the defective underside of their ideal—is reproductive medicine's ability to define and imprint the imperfect fetus as Other. As individual decisions in prenatal practice aggregate, the contours of both the imperfect, unacceptable child and the ideal, wanted child emerge. Reflecting currently dominant values and beliefs, imperfect and perfect images bear similar kinds of biases of class, race, culture, ethnicity, and gender that characterized perfectibility discourse over its changing history. Despite the egalitarian vision of a Condorcet, the Perfectibility of Man as it was to be achieved through science, medicine, and progress emerged as elitist, Eurocentric, and embodying universalized absolutes. Western dualisms privilege the rational, the scientific, and the abstract among these absolutes, which are male-identified. Reflecting an adversarial, disconnected mode of interaction among competing, atomized individuals, perfectibility is a masculinized discourse. The male science fiction fantasies of the 1920s and '30s, with their ectogenically produced, eugenically perfect beings, prefigured the objectified, and separated, woman and fetus of today's reproductive practice. As woman becomes a container for her fetus, which increasingly can be programmed and manipulated, we recall Haldane's scheme to conceive and gestate superior offspring in wombs detached from superior women. J. D. Bernal dispensed with the body altogether, his ideal a mind without body, yet somehow able to reproduce itself.[40] Late-twentieth- and early-twenty-first-century man-machine warrior cyborgs and robots carry on the vision of an asexual, controlled reproduction, an engineered replacement for human procreation.

Feminist visions of the future, by contrast, strive for connection even when imagining *ex utero* reproduction. Writes Hilary Rose, much of feminist utopian science fiction is centrally concerned with sexuality and reproduction.[41] Whether it opts for female conception without males, as in Charlotte Perkins Gilman's *Herland* or Sally Gearhart's *Wanderground;* for the ingenious method of childbearing by changing genders in Ursula LeGuin's *Left Hand of Darkness;* or for the collectively planned, machine-gestated babies of Marge Piercy's *Woman on the Edge of Time,* procreation in feminist futures has liberatory goals.[42] Projecting societies freed from gender-based strictures and oppressions, and that empower women, feminist procreative modes are built on a relational and caring ethic. The aim is not to create superior or even better people, but to create a better society. Even Shulamith Firestone's somewhat naive and seemingly non-nurturant proposal for a total system of artificial reproduction had as its goal a freer, egalitarian, de-gendered society for women, men, and children.[43] In Piercy's future Mattapoisett the collectivity chooses the characteristics of the child to be produced in the "brooder"—to be nurtured by three people who wish to parent—according to community-determined needs for balance. Although produced technologically, in a society with highly sophisticated technology, such children are "special" only in the sense that they are wanted and will be the responsibility of the entire community. As Patsy Schweickart has pointed out, rather than rejecting technology, Piercy's utopia provides a positive example of how feminist aims and values and advanced technology can be joined.[44]

Schweickart's comment on Piercy is critical. In order for women to have control of their own reproduction, to be able to have healthy, wanted children, and to widen and enhance their range of choices, we need not opt out of reproductive technologies and their benefits, as some feminists would have it. Rather, we need to develop a procreative discourse and practice that poses alternatives based on these feminist values and goals.

What we need to keep in mind is the common framework which gives birth to both the dominant discourse and resistances to it. The discourse of the perfect child is neither scientific-medical conspiracy nor male plot. It is sustained, rather, by our shared desire for healthy children. Deconstructing reproductive medical practice reveals how technology, medicine, and parental expectations intersect to distort the desire for normal, healthy babies into the dream of perfect ones. Revealed is the cultural legacy that labels and stigmatizes the imperfect. The dream we discover is founded on a nightmare, on deep-seated fears of a child that is far less than perfect. As prenatal diagnosis decisions aggregate to define criteria for this feared, unwanted child, they also begin to define the hoped-for, wanted child, revealing and shaping standards for what constitutes health, intelligence, beauty, and success. These standards reflect prevailing class, race, ethnic, and gendered beliefs, reinforcing those beliefs and an emerging health hierarchy of birth. Resistances to the discourse, sharing as they do the common desire for healthy children to be born, project contrasting sets of values to underwrite a reproductive medical practice dedicated to realizing that desire. Feminist approaches, joining and participating in these resistances, provide frameworks to articulate these values so as to reshape practice and transform procreative discourse.

Based on the experiences of real human beings in reproductive practice, a transformed discourse replaces the dream of "perfect babies" with the goal of health and well-being for all children born, with images of children who are wanted and cared for. The transformed vision is that they be born into a society which will nurture its children in all their differences and diversity.

NOTES

INTRODUCTION

1. "A Message from Beverly Sills," national chairman of the March of Dimes Birth Defects Foundation, in *Perfectly Beautiful, New York Times Magazine,* March 28, 1993, p. 4A. In a phone conversation on February 28, 1994, the *Times* advertising contact for the section attributed the phrase "perfectly beautiful" to Ms. Sills, who has long been an eloquent activist for people with disabilities. Both of the former opera diva's children were born deaf; one child is autistic, the other has multiple difficulties. I intend no criticism of Ms. Sills in quoting her. Rather, her words are important because they illustrate how language can play us false, how it can be recontextualized to convey meanings very different from the original intent.

2. *New York Times,* January 16, 1994, sec. 9, p. 6.

3. Lawrence J. Aiken, president of the Greater New York chapter of the March of Dimes Birth Defects Foundation and president and CEO of Sanofi Beauté, Inc., makers of Perry Ellis and other perfumes, was cited in the 1993 supplement as "a fragrance industry leader" for raising over $4 million in four years for the March of Dimes. He co-signed the "Message" with Ms. Sills in the April 3, 1994, supplement.

4. Twelve of the March 28, 1993, supplement's 20 pages carried these beauty ads; the April 3, 1994, section carried eight such ad pages out of 16. Text occupied much less than half the space in each. In each, the *Times* noted that the supplement was prepared by the March of Dimes and "did not involve the reporting or editing staff" of the *Times.* The March of Dimes Foundation's Greater New York chapter received 15 percent of the advertising revenue from each section. The cover title for the 1994 supplement was not "Perfectly Beautiful," but "Together We Can Deliver Small Miracles," featuring three color "snapshots" of babies: one African American, one Asian, and one White. The 1995 supplement in the April 2 *New York Times Magazine* was called "Marching toward a Future without Birth Defects"; its cover showed six babies (five White, from blond to brunette, and one African American). Focusing on the history of the March of Dimes since the 1930s—when it was founded to eradicate polio—the supplement was not paginated separately and was only eight pages long (against 16 the year before); four of those eight pages, however, were ads for Clinique (double-page spread), Lancôme, and Chanel. I have been unable to determine whether there had been any negative response to the phrase "perfectly beautiful" and, if so, whether it influenced the supplement's changes in language and message.

5. Chanel's ad in the 1994 supplement for "Lift Serum Extreme," which pictured a spray bottle instead of a model, promised that "you'll see your wrinkles reduced as much as 45%!" (p. 6A).

6. "Defect" is unfortunately the term in widespread use, with all its negative connotations. See further discussion in part 2 about the problems of using this term, and the reasons "diagnosable conditions" is a better choice.

7. The intent here is not to criticize the March of Dimes Foundation and its work. The text of these supplements emphasizes the Foundation's support for programs to reverse the major causes of birth defects, such as low birthweight and poor nutrition, often the result of inadequate prenatal care, and recent mailings and materials from the March of Dimes continue to pay major attention to these critical issues. The message of these supplements, and promotions since the mid-1990s, however, also serves to reinforce the role and power of genes, and for medicine and technology, to deliver "small miracles." Birth defects remain the enemy—no matter the causes—of achieving the goal of a blemish-free, "perfectly beautiful" child.

8. Joan W. Scott, "Deconstructing Equality-versus-Difference: Or, the Uses of Poststructuralist Theory for Feminism," *Feminist Studies* 14, no. 1 (Spring 1988): 35.

9. See, for example, Michel Foucault, *Discipline and Punish: The Birth of the Prison,* trans. Alan Sheridan (New York: Pantheon, 1977).

10. Michel Foucault, *The History of Sexuality, Volume 1: An Introduction,* trans. Robert Hurley (New York: Vintage, 1980), pp. 94–96.

11. Simone de Beauvoir, *The Second Sex,* ed. and trans. H. M. Parshley (New York: Alfred A. Knopf, 1953).

12. Susan Bordo writes that Foucault shows "our bodies are trained, shaped, and impressed with the stamp of prevailing historical forms of selfhood, desire, masculinity, femininity," and that this occurs "through the organization and regulation of the time, space, and movements of our daily lives." Susan R. Bordo, "The Body and the Reproduction of Femininity: A Feminist Appropriation of Foucault," in *Gender/Body/Knowledge: Feminist Reconstructions of Being and Knowing,* ed. Alison M. Jaggar and Susan R. Bordo (New Brunswick, N.J.: Rutgers University Press, 1989), p. 14.

13. See chapter three for the masculinist visions of J. D. Bernal, J. B. S. Haldane, and others.

1. THE PERFECTIBILITY OF MAN

1. John Passmore, *The Perfectibility of Man* (New York: Charles Scribner's Sons, 1970); and Arthur O. Lovejoy, *The Great Chain of Being: A Study of the History of an Idea* (1936; reprint, Cambridge, Mass.: Harvard University Press, 1964).

2. According to Passmore (*Perfectibility of Man,* p. 158), this separation occurred by the late eighteenth century, with William Godwin.

3. Jean-Antoine-Nicolas de Caritat, Marquis de Condorcet, *Sketch for a His-*

torical Picture of the Progress of the Human Mind, trans. June Barraclough (New York: Noonday, 1955). The work was first published in France in 1795, the year after Condorcet's death in prison following his arrest by the Revolutionary authorities.

4. Frank E. Manuel, *The Prophets of Paris* (1962; reprint, New York: Harper & Row, 1965), p. 78.

5. Condorcet, *Progress of the Human Mind,* p. 183.

6. For the development of the concept of atomized individualism in the English and American social and political contexts, see C. B. Macpherson, *The Political Theory of Possessive Individualism: Hobbes to Locke* (Oxford: Clarendon, 1962); and Louis Hartz, *The Liberal Tradition in America* (New York: Harcourt, Brace & World, 1955).

7. Condorcet, *Progress of the Human Mind,* pp. 196–97, 17–18.

8. Ibid., p. 105.

9. Ibid., p. 142.

10. Ibid., pp. 161ff. Almost three decades earlier Joseph Priestley had written that the instrument of perfection and continuous progress in arts and sciences was society and government. See Arthur A. Ekirch, Jr., *The Idea of Progress in America, 1815–1860* (New York: Columbia University Press, 1944), p. 17. Ekirch is referring to Priestley's *Essay on the First Principles of Government,* first published in 1768.

11. Condorcet, *Progress of the Human Mind,* pp. 199–200.

12. Ibid., p. 201.

13. Barbara M. Stafford, John La Puma, and David L. Schiedermayer, "One Face of Beauty, One Picture of Health: The Hidden Aesthetic of Medical Practice," *Journal of Medicine and Philosophy* 14, no. 2 (April 1989): 213–30. See also art historian Stafford's *Body Criticism: Imaging the Unseen in Enlightenment Art and Medicine* (Cambridge, Mass.: MIT Press, 1991). Dr. La Puma and Dr. Schiedermayer are both associated with centers for medical ethics or bioethics.

14. Charles Frankel, *The Faith of Reason: The Idea of Progress in the French Enlightenment* (New York: Octagon, 1969), pp. 172–73.

15. Condorcet, *Progress of the Human Mind,* p. 193.

16. Carl L. Becker, *The Heavenly City of the Eighteenth-Century Philosophers* (New Haven: Yale University Press, 1932); Frankel, *Faith of Reason.*

17. Quoted in Frederick J. Teggart, *The Idea of Progress: A Collection of Readings,* rev. ed. with an introduction by George H. Hildebrand (Berkeley: University of California Press, 1949), pp. 242, 15.

18. I am indebted to Garland Allen for sending me his article, which makes and applies these distinctions so clearly. Garland E. Allen, "The Misuse of Biological Hierarchies: The American Eugenics Movement, 1900–1940," *History and Philosophy of the Life Sciences,* section 2 of *Pubblicazioni della Stazione Zoologica di Napoli* 5, no. 2 (1983): 105–28. Allen attributes the identification and definition of constitutive and aggregational hierarchies to evolutionary biologist Ernst Mayr.

19. Lovejoy, *Great Chain of Being.*

20. George H. Hildebrand, introduction to Teggart, *Idea of Progress,* p. 15.

21. John C. Greene, *The Death of Adam: Evolution and Its Impact on Western Thought* (Ames: Iowa State University Press, 1959), pp. 144, 154.

22. Ibid., pp. 222ff.

23. Ibid., p. 242.

24. Francesca Rigotti, "Biology and Society in the Age of Enlightenment," *Journal of the History of Ideas* 47, no. 2 (April–June 1986): 223.

25. Manuel, *Prophets of Paris*, p. 77; and Charles Van Doren, *The Idea of Progress* (New York: Frederick A. Praeger, 1967).

26. According to Frank Manuel, however, "In filial deference to Turgot, the title of the *Esquisse* retained an intellectualist and elitist bias, but in the working out of the historical process the concept was weighted heavily in the direction of the social." Ibid., p. 63.

27. Stafford, La Puma, and Schiedermayer, "One Face of Beauty," p. 216.

28. Ibid., pp. 219–22.

29. In *Body Criticism,* Stafford writes that Camper was the "linchpin in the development and dissemination of a body calculus" (p. 111).

30. See Susan Bordo, "Feminism, Postmodernism, and Gender-Scepticism," in *Feminism/Postmodernism,* ed. Linda J. Nicholson (New York: Routledge, 1990), p. 137.

31. See Genevieve Lloyd, *The Man of Reason: "Male" and "Female" in Western Philosophy* (Minneapolis: University of Minnesota Press, 1985).

32. Stafford, *Body Criticism,* p. 33.

33. See Michel Foucault, "The Birth of the Asylum," from chapter 9 of *Madness and Civilization,* reprinted in Paul Rabinow, ed., *The Foucault Reader* (New York: Pantheon, 1984), pp. 141–67. Even though he criticized Foucault for his rejection of bourgeois therapeutic measures, especially those of Pinel, see Gerald Weissman, "Foucault and the Bag Lady," in *The Woods Hole Cantata: Essays on Science and Society* (New York: Dodd, Mead, 1985), pp. 26–39.

34. Manuel, *Prophets of Paris,* pp. 43–45, 92–96.

35. Manuel, *Prophets of Paris;* Krishan Kumar, *Prophecy and Progress: The Sociology of Industrial and Post-industrial Society* (Harmondsworth: Penguin, 1978), pp. 21–26.

36. Kumar, *Prophecy and Progress,* chapter 1.

37. Frankel, *Faith of Reason,* p. 173.

38. Rigotti, "Biology and Society," pp. 232–33.

39. Virginia Muller offers only this side of Condorcet's legacy in her uncritical celebration of human perfectibility as the hope for a revitalized democratic liberal thought. Virginia L. Muller, *The Idea of Perfectibility* (Lanham, Md.: University Press of America, 1985).

40. Alexis de Tocqueville, *Democracy in America,* vol. 2 (New York: Vintage, 1945), pp. 34, 35, 11.

41. Reflecting the influence of Enlightenment thought in the U.S., Alexander Everett, writing in 1833 in the *North American Review* (which he owned and edited), linked American progress to the post–French Revolution concept of

progress that was identified with the Perfectibility of Man theories of Condorcet, William Godwin, Robert Owen, and Frances Wright. See Ekirch, *Idea of Progress,* pp. 254–55.

2. THE "PERFECT RACE"

1. Kenneth M. Ludmerer, *Genetics and American Society: A Historical Appraisal* (Baltimore: Johns Hopkins University Press, 1972), pp. 9–10; and Ekirch, *Idea of Progress,* pp. 35–37.

2. Tocqueville, *Democracy in America,* p. 34.

3. Erasmus Darwin, *Zonomia* (1794), quoted in Greene, *Death of Adam,* p. 168.

4. Jean-Baptiste de Lamarck, *Philosophie Zoologique* (1809), quoted in ibid., p. 161.

5. Robert Chambers, *Vestiges of the Natural History of Creation* (London: George Routledge and Sons, 1890), pp. 204–205. *Vestiges* was originally published anonymously in 1844. A new edition published in the U.S. in 1994 contains the *Vestiges* and others of Chambers's writings, plus "Explanations: A Sequel," Chambers's autobiographical preface to the 1853 edition (though he was not revealed as its author until 1884). See Robert Chambers, *Vestiges of the Natural History of Creation and Other Evolutionary Writings,* ed. James A. Secord (Chicago: University of Chicago Press, 1994); and James A. Secord, *Victorian Sensation: The Extraordinary Publication, Reception, and Secret Authorship of "Vestiges of the Natural History of Creation"* (Chicago: University of Chicago Press, 2001).

6. Chambers, *Vestiges,* pp. 227, 220.

7. John S. Haller, Jr., *Outcasts from Evolution: Scientific Attitudes of Racial Inferiority, 1859–1900* (Urbana: University of Illinois Press, 1971), pp. 73–74, viii–x, 77–78.

8. Auguste Comte, *Auguste Comte and Positivism: The Essential Writings,* ed. Gertrude Lenzer (1975; reprint: Chicago: University of Chicago Press, 1983), p. 279.

9. Herbert Spencer, *On Social Evolution: Selected Writings,* ed. J. D. Y. Peel (Chicago: University of Chicago Press, 1972), pp. 40–41. The twin assumptions that evolution progresses toward complexity and that the more complex an organism is, the better—assumptions that have lingered long into the twentieth century —are now being seriously questioned and refuted. See Stephen Jay Gould, *Full House: The Spread of Excellence from Plato to Darwin* (New York: Harmony, 1996); and Carol Kaesuk Yoon, "Biologists Deny Life Gets More Complex," *New York Times,* March 30, 1993, pp. C1, C11.

10. Spencer, *On Social Evolution,* pp. 167–74. See also John C. Greene, *Darwin and the Modern World View* (Baton Rouge: Louisiana State University Press, 1961), pp. 92–95.

11. Haller, *Outcasts from Evolution,* pp. 127, 121–38 passim.

12. In *The Descent of Man* (London: John Murray, 1871), Darwin pictured evolution as a many-branched bush. Taking up this image, Mary Midgely writes

that he "developed his own view of selection on the humbler model of a bush—a rich radiation of varying forms, in which human qualities cannot . . . determine a general direction for the whole." Mary Midgely, *Evolution as a Religion: Strange Hopes and Stranger Fears* (London: Methuen, 1985), p. 6. Both she and Greene (in *Death of Adam*) point out that Darwin specifically rejected the metaphor of an evolutionary "ladder."

13. Greene, *Death of Adam,* pp. 300, 328–29.

14. Darwin, *The Descent of Man,* as discussed in Teggart, *Idea of Progress,* pp. 448–50.

15. Greene, *Death of Adam,* p. 300.

16. See chapter seven for further discussion of Darwin's dilemma.

17. Comte, *Positivism,* pp. 193, 253–55, 75–77, 87–101.

18. Lenzer, introduction to ibid., p. lvi. Social Darwinists would later bring evolutionary theory to bear on positivist views of human nature and natural laws to create a "science of man" that could predict and control behavior. Hamilton Cravens, *The Triumph of Evolution: American Scientists and the Heredity-Environment Controversy, 1900–1941* (Baltimore: Johns Hopkins University Press, 1978), p. 7.

19. Greene, *Darwin and the Modern World View,* p. 92.

20. Herbert Spencer, *Principles of Sociology,* quoted in ibid., p. 94. Greene notes (pp. 94–95) that Spencer would later draw back from the militaristic implications of this struggle.

21. Ibid., p. 100.

22. Young argues, perhaps naively, that the study of the brain's relation to human behavior could have remained isolated from the ideological uses to which Social Darwinists or others might put it. Robert Maxwell Young, *Mind, Brain and Adaptation in the Nineteenth Century: Cerebral Localization and Its Biological Context from Gall to Ferrier* (Oxford: Clarendon, 1970).

23. Stephen Jay Gould, *The Mismeasure of Man* (New York: W. W. Norton, 1981), esp. chapter 3, "Measuring Heads: Paul Broca and the Heyday of Craniometry."

24. See esp. Gould, *Mismeasure of Man.*

25. Haller, *Outcasts from Evolution,* pp. vii–xi.

26. Cravens, *Triumph of Evolution,* pp. 37–38; and Ludmerer, *Genetics and American Society,* p. 39.

27. Ludmerer, *Genetics and American Society,* p. 13.

28. Cravens, *Triumph of Evolution,* pp. 159ff.; and Thomas Hunt Morgan, "Chromosomes and Heredity," *American Naturalist* 44, no. 524 (August 1910): 449–96 passim.

29. Francis Galton, *Hereditary Genius: An Inquiry into Its Laws and Consequences,* rev. ed. (New York: D. Appleton, 1900), pp. 339–43.

30. Daniel J. Kevles, *In the Name of Eugenics: Genetics and the Uses of Human Heredity* (Berkeley: University of California Press, 1985), chapters 1 and 2.

31. Karl Pearson, *The Groundwork of Eugenics* (London: Dulau, 1912), pp. 10, 19–20.

32. Karl Pearson, *National Life from the Standpoint of Science* (London: Black, 1901), quoted in W. Warren Wagar, ed., *The Idea of Progress since the Renaissance* (New York: John Wiley & Sons, 1969), pp. 109–12.

33. Ludmerer, *Genetics and American Society,* pp. 45–46. For a social analysis of the rise, development, and demise of the Eugenics Record Office, see Garland E. Allen, "The Eugenic Record Office at Cold Spring Harbor, 1910–1940: An Institutional History," *Osiris,* 2nd series, 2 (1986): 225–64.

34. Charles Benedict Davenport, *Heredity in Relation to Eugenics* (New York: H. Holt, 1911), pp. 241ff.

35. Sheldon C. Reed, "A Short History of Human Genetics in the USA," *American Journal of Medical Genetics* 3, no. 3 (1979): 282–95. See also Arthur Caplan, "Genetic Counseling, Medical Genetics and Theoretical Genetics: An Historical Overview," in *Genetic Counseling: Facts, Values, and Norms,* ed. Alexander Morgan Capron, Marc Lappé, Robert F. Murray, Jr., Tabitha M. Powledge, Sumner B. Twiss, and Daniel Bergsma (New York: Alan R. Liss, 1979), pp. 21–31; Victor A. McCusick, *Human Genetics,* 2nd ed. (Englewood Cliffs, N.J.: Prentice Hall, 1969); and Charles E. Rosenberg, *No Other Gods: On Science and American Social Thought* (Baltimore: Johns Hopkins University Press, 1976), pp. 96–97.

36. Davenport, *Heredity,* pp. 10–23.

37. Kevles, *In the Name of Eugenics,* chapter 3.

38. Rosenberg, *No Other Gods,* p. 95.

39. Barbara Ehrenreich and Deirdre English, *For Her Own Good: 150 Years of the Experts' Advice to Women* (Garden City, N.Y.: Anchor/Doubleday, 1979), pp. 118–19, 120–25.

40. Davenport, *Heredity,* p. 7.

41. Karl Pearson, *The Scope and Importance to the State of the Science of National Eugenics,* 3rd ed. (London: Dulau, 1911), pp. 43–44.

42. Anne Finger, "Claiming *All* of Our Bodies: Reproductive Rights and Disability," in *Test-Tube Women,* ed. Rita Arditti, Renate Duelli Klein, and Shelley Minden (London: Pandora 1984), pp. 284–85; and *Oxford English Dictionary,* 2nd ed., s.v. "defective."

43. Seymour S. Sarason and John Doris, *Psychological Problems in Mental Deficiency,* 4th ed. (New York: Harper & Row, 1969), pp. 238–43.

44. Ibid., p. 220, quoting A. F. Tredgold's "classic text," *Mental Deficiency (Amentia),* published in 1908.

45. Charles Rosenberg, "Disease and Social Order in America: Perceptions and Expectations," *Milbank Quarterly* 64, supplement 1 (1986): 44 and passim.

46. Harry H. Laughlin, *Report of the Committee to Study and to Report on the Best Practical Means of Cutting Off the Defective Germ-Plasm in the American Population. 1. The Scope of the Committee's Work,* bulletin no. 10A (Cold Spring Harbor, N.Y.: Eugenics Record Office, February 1914), p. 17.

47. *Oxford English Dictionary,* 2nd ed., s.v. "cacogenesis."

48. Pearson, *Groundwork of Eugenics,* p. 27.

49. See, for example, Robert Bogdan, *Freak Show: Presenting Human Oddities for Amusement and Profit* (Chicago: University of Chicago Press, 1988).

50. Greene, *Death of Adam,* pp. 223–24.

51. Quoted in Diane B. Paul, " 'In the Interests of Civilization': Marxist Views of Race and Culture in the Nineteenth Century," *Journal of the History of Ideas* 42, no. 1 (January–March 1981): 115–21.

52. Haller, *Outcasts from Evolution,* pp. 5, 9.

53. Galton, *Hereditary Genius,* pp. 349–50.

54. Davenport, *Heredity,* pp. 264–66.

55. Kevles, *In the Name of Eugenics,* p. 107.

56. Davenport, *Heredity,* p. 2.

57. Galton, *Hereditary Genius,* p. 346. See also chapter 8.

58. Donald MacKenzie, "Karl Pearson and the Professional Middle Class," *Annals of Science* 36, no. 2 (March 1979): 137.

59. Diane B. Paul, "Eugenics and the Left," in Diane B. Paul, *The Politics of Heredity: Essays on Eugenics, Biomedicine, and the Nature-Nurture Debate* (Albany: State University of New York Press, 1998), pp. 11–35. Biologist J. B. S. Haldane, however, believed in the genetic superiority of the upper classes. See chapter 3. Paul further observes that not all eugenicists valued intelligence to the same degree as a desirable trait for race progenitors. Some worried that eugenic policies would produce more intelligent people than society could absorb, Paul noting that this "was a major topic of debate" in the 1920s. Galton had earlier come down clearly on the side of intelligence, calling "for more brains and mental stamina than the average of our race possesses." Galton, *Hereditary Genius,* p. 345.

60. Cravens, *Triumph of Evolution,* p. 48.

61. Garland Allen's class analysis of the American eugenics movement focuses on its upper-middle-class backers who, as heirs to business fortunes, sought to promote measures of social control to preserve their own capitalist self-interests. See Allen, "Eugenic Record Office," and his earlier "Genetics, Eugenics, and Class Struggle," *Genetics* 79 (1975): S29–S45.

62. See, for example, Rosenberg, *No Other Gods,* chapter 2 (co-authored with Carroll Smith-Rosenberg). See also Cynthia Russett, *Sexual Science: The Victorian Construction of Womanhood* (Cambridge, Mass.: Harvard University Press, 1989).

63. Rosenberg, *No Other Gods,* pp. 37–38. Mounting pressures on women to hold to such regimens prefigured attempts today to prescribe and proscribe a pregnant woman's habits—as in surrogacy contracts—lest she "harm" her fetus.

64. D. Colin Wells, "Social Darwinism," *American Journal of Sociology* 12 (March 1907): 716.

65. Rosaleen Love, " 'Alice in Eugenics-Land': Feminism and Eugenics in the Scientific Careers of Alice Lee and Ethel Elderton," *Annals of Science* 36, no. 2 (March 1979): 155–56.

66. Galton, *Hereditary Genius,* pp. 324–26.

67. Ibid., p. 3.

68. Mrs. Harriman, widow of railroad magnate Edward Henry Harriman, was the first donor to the Eugenics Office and its main support in its first seven years. See Allen, "Eugenic Record Office," pp. 234–35; and Kevles, *In the Name of Eugenics,* pp. 54–56.

69. Love, " 'Alice in Eugenics-Land.' "

70. See, for example, Paul, " 'Interests of Civilization.' "

71. Philip Reilly, *The Surgical Solution: A History of Involuntary Sterilization in the U.S.* (Baltimore: Johns Hopkins University Press, 1991), p. 29. Unless otherwise noted, the following discussion of sterilization history is drawn from Reilly's book.

72. *Buck v. Bell,* 274 U.S. 200 (1927).

73. Jonas Robitscher, *The Powers of Psychiatry* (Boston: Houghton Mifflin, 1980), p. 270. See also the collection he compiled and edited, *Eugenic Sterilization* (Springfield, Ill.: Charles C. Thomas, 1973).

74. Reilly, *Surgical Solution,* pp. 94–95; and Robitscher, *Powers of Psychiatry.*

75. Rex Dunn, "Eugenic Sterilization Statutes: A Constitutional Re-evaluation," *Journal of Family Law* 14, no. 2 (1975): 289–90; and Robitscher, *Powers of Psychiatry,* p. 268.

76. European countries with sterilization laws, such as Denmark and Sweden, which had far more rigorous safeguards than did U.S. states, advanced similar reasoning, but explicitly rejected eugenics. See Allan Chase, *The Legacy of Malthus: The Social Costs of the New Scientific Racism* (New York: Alfred A. Knopf, 1977).

77. Stanley Davies, *Social Control of the Mentally Deficient* (New York: Thomas Y. Crowell, 1930), pp. 368–78 passim.

78. The Rockefeller Foundation was a major supporter of eugenic research, starting in the period before World War I and continuing through the 1920s. See Kevles, *In the Name of Eugenics,* pp. 208–209; and Allen, "Eugenic Record Office."

79. Alexis Carrel, *Man, the Unknown* (1935; reprint, New York: MacFadden, 1961), pp. 318–19.

80. Ibid., pp. 299–303.

81. Marian S. Olden, "Present Status of Sterilization in the United States," *Eugenical News* 31, no. 1 (March 1946): 3.

82. Ibid.

83. *Eugenical News* (June 1944): 34.

84. *Skinner v. Oklahoma,* 316 U.S. 535 (1942). The Court held that the Oklahoma statute providing for sterilization of certain habitual criminals violated the equal protection clause of the Fourteenth Amendment.

85. See, for example, Frederick Osborn, "The Eugenic Hypothesis: Part II: Negative Eugenics," *Eugenical News* 37, no. 1 (March 1952): 9.

86. E. Sabagh and R. B. Edgerton, "Sterilized Mental Defectives Look at Eugenic Sterilization," *Eugenics Quarterly* 9, no. 4 (December 1962): 213–22.

87. Olden, "Present Status of Sterilization," p. 13; and Lee R. Dice, "Resources of Mental Ability: How Can the Supply of Superior Ability Be Conserved and

Perhaps Increased?" *Eugenics Quarterly* 7, no. 1 (March 1960): 18. The exact figure given was 15,799. Dice, a zoologist and founder of an early heredity counseling clinic at the University of Michigan, noted that the sterilization of mentally deficient persons was "only slightly successful," even though the elimination of genes contributing to mental or physical defects was "highly desirable." But, he added, little increase in such programs could be expected in a democracy.

88. See Chase, *Legacy of Malthus;* and Robert G. Weisbord, *Genocide? Birth Control and the Black American* (Westport, Conn.: Greenwood, 1975).

89. National Conference on Race Betterment, *Proceedings of the Third Race Betterment Conference, January 2–6, 1928* (Battle Creek, Mich.: The Race Betterment Foundation, 1928), p. ii.

3. REFORMED EUGENICS AND MEDICAL GENETICS

1. Among the other signatories were J. B. S. Haldane, Lancelot Hogben, Julian Huxley, Joseph Needham, Gunnar Dahlberg, Theodosius Dobzhansky, and Conrad Hal Waddington. See Paul, "Eugenics and the Left," p. 23.

2. Ludmerer, *Genetics and American Society,* p. 133. The Manifesto was reprinted in the *Eugenics Quarterly.* Paul, "Eugenics and the Left," p. 23.

3. Writes Haldane, "ectogenesis is . . . universal." After women's ovaries are removed, they are kept alive and "growing in a suitable fluid for as long as twenty years." The ovary produces "a fresh ovum each month, of which 90 percent can be fertilized, and the embryos grown successfully for nine months, and then brought out into the air." Women are injected to lactate, thus to "conserve much of what was best in the former instinctive cycle." To compensate for the "unpleasant" ovary-removal operation and for premature aging, women receive that "chemical substance" (presumably hormones) produced by the ovaries so as to stay youthful! J. B. S. Haldane, *Daedalus, or Science and the Future* (New York: E. P. Dutton, 1924), pp. 64–74. Hormone research was underway in the 1920s; the female hormone estrone was isolated at the end of the decade. See Naomi Pfeffer, *The Stork and the Syringe* (London: Blackwell, 1994); and the obituary of Adolf Butenandt, a Nobel Prize winner for his work on hormones, *New York Times,* January 19, 1995, p. B11.

4. Hermann J. Muller, *Out of the Night: A Biologist's View of the Future* (1935; reprint, New York: Garland, 1984), p. 113.

5. Kevles, *In the Name of Eugenics,* pp. 190–91.

6. While one could argue that selected men are relegated to being sperm factories, women for Haldane are disembodied objects reduced to and valuable only for their procreative organs and as wet nurses. In the 1920s the elite women Haldane was concerned with presumably had access to the forms of contraception then available, as well as the means to obtain abortions, and therefore could exercise some degree of control over their fertility. Haldane obviously assumed that such women would be willing participants in the name of creating the new society. He does not specify how the fertility of other women—and men—is to be curbed; perhaps by voluntary sterilization?

7. The extreme of the male super-scientist, finally achieving masculine, disembodied procreation and a bodiless ideal, finds full expression in physicist J. D. Bernal's *The World, the Flesh and the Devil: An Inquiry into the Future of the Three Enemies of the Rational Soul* (1929; reprint, London: Jonathan Cape, 1970). See discussion in Brian Easlea, *Fathering the Unthinkable: Masculinity, Scientists and the Nuclear Arms Race* (London: Pluto, 1983), pp. 150–55.

8. Critics did not necessarily reject negative eugenics out of hand. Rather, they maintained that sterilization was not effective to curb the spread of defective traits. Haldane, who opposed compulsory measures in the U.S., used this rationale to argue against a proposed law to permit voluntary sterilization in Britain in the 1930s. Only those conditions caused by dominant genes, not those due to recessives or mutations, would be prevented. Nor would sterilization prevent the many conditions that are not inherited. Further (along with other geneticists on the left), Haldane argued sterilization would be an unwarranted restriction on liberty and could result in class discrimination. For mental defectives, he favored more "humane" measures such as sexual segregation (though he does not say how this would be accomplished without compulsion), discouraging inbreeding, and providing simple jobs. Noting that advocates of harsher measures may be motivated by hatred or horror of defectives, Haldane wrote, "I must confess to a certain liking for them." He quoted Sutherland, who worked with them: " 'The smiling face of the Mongolian imbecile suggests the possession of a secret source of joy.' " J. B. S. Haldane, *Heredity and Politics* (New York: W. W. Norton, 1938), p. 92.

9. I will use "evolutionary biologists" and "evolutionary scientists" as inclusive terms for those scientists in the middle third of the century—roughly 1930s–1960s—whose work in the life sciences related to evolutionary theory. They are distinguished from "research geneticists," whose work more directly concerned medical applications.

10. A few, such as geneticist Theodosius Dobzhansky and zoologist Ernst Mayr, continued their writings into the next few decades.

11. Sol Tax and Charles Callender, eds., *Issues in Evolution*, vol. 3 of *Evolution after Darwin: The University of Chicago Centennial*, ed. Sol Tax (Chicago: University of Chicago Press, 1960), pp. 278ff. Almost all participants were male. The two females were a representative from the USSR Academy of Medical Sciences, who was then at the University of Chicago, and a research scientist from Australia.

12. This is not to suggest that all evolutionary scientists—even those extremely sympathetic to the eugenics movement—had completely dismissed environmental influences on heredity and species change and adaptation. Some early on had cautioned against ignoring the role of the environment. In 1925 zoologist Herbert Jennings argued that environmental factors, as well as genetics, were critical to producing "superior" or "inferior" children. Herbert S. Jennings, *Prometheus, or Biology and the Advancement of Man* (New York: E. P. Dutton, 1925).

13. Julian Huxley, "The Evolutionary Vision," in Tax and Callender, *Issues in Evolution*, pp. 249–61.

14. Cravens, *Triumph of Evolution.*

15. Julian Huxley, *Evolution: The Modern Synthesis* (New York: Harper & Brothers, 1942; 3rd ed., New York: Hafner, 1974).

16. For example, Dobzhansky, Mayr, and anthropologist Gaylord Simpson argued that biological and cultural evolution still interacted and had to continue to do so to ensure evolutionary change and human improvement. See Theodosius Dobzhansky, *Mankind Evolving* (New Haven: Yale University Press, 1962), pp. 319ff., 18–20; Ernst Mayr, "Comments on Genetic Evolution," in *Evolution and Man's Progress,* ed. Hudson Hoagland and Ralph W. Burhoe (New York: Columbia University Press, 1962), pp. 50–51; and George Gaylord Simpson, *The Meaning of Evolution: A Study of the History of Life and of Its Significance for Man* (1949; rev. ed., New Haven: Yale University Press, 1967), pp. 59–60.

17. Huxley, "Evolutionary Vision," p. 250.

18. Huxley, *Modern Synthesis,* p. 578.

19. Simpson, *Meaning of Evolution,* pp. 259–63.

20. Dobzhansky, *Mankind Evolving,* pp. 345–48.

21. Theodosius Dobzhansky, *Heredity and the Nature of Man* (New York: Harcourt, Brace & World, 1964), p. 138.

22. Although the Modern Synthesis might have suggested that environment contributed to producing intelligence, Huxley in his Galton lecture in 1962 held "that the human I.Q. . . . is largely a measure of genetic endowment." In a nod to Galton, he stated that advances in human affairs come through the highly gifted and true geniuses. Julian Huxley, *Essays of a Humanist* (New York: Harper & Row, 1964), pp. 254–55. H. J. Muller, noting that intelligence is caused by multiple genetic factors, its inheritance therefore highly variable, still named "outstanding mental ability" as the main criterion for his "superior sperm donors." Hermann J. Muller, "The Guidance of Human Evolution," in *The Evolution of Man,* vol. 2 of *Evolution after Darwin: The University of Chicago Centennial,* ed. Sol Tax (Chicago: University of Chicago Press, 1960), pp. 450–51. J. B. S. Haldane, however, had much earlier criticized the view that intelligence was largely inherited. Haldane, *Heredity and Politics,* pp. 121–37 passim.

23. Huxley, *Modern Synthesis,* pp. 570–71.

24. Simpson, *Meaning of Evolution,* pp. 266, 299.

25. Robert Hutchins, president of the University of Chicago, promoted the "Great Books" curriculum in his fifty-four-volume *Great Books of the Western World* (1954).

26. Huxley, *Modern Synthesis,* p. 562.

27. Ibid., p. 572.

28. Huxley, *Essays of a Humanist,* p. 263. Choosing from the "enormous range of variation," stated Huxley at the Centennial, we "should give most attention to improving our genetic heritage." Huxley, "Evolutionary Vision," pp. 242–43.

29. Dobzhansky, *Mankind Evolving,* pp. 330ff.

30. Muller, "Guidance of Human Evolution," p. 433.

31. Ibid., pp. 424−25, 433; Huxley, "Evolutionary Vision," pp. 242−43; and Huxley, *Essays of a Humanist,* p. 266.

32. Huxley, *Essays of a Humanist,* pp. 51−52.

33. Muller, "Guidance of Human Evolution," pp. 430−33. Muller was criticized by some of his colleagues for fastening on an ideal and for where his scheme of super-intelligent donors might lead. Unless this perfect specimen had a "perfect set of genes," noted behavioral scientist J. Paul Scott, his injurious genes, if not countered by his "good genes," would spread through the population. J. Paul Scott, "Comments . . . ," in Hoagland and Burhoe, *Evolution and Man's Progress,* p. 48. Dobzhansky, owning that "mankind would profit immeasurably from the birth of more persons with the mental stamina of Einstein, Pasteur, and even Lenin," went on to ask, "do we really want to live in a world with millions of Einsteins, Pasteurs, and Lenins?" He criticized Muller's "implied assumption that there is, or can be, *the* ideal genotype . . . to bestow upon everybody" as "not only unappealing but almost certainly wrong—it is human diversity" that is a "leaven of creative effort." Dobzhansky, *Mankind Evolving,* p. 330. Robert Morison, director of medical and natural sciences at the Rockefeller Foundation, had commented that it may be "much easier to agree on minimizing the 'bad' than on maximizing the 'good.' " He warned against looking for one "best," opting rather for the Greek golden mean. Robert S. Morison, "Comments . . . ," in Hoagland and Burhoe, *Evolution and Man's Progress,* pp. 42−43.

34. Diane Paul points out the tension in Muller between positive and negative eugenics. While he sought a radical improvement in intellect and character, he also worried about the deleterious effects of mutant genes. Diane B. Paul, " 'Our Load of Mutations' Revisited," *Journal of the History of Biology* 20, no. 3 (Fall 1987): 321−35. See also H. J. Muller, "Our Load of Mutations," *American Journal of Human Genetics* 2 (1950): 111−76.

35. Huxley, *Essays of a Humanist,* pp. 268−71.

36. Dobzhansky, *Mankind Evolving,* p. 333.

37. James F. Crow, "Mechanisms and Trends in Human Evolution," in Hoagland and Burhoe, *Evolution and Man's Progress,* pp. 16−17.

38. Dobzhansky, *Mankind Evolving,* pp. 14−15.

39. Muller, "Guidance of Human Evolution," pp. 434−35.

40. Reed, "Short History of Human Genetics," p. 287; Ludmerer, *Genetics and American Society.*

41. The American Society of Human Genetics and its journal, the *American Journal of Human Genetics,* were co-founded by Herluf Strandskov, H. J. Muller, Laurence H. Snyder, and C. W. Cotterman in 1949. See Caplan, "Genetic Counseling," pp. 21−22.

42. Ludmerer, *Genetics and American Society,* p. 71.

43. Madge Thurlow Macklin, "The Need of a Course in Medical Genetics in the Medical Curriculum: A Pivotal Point in the Eugenic Program," in *A Decade of Progress in Eugenics: Scientific Papers of the Third International Congress of Eu-*

genics, American Museum of Natural History, New York, August 21–23, 1932 (Baltimore: Williams and Wilkins, 1934), pp. 157–58. See also M. T. Macklin, "Medical Genetics: An Essential Part of the Medical Curriculum from the Standpoint of Prevention," *Journal of the Association of American Medical Colleges* 8 (1933): 291–301.

44. Haven Emerson, "Eugenics in Relation to Medicine," *Eugenical News* 24, no. 4 (December 1939): 67–70. Dr. Emerson was a former New York City commissioner of health. See the obituary of his daughter, Dr. Ethel Emerson Wortis, *New York Times,* July 12, 1995, p. B7.

45. Morton D. Schweitzer, "What Can the Physician Make of Medical Genetics?" *Eugenical News* 6, no. 2 (May 1941): 34–35.

46. Ludmerer, *Genetics and American Society,* pp. 63–73.

47. Ibid., pp. 184, 168–69.

48. Ibid., pp. 185–88.

49. Reed, "Short History of Human Genetics," p. 288.

50. H. Warner Kloepfer, "Genetic Signposts of Preventive Medicine," *Eugenics Quarterly* 7, no. 2 (June 1960): 72.

51. In the journal's initial issue, editor in chief John M. Opitz noted that he had unsuccessfully proposed such a journal to a publishing house 12 years earlier. In the "lively title debate" at the founding of the *American Journal of Human Genetics* in 1949, the term "medical" rather than "human" genetics was "turned down emphatically." J. M. Opitz, "The American Journal of Medical Genetics—Forward," *American Journal of Medical Genetics* 1, no. 1 (1977): 1–2.

52. Ludmerer, *Genetics and American Society,* pp. 187–88.

53. Regina H. Kenen, "Genetic Counseling: The Development of a New Interdisciplinary Occupational Field," *Social Science and Medicine* 18, no. 7 (1984): 543.

54. Ludmerer, *Genetics and American Society,* pp. 187–88.

55. Lee R. Dice, "Heredity Clinics, Their Value for Public Service and for Research," *American Journal of Human Genetics* 4, no. 1 (1952): 1–13.

56. The second edition, in 1960, of Curt Stern's widely used text, *Principles of Human Genetics,* used the terms "eugenic counseling" and "genetic counseling" interchangeably (San Francisco: W. H. Freeman, 1960). See Ludmerer, *Genetics and American Society,* pp. 178–79, 187–88. Chapter 29, "Selection in Civilization," and chapter 30, "Aspects of Medical Genetics," of Stern's text carried clear eugenic messages. (In 1949, *Science,* the journal of the American Association for the Advancement of Science, had published a condensed version of the first edition's "Selection and Eugenics" chapter: "Selection and Eugenics," *Science* 110 [August 26, 1949]: 201–208.)

57. Frederick Osborn, "The Eugenic Hypothesis: Part I: Positive Eugenics," *Eugenical News* 36, no. 2 (June 1951): 19–21; and Osborn, "Part II: Negative Eugenics."

58. *Eugenics Quarterly* 5, no. 1 (March 1958), inside front cover.

59. O. J. Miller, H. L. Cooper, and Kurt Hirschhorn, "Recent Developments in Human Cytogenetics," *Eugenics Quarterly* 8, no. 1 (March 1961): 23–33.

60. Dobzhansky's chairmanship of the board of the American Eugenics Society in 1969 coincided with the change of the journal's name from *Eugenics Quarterly* to *Social Biology*. In 1971, geneticists Victor McCusick and James Crow joined the board. Two years later, the American Eugenics Society became the Society for the Study of Social Biology, making the transition complete. Page 1 of the journal's first issue published under the auspice of the newly named society explained the change this way, under the heading "A New Name: Society for the Study of Social Biology (formerly The American Eugenics Society)":

> Four years ago the name of this journal was changed because the word eugenics had a meaning too narrow to characterize the contexts of the journal. The American Eugenics Society, as sponsor of the journal, elected at that time to retain its old name for historical reasons and because eugenics remained the ultimate focus of interest.
>
> As proximate goals became more diverse and more clearly perceived, dissatisfaction with the old name increased. . . . The final choice, *Society for the Study of Social Biology*, was prompted mainly by the new name of the journal. . . .
>
> The change of name of the Society does not coincide with any change of its interests or policies. Such a change was marked rather by the founding of this journal twenty years ago [meaning the *Eugenics Quarterly*]. The common interests that have long united the membership, and to which their scientific disciplines are relevant, are the trends of human evolution and the biological, medical, and social forces that determine these trends. (*Social Biology* 20, no. 1 [March 1973]: 1)

61. "Editorial Comment," *Eugenics Quarterly* 1, no. 1 (March 1954): 1. This was the first issue of the association's renamed and transformed journal, the former *Eugenical News*.

62. C. Nash Herndon, "III. Heredity Counseling," *Eugenics Quarterly* 2, no. 2 (June 1955): 88–89.

63. Frederick Osborn, *Preface to Eugenics*, rev. ed. (New York: Harper & Brothers, 1951).

64. Frederick Osborn, in "Proceedings of the Heredity Counseling Symposium Held at the New York Academy of Medicine Building. Nov. 1, 1957: Sponsored by the American Eugenics Society," *Eugenics Quarterly* 5, no. 1 (March 1958): p. 62. The proceedings were subsequently published as a book: Helen G. Hammons, ed., *Heredity Counseling* (New York: Paul B. Hoeber, 1959).

65. Kenen, "Genetic Counseling," p. 543.

66. In this connection, see Diane Paul, "From Reproductive Responsibility to Reproductive Autonomy," in *Mutating Concepts, Evolving Disciplines: Genetics, Medicine, and Society*, ed. Lisa S. Parker and Rachel A. Ankeny (Boston: Kluwer Academic Publishers, 2002), pp. 87–105. Paul points out how the discourse changed from reproduction as a social responsibility—and thus the view of eugenicists that it could be restricted—to one of reproductive autonomy, that pro-

creation was a private matter to be freely exercised. Yet she notes that while the rhetoric changed so as to reject eugenics, an underlying agreement remained that one should not bring a defective child into the world. See further discussion of reproductive autonomy in this volume, especially chapters 5, 6, and 10.

67. Although the overt misogyny of an earlier day, which openly upbraided educated women for not having babies and for thus failing to promote the eugenic cause, had become unfashionable, women continued to be either ignored or objectified. Whether it was Muller considering only the sperm of great men to create his race of mental giants or the disembodied proposals of J. B. S. Haldane for artificial selection, perfectibility discourse remained quintessentially male and masculine. This mindset would not change appreciably in the perfectibility discourse of reproductive medicine.

68. Dobzhansky, for example, did not hesitate to discuss genetic fitness and to relate genetic fitness to social fitness. Dobzhansky, *Mankind Evolving*, pp. 333–35.

69. Muller, *Out of the Night*, p. 108. Muller says that these techniques have succeeded with "the rodent." (Such transplanting has, of course, since occurred among humans.) Like Haldane, he wanted to gestate fetuses in an alternative womb so as to "reach that ideal condition of complete ectogenesis" and thus greatly enhance the "degree of control over our choice" of the kinds of children produced (p. 110).

70. Dobzhansky, *Mankind Evolving*, pp. 332–33.

4. THE TOOLS

1. See "Genome's Riddle: Few Genes, Much Complexity," Science Times, *New York Times*, February 13, 2001, pp. F1, F4, F5.

2. Nicholas Wade, "Gene Sweepstakes Ends, but Winner May Well Be Wrong," *New York Times*, June 3, 2003, pp. F1, F2. The scientists, meeting in Cold Spring Harbor, agreed to extend their sweepstakes for another five years, with bets remaining at $20.

3. *Genome:* literally, gene + chromosome; a complete set of chromosomes containing all the genes of an organism, that is, the organism's total genetic material.

4. James D. Watson and Francis Crick, "Molecular Structure of Nucleic Acids: Structure for Deoxyribose Nucleic Acid," *Nature* 171 (25 April 1953): 737–38. The fiftieth anniversary of the discovery of the double helix in 2003 prompted a special section of the *New York Times*'s Science Times: "A Revolution at 50: DNA Changed the World. Now What?" (February 25, 2003, sec. F), and the publication of several books, among them James D. Watson with Andrew Berry, *DNA: The Secret of Life* (New York: Alfred A. Knopf, 2003); and Victor K. McElheny, *Watson and DNA: Making a Scientific Revolution* (Cambridge, Mass.: Perseus, 2003). See also Jerry A. Coyne, "Doing Acid," review of *DNA: The Secret of Life* and *Watson and DNA*, *New York Times Book Review*, June 15, 2003, pp. 11–12.

5. A draft sequence and initial analysis was published in February 2001. National Human Genome Research Institute, National Institutes of Health, "In-

ternational Human Sequencing Consortium Publishes Sequence and Analysis of the Human Genome" (Washington, D.C.: National Human Genome Research Institute, National Institutes of Health, February 12, 2001). See also articles in *Nature*, February 15, 2001; *Science*, February 16, 2001. On the 2003 announcement, see E. Pennisi, "Human Genome. Reaching Their Goal Early, Sequencing Labs Celebrate," *Science* 300, no. 5618 (April 18, 2003): 409; and Nicholas Wade, "Once Again, Scientists Say Human Genome Is Complete," *New York Times*, April 15, 2003, pp. F1, F4. Genome research was originally a publicly funded enterprise, conducted by the international Human Genome Organization (HUGO), conceived in the late 1980s, and the U.S. Human Genome Project (HGP), officially launched in 1990. Private companies took up the effort to sequence the genome in the mid- and late 1990s, and the ensuing competition was partly responsible for the sequencing's being finished at least two years ahead of schedule.

6. Cecie Starr and Ralph Taggart, *Biology: The Unity and Diversity of Life*, 4th ed. (Belmont, Calif.: Wadsworth, 1987), p. 178.

7. Ibid., pp. 213–15.

8. Jeffrey R. Sawyer, Mark Paul Johnson, and Orlando J. Miller, "Traditional and Molecular Cytogenetics," *Journal of Reproductive Medicine* 37, no. 6 (June 1992): 485–98.

9. "In this Review Issue of *Prenatal Diagnosis* we celebrate the pre-eminence of DNA analysis in the differential diagnosis of many types of serious fetal abnormality *in utero*." M. A. Ferguson-Smith, "DNA for Diagnosis," editorial introduction, *Prenatal Diagnosis* 16, no. 13 (December 1996): 1175.

10. Detection and treatment of PKU, for example, have a long history: see chapter three.

11. See list in Mark I. Evans, Mary Helen Quigg, Frederick C. Koppitch III, and Joseph D. Schulman, "Prenatal Diagnosis of Chromosomal and Mendelian Disorders," in *Fetal Diagnosis and Therapy: Science, Ethics and the Law*, ed. Mark I. Evans, John C. Fletcher, Alan O. Dixler, and Joseph D. Schulman (Philadelphia: J. B. Lippincott, 1989), pp. 21–27.

12. This discussion has been drawn from the following accounts: Theodore Friedmann, "The Human Genome Project—Some Implications of Extensive 'Reverse Genetic' Medicine," *American Journal of Human Genetics* 46, no. 3 (March 1990): 407–14; H. Galjaard, "Fetal Diagnosis of Inborn Errors of Metabolism," in *Fetal Diagnosis of Genetic Defects*, ed. Charles H. Rodeck (London: Baillière Tindall, 1987), 547–67; and Marcus E. Pembrey, "Impact of Molecular Biology on Clinical Genetics," *British Medical Journal* 295, no. 6600 (September 19, 1987): 711–13.

13. Anne Maddalena, David P. Bick, and Joseph D. Schulman, "Molecular Diagnosis of Genetic Disease," *Journal of Reproductive Medicine* 37, no. 5 (May 1992): 439. See also R. K. Saiki, "Primer-Directed Enzymatic Amplification of DNA with a Thermostable DNA Polymerase," *Science* 239, no. 4839 (January 29, 1988): 487–91. For an early description of the discovery of the procedure, see R. K. Saiki, S. Scharf, F. Faloona, K. B. Mallis, J. T. Horm, H. S. Erlich, and N. Arnheim,

"Enzymatic Amplification of Beta-globin Genomic Sequences and Restriction Site Analysis for Diagnosis of Sickle Cell Anemia," *Science* 230, no. 4732 (December 20, 1985): 1350–54.

14. See description in Ferguson-Smith, "DNA for Diagnosis," p. 1176.

15. Ibid., p. 1175.

16. Povl Riis and Fritz Fuchs, "Antenatal Determination of Foetal Sex in Prevention of Hereditary Disease," *Lancet* 276, no. 7143 (July 23, 1960): 180–82; Fritz Fuchs and Povl Riis, "Antenatal Sex Determination," *Nature* 177, no. 403 (February 18, 1956); E. L. Makowski, K. A. Prem, and I. H. Kaiser, "Detection of Sex of Fetuses by the Incidence of Sex Chromatin Body in Nuclei of Cells in Amniotic Fluid," *Science* 123, no. 3196 (March 30, 1956): 542–43; C. J. Dewhurst, "Diagnosis of Sex before Birth," *Lancet* 270, no. 6921 (April 21, 1956): 471–72; Landrum B. Shettles, "Nuclear Morphology of Cells in Human Amniotic Fluid in Relation to Sex of Infant," *American Journal of Obstetrics and Gynecology* 71, no. 4 (April 1956): 834–38; and Eduardo Keymer, Edna Silva-Inzunza, and Waldeman E. Coutts, "Contribution to the Antenatal Determination of Sex," *American Journal of Obstetrics and Gynecology* 74, no. 5 (November 1957): 1098–1101.

17. Riis and Fuchs, "Antenatal Determination of Foetal Sex." In Denmark, a legal abortion could be obtained in such cases on "eugenic grounds" (p. 181).

18. Dr. Fuchs died in February 1995. Although born and trained in Denmark, he was associated with Cornell University Medical College in New York from the mid-1960s on, where he established the New York–Cornell amniocentesis laboratory. See his obituary in the *New York Times*, March 4, 1995, p. 26.

19. Riis and Fuchs, "Antenatal Determination of Foetal Sex," 182. During this very early phase the emphasis was on severe or fatal disorders. Most could not be treated, and if the fetus was at risk, the pregnancy was terminated. But in some cases, such as RH blood incompatibility and a postnatally treatable enzyme deficiency, the diagnosis could prevent fetal death or severe disabilities. John T. Queenan, "Amniocentesis and Transamniotic Fetal Transfusion for RH Disease," *Clinical Obstetrics and Gynecology* 9, no. 2 (June 1966): 491–507; T. N. A. Jeffcoate, J. C. Davis, A. P. Wade, J. R. H. Fliegner, and Shona H. Russell, "Diagnosis of the Adrenogenital Syndrome before Birth," *Lancet* 286, no. 7412 (September 18, 1965): 553–55; and Henry L. Nadler, "Antenatal Detection of Hereditary Disorders," *Pediatrics* 42, no. 6 (December 1968): 912–18.

20. Anthony Johnson and Lynn Godmilow, "Genetic Amniocentesis at 14 Weeks or Less," *Clinical Obstetrics and Gynecology* 31, no. 2 (June 1988): 345.

21. Cecil B. Jacobson and Robert H. Barter, "Intrauterine Diagnosis and Management of Genetic Defects," *American Journal of Obstetrics and Gynecology* 99, no. 6 (November 15, 1967): 796–807.

22. Nadler, "Antenatal Detection," pp. 916–17. Perhaps because of the rate of fetal loss and the pregnancy difficulties that occurred when the procedure was done at the end of the first trimester, Dr. Fuchs held that later amniocentesis was safer for both mother and fetus. Fritz Fuchs, "Symposium on Amnio Fluid: Foreword," *Clinical Obstetrics and Gynecology* 9, no. 2 (June 1966): 425–26.

23. Mark I. Evans and Mark Paul Johnson, "Prenatal Diagnosis in the '90s: A Symposium," *Journal of Reproductive Medicine* 37, no. 5 (May 1992): 387–88; George P. Henry and Wayne A. Miller, "Early Amniocentesis," *Journal of Reproductive Medicine* 37, no. 5 (May 1992): 396–402; and R. Douglas Wilson, "Early Amniocentesis: A Clinical Review," *Prenatal Diagnosis* 15, no. 13 (December 1995): 1259–73.

24. Miguel Diaz Vega, P. De La Cueva, C. Leal, and F. Aisa, "Early Amniocentesis at 10–12 Weeks' Gestation," *Prenatal Diagnosis* 16, no. 4 (April 1996): 307.

25. Jacobson and Barter, "Intrauterine Diagnosis and Management," p. 797; and Nadler, "Antenatal Detection."

26. National Down Syndrome Society, "Down Syndrome Fact Sheet," http://www.ndss.org/content.cfm?fuseaction=NwsEvt.PressDSFS, accessed September 20, 2004.

27. The syndrome is named after a British physician, John Langdon Haydon Down, who first systematically described the condition in 1866. He labeled those affected throwbacks to Asian Mongols, whom he thought represented an earlier human type: hence the persisting use of the terms "mongolism" and "mongolian idiot" or "imbecile." Kevles, *In the Name of Eugenics,* p. 160.

28. James E. Haddow and Glenn E. Palomaki, "Prenatal Screening for Down Syndrome," in *Essentials of Prenatal Diagnosis,* ed. Joe Leigh Simpson and Sherman Elias (New York: Churchill Livingstone, 1993), p. 188.

29. Some have argued for correlation with paternal age, too. In 1980 Laurence Karp noted mounting evidence that genetic mutations are related to paternal as well as maternal age. Laurence E. Karp, "Older Fathers and Genetic Mutations," *American Journal of Medical Genetics* 7, no. 4 (1980): 405–406. However, in 1991 a team of two dozen scientists from several countries, including the U.S., reported research that showed that the extra chromosome causing Down syndrome comes from the mother's egg about 95 percent of the time. Further, the error occurs when the egg is formed, before the woman is even born. Gina Kolata, "Cell Error Pinpointed in Down Syndrome," *New York Times,* May 28, 1991, p. C3. See also L. Wilkins-Haug, "The Emerging Genetic Theories of Unstable DNA, Uniparental Disomy, and Imprinting," *Clinical Obstetrics and Gynecology* 5, no. 2 (April 1993): 179–85.

30. Evans, Quigg, et al., "Prenatal Diagnosis," p. 19. See also Haddow and Palomaki, "Prenatal Screening," p. 189; the age incidence figures here vary slightly but tell the same story.

31. Joe Leigh Simpson, "Pregnancies in Women with Chromosomal Abnormalities," in *Genetic Diseases in Pregnancy: Maternal Effects and Fetal Outcome,* ed. Joseph D. Schulman and Joe Leigh Simpson (New York: Academic Press, 1981), pp. 448–49.

32. Mark I. Evans, Mark Paul Johnson, and Wolfgang Holzgreve, "Chorionic Villus Sampling," *Journal of Reproductive Medicine* 37, no. 5 (May 1992): 390.

33. Haddow and Palomaki, "Prenatal Screening," 187. In a table listing indications for amniocentesis and the risk of genetic disorders, published in 1997,

the highest risk, 25–50 percent, is present when parents carry Mendelian traits. The next highest, 25–30 percent, is present when major fetal malformations have been diagnosed by ultrasound. Certain kinds of translocations in the parents' chromosomes bring a risk of 12–15 percent; and other indictors bear risks from 6 down to 1 percent. At the bottom of the list is advanced maternal age, with less than 0.5 percent risk. Arie Drugan, Mark P. Johnson, Roderick F. Hume, Jr., and Mark I. Evans, "Amniocentesis," in *Invasive Outpatient Procedures in Reproductive Medicine,* ed. Mark I. Evans, Mark P. Johnson, and Kamran S. Moghissi (Philadelphia: Lippincott-Raven, 1997), p. 4.

34. Mark I. Evans, Robin L. Belsky, Anne Greb, Nancy Clementino, and Frank N. Syner, "Alpha-Fetoprotein: Maternal Serum and Amniotic Fluid Analysis," in Evans, Fletcher, et al., *Fetal Diagnosis and Therapy,* pp. 44–45.

35. Arie Drugan, Joseph E. O'Brien, Raymond S. Gambino, and Mark I. Evans, "Prenatal Biochemical Screening," *Journal of Reproductive Medicine* 37, no. 5 (May 1992): 403.

36. Most of my description of MSAFP is drawn from ibid., 403–409, and Evans, Belsky, et al., "Alpha-Fetoprotein."

37. A 1987 editorial in *Obstetrics and Gynecology* recommended that MSAFP screening for NTDs be made available to pregnant women at centers where follow-up procedures were available. Joe Leigh Simpson and Henry Nadler, "Maternal Serum Alpha-Fetoprotein Screening in 1987," *Obstetrics and Gynecology* 69, no. 1 (January 1987): 134–35. Drugan et al., "Prenatal Biochemical Screening," stated that "(MSAFP) screening should be offered to *all* pregnant women" (p. 404, emphasis in original). See discussion in chapter 5.

38. Evans, Belsky, et al., "Alpha-Fetoprotein," p. 44; and Devereux N. Saller, Jr., and Jacob A. Canick, "Maternal Serum Screening for Fetal Down Syndrome: The Detection of Other Pathologies," *Clinical Obstetrics and Gynecology* 39, no. 4 (December 1996): 793–800.

39. Devereux N. Saller, Jr., and Jacob A. Canick, "Maternal Serum Screening for Fetal Down Syndrome: Clinical Aspects," *Clinical Obstetrics and Gynecology* 39, no. 4 (December 1996): 783–92. In 1995 researchers were considering extending serum screening for Down syndrome to the first trimester, at 10 weeks. N. J. Wald, A. Kennard, and A. K. Hackshaw, "First Trimester Serum Screening for Down's Syndrome," *Prenatal Diagnosis* 15, no. 13 (December 1995): 1227–40.

40. The sample protocol shows that in every thousand pregnancies tested, there would be one case of anencephaly, one or two neural tube defects, and one chromosome abnormality. Evans, Belsky, et al., "Alpha-Fetoprotein," p. 51. Figures are similar in a protocol described by Roger A. Williamson, "Abnormalities of Alpha-Fetoprotein and Other Biochemical Tests," in *High Risk Pregnancy: Management Options,* ed. D. K. James, P. J. Steen, C. P. Weiner, and B. Gonik (London: W. B. Saunders, 1994), pp. 645–46. See further discussion in chapter 6.

41. I thank Barbara Katz Rothman for helping me to view "risk" from this perspective, in a conversation in July 1990.

42. Ann Oakley, *The Captured Womb* (Oxford: Basil Blackwell, 1984), pp.

155–86; and Rosalind Pollack Petchesky, "Foetal Images: The Power of Visual Culture in the Politics of Reproduction," in *Reproductive Technologies: Gender, Motherhood and Medicine,* ed. Michelle Stanworth (Minneapolis: University of Minnesota Press, 1987), pp. 65–66.

43. Frank A. Chervenak and Glenn Isaacson, "Ultrasound Detection of Fetal Anomalies," in Evans, Fletcher, et al., "Fetal Diagnosis and Therapy," p. 60. See also discussion in Dru E. Carlson and Lawrence D. Platt, "Ultrasound Detection of Genetic Anomalies," *Journal of Reproductive Medicine* 37, no. 5 (May 1992): 419–27.

44. See further discussion in chapter 5.

45. John W. Seeds, "The Routine or Screening Obstetrical Ultrasound Examination," *Clinical Obstetrics and Gynecology* 39, no. 4 (December 1996): 829.

46. Richard W. Wertz and Dorothy C. Wertz, *Lying-In: A History of Childbirth in America,* expanded ed. (New Haven: Yale University Press, 1989), p. 246. See also discussion in Lyn S. Chitty, "Ultrasound Screening for Fetal Abnormalities," *Prenatal Diagnosis* 15, no. 13 (December 1995): 1251–52.

47. See, for example, Caroline Whitbeck, "Fetal Imaging and Fetal Monitoring: Finding the Ethical Issues," in *Embryos, Ethics, and Women's Rights: Exploring the New Reproductive Technologies,* ed. Elaine Hoffman Baruch, Amadeo F. D'Adamo, Jr., and Joni Seager (New York: Harrington Park, 1988), pp. 47–57.

48. Chitty, "Ultrasound Screening"; and Seeds, "Obstetrical Ultrasound Examination." See further discussion in chapters 5 and 9, especially relating to the RADIUS study (Routine Antenatal Diagnostic Imaging Ultrasound Study), published in 1993.

49. Yves Dumez, Jean-Francois Oury, and Marc Dommergues, "Embryoscopy," in Evans, Johnson, and Moghissi, *Invasive Outpatient Procedures,* p. 51. The use of military language, such as the word *armamentarium,* is not uncommon. See the discussion of CVS and further use in chapter 5.

50. Ronald J. Wapner and Laird Jackson, "Chorionic Villus Sampling," *Clinical Obstetrics and Gynecology* 31, no. 2 (June 1988): 329. Although Wapner and Jackson do not specify, given the bias toward males in Chinese society we can assume that most, perhaps all, of the aborted fetuses were female. My discussion of CVS is drawn from their article; R. H. T. Ward, "Techniques of Chorionic Villus Sampling," in Rodeck, *Fetal Diagnosis,* 489–511; and Evans, Quigg, et al., "Prenatal Diagnosis."

51. Wapner and Jackson, "Chorionic Villus Sampling," p. 329.

52. Interviews with medical personnel, both pro and con, in the Boston area, June 1990.

53. Evans, Quigg, et al., "Prenatal Diagnosis," p. 30.

54. Stephen Abbs, "Prenatal Diagnosis of Duchenne and Becker Muscular Dystrophy," *Prenatal Diagnosis* 16, no. 13 (December 1996): 1187. It is associated with progressive muscle weakness at about age three, eventual loss of the ability to walk, and death usually by age 20.

55. John Old, "Haemoglobinopathies," *Prenatal Diagnosis* 16, no. 13 (December 1996): 1181–86.

56. Males are more vulnerable to fragile X syndrome because they have only one X chromosome; if only one of a female's two X chromosomes carries the defective gene, she will not develop the syndrome. Brenda Finucane, "Should All Pregnant Women Be Offered Carrier Testing for Fragile X Syndrome?" *Clinical Obstetrics and Gynecology* 39, no. 4 (December 1996): 772–82. See the references to Finucane's article for further discussion of fragile X.

57. Teresa Doksum and Barbara A. Bernhardt, "Population-Based Carrier Screening for Cystic Fibrosis," *Clinical Obstetrics and Gynecology* 39, no. 4 (December 1996): 763–71. The gene mutation causing up to 70 percent of the cases of cystic fibrosis was discovered in 1989. In CF a heavy mucus interferes with the functioning of the lungs, the pancreas, and the sweat glands, as well as other organs.

58. Ian Findlay, Glenn Atkinson, Michaela Chambers, Philip Quirke, James Campbell, and Anthony Rutherford, "Rapid Genetic Diagnosis at 7–9 Weeks Gestation: Diagnosis of Sex, Single Gene Defects and DNA Fingerprint from Coelomic Samples," *Human Reproduction* 11, no. 11 (1996): 2448–53.

59. See, for example, Finucane, "Should All Pregnant Women," and Doksum and Bernhardt, "Population-Based Carrier Screening," for discussions of carrier screening.

60. These focused particularly on limb abnormalities. See discussion of the safety of CVS in chapter 5.

61. C. Danae Steele, Ronald J. Wapner, J. Bruce Smith, Mark K. Hanes, and Laird G. Jackson, "Prenatal Diagnosis Using Fetal Cells Isolated from Maternal Peripheral Blood: A Review," *Clinical Obstetrics and Gynecology* 39, no. 4 (December 1996): 801.

62. Ibid., p. 811.

63. S. S. Wachtell, L. P. Shulman, and D. Sammons, "Fetal Cells in Maternal Blood," *Clinical Genetics* 59, no. 2 (February 2001): 74–79.

64. M. Rodriguez de Alba, P. Palomino, C. Gonzalez-Gonzalez, I. Lorda-Sanchez, M. A. Ibanez, R. Sanz, J. M. Fernandez-Moya, C. Ayuso, J. Diaz-Recasens, and C. Ramos, "Prenatal Diagnosis on Fetal Cells from Maternal Blood: Practical Comparative Evaluation of the First and Second Trimesters," *Prenatal Diagnosis* 21, no. 3 (March 2001): 165 (abstract).

65. The British effort resulted first in the Warnock Report in 1984, which established definitions and guidelines for embryo research, and subsequently, as the tenor of the debates changed further, in passage of the Human Fertilization and Embryology Act of 1990, which clarified the boundaries and social mechanisms to maintain them. See Michael Mulkay, "Rhetorics of Hope and Fear in the Great Embryo Debate," *Social Studies of Science* 23, no. 4 (November 1993): 721–42; Michael Mulkay, "Embryos in the News," *Public Understanding of Science* 3, no. 1 (January 1994): 33–51; and Michael Mulkay, "Changing Minds about Embryo Research," *Public Understanding of Science* 3, no. 2 (April 1994): 195–213. Although U.S. researchers also limit work to embryos under 14 days old, this restriction is voluntary and applies only to private research, since it is not done

under government-funded programs and government rules or guidelines. Embryo research in the U.S. remains highly controversial, subject to the political winds and the policies of the administration in power.

66. R. G. Edwards and Patrick Steptoe, *A Matter of Life: The Story of a Medical Breakthrough* (New York: William Morrow, 1980). Edwards, an embryologist now affiliated with Hammersmith Hospital in London, is one of the leaders in embryo research. Dr. Steptoe died in 1988. See his obituary in the *New York Times,* March 23, 1988, p. D27.

67. Although some descriptions use the term *partner* rather than *husband,* the IVF procedure followed to produce these embryos for testing is almost exclusively confined to married couples.

68. Accurate figures for success rates for IVF in particular, and assisted reproductive technologies generally, are hard to come by. Reports have ranged from a low of about 10 percent to claims of over 30 percent. Centers can vary widely, and methods and bases of accounting and reporting are by no means uniform. Combining statistics from three U.S. sources—the Society for Assisted Reproduction Technology, the Centers for Disease Control and Prevention, and the Department of Health and Human Services—a 2003 article gave a figure of 35,000 live births for the year 2000, or a 35 percent success rate, noting a rapid rise from 12 percent in 1988. Mary Duenwald, "After 25 Years, New Ideas in the Prenatal Test Tube," *New York Times,* July 15, 2003, pp. F5, F8. This figure, however, included all types of assisted reproduction, not just IVF, and pregnancies using donor eggs as well as eggs from the mothers themselves.

69. A. H. Handyside, F. H. Kontogianni, K. Hardy, and R. M. L. Winston, "Pregnancies from Biopsied Human Preimplantation Embryos Sexed by Y-Specific DNA Amplification," *Nature* 344, no. 6268 (April 19, 1990): 768; and "Scientists Identify Sex of 3-Day-Old Embryos," *New York Times,* April 19, 1990, p. A19.

70. In 1989, even before cells had been successfully isolated and analyzed, researchers predicted that DNA analysis techniques would be able to detect chromosomal, genetic, and enzyme disorders in embryos ranging from 4 to 64 cells (i.e., a "pre-embryo"). Matteo Adinolfi and Paul E. Polani, "Prenatal Diagnosis of Genetic Disorders in Preimplantation Embryos: Invasive and Non-Invasive Approaches," *Human Genetics* 83, no. 1 (August 1989): 16–19.

71. Alan H. Handyside, John G. Lesko, Juan J. Tarin, Robert M. L. Winston, and Mark R. Hughes, "Birth of a Normal Girl after In Vitro Fertilization and Preimplantation Diagnostic Testing for Cystic Fibrosis," *New England Journal of Medicine* 327, no. 13 (September 24, 1992): 905–909.

72. Manal Morsy, Kazuhiro Takeuchi, Robert Kaufmann, Lucinda Veeck, Gary D. Hodgen, and Stephen J. Beebe, "Preclinical Models for Human Pre-embryo Biopsy and Genetic Diagnosis. II. Polymerase Chain Reaction Amplification of Deoxyribonucleic Acid from Single Lymphoblasts and Blastomeres with Mutation Detection," *Fertility & Sterility* 57, no. 2 (February 1992): 431–38. The lymphoblasts (immature white blood cells) were human cells; the blastomeres (early embryonic cells) were from mice.

73. J. D. Delhanty and J. C. Harper, "Pre-implantation Genetic Diagnosis," *Baillière's Best Practices Research: Clinical Obstetrics and Gynaecology* 14, no. 4 (August 2000): 691 (abstract).

74. Sergio Oehninger, Suheil J. Muasher, and Herbert E. Bevan, "Current Status of Preimplantation Diagnosis," *Journal of Assisted Reproduction and Genetics* 14, no. 2 (February 1997): 72. These figures were presented at the Sixth Annual Meeting of the International Working Group on Preimplantation Genetics, held in Rio de Janeiro in August 1996 in connection with the Ninth International Congress on Human Genetics.

75. Joyce C. Harper, "Preimplantation Diagnosis of Inherited Disease by Embryo Biopsy: An Update of the World Figures," *Journal of Assisted Reproduction and Genetics* 13, no. 2 (February 1996): 90–95. The figures were as of February 28, 1995. This special issue of the *Journal of Assisted Reproduction and Genetics* was devoted to selected papers from the Fifth Annual Meeting of the International Working Group on Preimplantation Genetics, Hamburg, Germany, June 28, 1995, the group founded in 1990. At the time, Harper was affiliated with Hammersmith Hospital as well as the Galton Laboratory in London.

76. Dr. Verlinksy edited the *Journal of Assisted Reproduction and Genetics*'s special issue on preimplantation diagnosis, cited above.

77. C. M. Strom, S. Strom, E. Levine, N. Ginsberg, J. Barton, and Y. Verlinsky, "Obstetric Outcomes in 102 Pregnancies after Preimplantation Genetic Diagnosis," *American Journal of Obstetrics and Gynecology* 182, no. 6 (June 2000): 1629–32.

78. Harper, "Preimplantation Diagnosis," p. 90.

79. The 35,000 babies born in 2000 through assisted reproduction represented less than 1 percent of all babies born in the U.S. that year. Duenwald, "New Ideas," F5.

80. Nazar N. Amso, "Potential Health Hazards of Assisted Reproduction Continued: Problems Facing the Clinician," *Human Reproduction* 10, no. 7 (July 1995): 1628–30. This article appeared in a section called "Debate," as part of a continuing discussion of various problems with IVF and other forms of assisted reproduction, including hazards to the developing fetus and hazards to women from the medications they are given.

81. Claire Snowden and Josephine M. Green, "Preimplantation Diagnosis and Other Reproductive Options: Attitudes of Male and Female Carriers of Recessive Disorders," *Human Reproduction* 12, no. 2 (February 1997): 341–50.

82. The numbers were two "healthy deliveries" and "three ongoing pregnancies confirmed to be unaffected by" CVS out of 119 oocytes which were fertilized, and a total of 155 tested. Y. Verlinsky, J. Cieslak, M. Freidine, V. Ivakhnenko, G. Wolf, L. Kovalinskaya, M. White, A. Lifchez, B. Kaplan, J. Moise, J. Valle, N. Ginsberg, C. Strom, and A. Kuliev, "Pregnancies following Pre-conception Diagnosis of Common Aneuploidies by Fluorescent In-Situ Hybridization," *Human Reproduction* 10, no. 7 (July 1995): 1923–27.

83. D. T. Carrell, A. L. Wilcox, L. C. Udoff, C. Thorp, and B. Campbell,

"Chromosome 15 Aneuploidy in the Sperm and Conceptus of a Sibling with Variable Familial Expression of Round-Headed Sperm Syndrome," *Fertility & Sterility* 76, no. 6 (Dec 2001): 1258–60.

84. See M. Kent-First, "The Critical and Expanding Role of Genetics in Assisted Reproduction," *Prenatal Diagnosis* 20, no. 7 (July 2000): 536–51.

85. Gina Kolata, "Biologists Stumble Across New Pattern of Inheritance," *New York Times,* July 16, 1991, pp. C1, C7; and correction July 18, 1991, 2; Kolata, "Cell Error Pinpointed," May 28, 1991, p. C3; and Wilkins-Haug, "Emerging Genetic Theories," 179–85. A study reported in 2000 showed that an extra chromosome 21 came from the father 11 percent of the time; the figure in the earlier study had been 7 percent. In either case, its origins remained overwhelmingly female. F. Muller, M. Rebiffe, A. Taillandier, J. F. Oury, and E. Mornet, "Parental Origin of the Extra Chromosome in Prenatally Diagnosed Fetal Trisomy 21," *Human Genetics* 106, no. 3 (March 2000): 340–44.

86. This argument, of course, does not apply to those who believe that life begins at conception and therefore regard discarding an embryo as murder. But medical personnel or prospective parents who share this view would probably not involve themselves in such procedures. Attitudes concerning abortion and prenatal diagnosis will be treated further in chapters 5 and 6.

87. Frank Costantini, Kiran Chada, and Jeanne Magram, "Correction of Murine-Beta-Thalassemia by Gene Transfer into the Germline," *Science* 233, no. 4769 (September 12, 1986): 1192–94; and Harold M. Schmeck, Jr., "Gene Transplant Causes Fertility," *New York Times,* December 5, 1986, p. A17. Scientists find the mouse genome a powerful research tool to apply to human genome research because the mouse genome carries virtually the same set of genes as the human, but can be used in laboratory research. The sequencing of the mouse genome was announced in December 2002. National Institutes of Health, "The Mouse Genome and the Measure of Man," http://www.genome.gov/10005831, accessed September 20, 2004.

88. "Points to Consider in the Design and Submission of Human Somatic-Cell Gene Therapy Protocols" (1986), available from National Institutes of Health (NIH), Rockville, Maryland.

89. The treatment involved transferring virus-treated genes into her bone marrow; it was reported in 1990 by the National Heart, Lung and Blood Institute of NIH. See Evelyn M. Karson, William Polvino, and W. French Anderson, "Prospects for Human Gene Therapy," *Journal of Reproductive Medicine* 37, no. 6 (June 1992): 508–14, for discussion of the techniques and their applications. See also Natalie Angier, "Doctors Have Success Treating a Blood Disease by Altering Genes," *New York Times,* July 28, 1991, p. 20.

90. Eugene Pergament and Morris Fiddler, "Prenatal Gene Therapy: Prospects and Issues," *Prenatal Diagnosis* 15, no. 13 (December 1995): 1303–1304.

91. Sharon R. Stephenson and David D. Weaver, "Prenatal Diagnosis—A Compilation of Diagnosed Conditions," *American Journal of Obstetrics and Gynecology* 141, no. 3 (October 1981): 319–43.

92. David D. Weaver, "A Survey of Prenatally Diagnosed Disorders," *Clinical Obstetrics and Gynecology* 31, no. 2 (June 1988): 253–69.

93. David D. Weaver, *Catalog of Prenatally Diagnosed Conditions* (Baltimore: Johns Hopkins University Press, 1989).

94. Evans, Quigg, et al., "Prenatal Diagnosis," p. 30.

95. David D. Weaver, *Catalog of Prenatally Diagnosed Conditions,* 2nd ed. (Baltimore: Johns Hopkins University Press, 1992).

96. David D. Weaver, with the assistance of Ira K. Brandt, *Catalog of Prenatally Diagnosed Conditions,* 3rd ed. (Baltimore: Johns Hopkins University Press, 1999), p. xxi, table 1.

97. As discussed above, some preimplantation screening for sex does have a medical purpose.

5. THE DOCTORS

1. On the power of professional socialization in medicine, see Eliot Freidson, *Profession of Medicine: A Study of the Sociology of Applied Knowledge* (1970; reprint, Chicago: University of Chicago Press, 1988).

2. William Ray Arney, *Power and the Profession of Obstetrics* (Chicago: University of Chicago Press, 1982), chapters 1, 2, and 3.

3. Wertz and Wertz, *Lying-In,* p. 135.

4. Ibid., p. 164; and Arney, *Power and the Profession of Obstetrics.*

5. Wertz and Wertz, *Lying-In,* p. 165.

6. Arney, *Power and the Profession of Obstetrics.*

7. Quoted in ibid., p. 136.

8. They include Wayne State University's Hutzel Hospital in Detroit, Thomas Jefferson University Hospital in Philadelphia, the University of Tennessee Medical School in Memphis, the UCLA School of Medicine, the Johns Hopkins University School of Medicine in Baltimore, and Weill Medical College of Cornell University in New York.

9. Obstetrics-gynecology is one of the five highest specialties for physicians in the U.S. Ninety-seven percent of ob/gyns are engaged in patient care as their primary professional activity. Seventy-nine percent are office-based. Of those who are hospital-based, 11.8 percent are residents or fellows (recent graduates receiving supervised training), and 5.8 percent are physician staff. Compare age groupings of male and female ob/gyns:

Age Range	% of Men	% of Women
under 35	8.8	32.9
35–44	21.3	36.4
45–54	29.6	21.4
55–64	23.0	6.9
65 and over	17.3	2.4

Thus, seven out of ten female ob/gyns are under 45, with almost one-third under 35, and just over one-third in the 35–44 age group. While 40 per cent of men ob/gyns are over 55, only 9 percent of women are. Twenty-four percent of female ob/gyns are hospital residents or fellows, in contrast to 6 percent of males. Statistics are from *Physician Characteristics and Distribution in the U.S., 2001–2002 Edition* (Chicago: American Medical Association, 2002). Data are as of December 31, 1999. The AMA updates this compilation annually.

10. Kenen, "Genetic Counseling," pp. 541–49, esp. table 1, p. 542. See B. Meredith Burke and Aliza Kolker, "Directiveness in Prenatal Genetic Counseling," *Women & Health* 22, no. 2 (1994): 31–53. In 1992, six genetic counselors concerned over a further lowering of status of the master's level genetic counselor, protested unsuccessfully against a "proposed disunion of physician and Ph.D. diplomates of the American Board of Medical Genetics (ABMG) from diplomates in genetic counseling," which would affect membership and certification. They asked, "Could the result be a two class system for medical genetics? Will genetic counselors lose some degree of the prestige accorded to them in the field of medicine?" (p. 33). The separation did take place, and since 1993 genetic counselors have been certified by the American Board of Genetic Counseling.

11. In 1981, in the preface to a volume of papers from a symposium on genetic issues in pediatrics and obstetrics, editor Michael Kaback, from the Harbor-UCLA Medical Center, noted that a decade earlier "fewer than 25% of the medical schools had any defined curriculum in human genetics" and therefore practicing physicians had little formal exposure to the "precepts of medical genetics." He stressed the need to educate such physicians. Michael M. Kaback, ed., *Genetic Issues in Pediatric and Obstetric Practice* (Chicago: Year Book Medical Publishers, 1981), p. xi. A report on the results of a 1985 survey of medical schools found that the position of human genetics in the curriculum was not much improved; the approach was still fragmented and medical students were not always being prepared for the "revolution" in human genetics. Vincent M. Riccardi and Roy D. Schmickel, "Human Genetics as a Component of Medical School Curricula: A Report to the American Society of Human Genetics," *American Journal of Human Genetics* 42 (April 1988): 639–43. In 1993 hospital residents in Philadelphia were found to be deficient in knowledge of genetics, the authors recommending postgraduate training for obstetricians in medical genetics, its application to prenatal diagnosis and genetic counseling, utilizing available services, and educating parents. Melissa A. Kershner, Elizabeth A. Hammond, and Alan E. Donnenfeld, "Knowledge of Genetics among Residents in Obstetrics and Gynecology," *American Journal of Human Genetics* 53, no. 6 (December 1993): 1356–58. The first section of a text edited by Dr. Mark I. Evans at Wayne State University in 1992, which was aimed at the practicing physician, included a lesson in the genetics of inheritance, genetic counseling, and principles of teratology, which readers were cautioned not to skip, even if the information seemed elementary. Mark I. Evans, *Reproductive Risks and Prenatal Diagnosis* (Norwalk, Conn.: Appleton and Lange, 1992), section 1, "General Principles."

12. Evans, Johnson, and Moghissi, *Invasive Outpatient Procedures,* p. xi.

13. Michael R. Harrison, Mitchell S. Golbus, and Roy A. Filly, *The Unborn Patient: Prenatal Diagnosis and Treatment* (Orlando, Fla.: Grune & Stratton, 1984), pp. 1, 7. Drs. Harrison, Golbus, and Filly dedicate the book to Gretchen, Antoinette, and Barbara (presumably their wives) "and to the courageous mothers who carry our unborn future." In the preface, the authors appropriate the language of pregnancy to describe the course of their project, moving from "conception" to "gestation" through the first, second, and third "trimester[s]" (p. xix).

14. Ibid., p. 9.

15. Asim Kurjak, ed. *The Fetus as a Patient* (New York: Excerpta Medica, distributed by Elsevier, 1985); Asim Kurjak and Frank A. Chervenak, eds., *The Fetus as a Patient: Advances in Diagnosis and Therapy* (New York: Parthenon, 1994); Frank A. Chervenak and Asim Kurjak, eds., *Current Perspectives on the Fetus as a Patient* (New York: Parthenon, 1996); Frank A. Chervenak, Asim Kurjak, and Zoltan Papp, eds., *The Fetus as a Patient: The Evolving Challenge* (Boca Raton, Fla.: Parthenon, 2002).

16. See Monica J. Caspar, *The Making of the Unborn Patient: A Social Anatomy of Fetal Surgery* (New Brunswick, N.J.: Rutgers University Press, 1998).

17. Chervenak and Kurjak, *Current Perspectives,* p. xiii.

18. Evans and Johnson, "Prenatal Diagnosis in the '90s," 388. The symposium appeared in two consecutive issues of the *Journal of Reproductive Medicine* 37, no. 5 (May 1992): 383–444, and 37, no. 6 (June 1992): 485–524. Describing the latest research and practice and future directions, the symposium contributions were from leaders in the field, mostly M.D.s at prestigious medical institutions.

19. George G. Rhoads et al., "The Safety and Efficacy of Chorionic Villus Sampling for Early Prenatal Diagnosis of Cytogenic Abnormalities," *New England Journal of Medicine* 320, no. 10 (March 9, 1989): 609–17.

20. Anver Kuliev et al., "Chorionic Villus Sampling Safety: Report of World Health Organization/EURO Meeting in Association with the Seventh International Conference on Early Prenatal Diagnosis of Genetic Diseases, Tel-Aviv, Israel, May 21, 1994," *American Journal of Obstetrics and Gynecology* 174, no. 3 (March 1996): 807–11.

21. Godelieve C. M. L. Christiaens and Nico J. Leschot, "Limb Deficiencies and Chorion Villus Sampling," letter to the editor, *American Journal of Medical Genetics* 45 (1993): 529. Christiaens and Leschot cite reports by others of such problems, as well as their own findings from as early as 1989.

22. Studies continue to show that women prefer amniocentesis to CVS, although the way physicians influence their choice is not clear. See, for example, P. S. Heckerling, M. S. Verp, and N. Albert, "The Role of Physician Preferences in the Choice of Amniocentesis or Chorionic Villus Sampling for Prenatal Genetic Testing," *Genetic Testing* 2, no. 1 (1998): 61–66.

23. Drugan et al., "Prenatal Biochemical Screening," p. 403. California had led the way in 1986 with a law that mandated offering MSAFP screening to all

pregnant women. See discussion by Robert Steinbrook, "In California, Voluntary Mass Prenatal Screening," *Hastings Center Report* 16, no. 5 (October 1986): 5–7.

24. Carlson and Platt, "Ultrasound Detection," 419, 425. Drs. Carlson and Platt were with the Division of Maternal-Fetal Medicine, Department of Obstetrics and Gynecology, UCLA School of Medicine, Los Angeles.

25. The RADIUS (Routine Antenatal Diagnostic Imaging with Ultrasound) study is discussed further in chapter 9. Dr. Seeds, of the Medical College of Virginia, states that the "most likely benefits of ultrasound" for the "low-risk patient" are "obstetrical": to confirm due dates, identify multiple fetuses, locate the placenta, and so on. "The detection of the unexpected major fetal malformation has always been the least likely benefit of routine ultrasound." He finds "diagnostic sensitivity . . . to be highest in high-risk patients examined by highly specialized experienced personnel," though such sensitivity "may be quite good . . . in low-risk patients" if certain content guidelines are followed and referred to "experienced referral resources." Seeds, "Obstetrical Ultrasound Examination," 828. See also Chitty, "Ultrasound Screening."

26. M. H. Graupe, C. S. Naylor, N. H. Greene, D. E. Carlson, and L. Platt, "Trisomy 21: Second-Trimester Ultrasound," *Clinical Perinatology* 28, no. 2 (June 2001): 303 (abstract).

27. V. L. Souter and D. A. Nyberg, "Sonographic Screening for Fetal Aneuploidy: First Trimester," *Journal of Ultrasound Medicine* 20, no. 7 (July 2001): 775–90.

28. Ibid.

29. Wolfgang Holzgreve, Henk S. P. Harritsen, and Dorothee Ganshirt-Ahlert, "Fetal Cells in the Maternal Circulation," *Journal of Reproductive Medicine* 37, no. 5 (May 1992): 410.

30. See Wachtell, Shulman, and Sammons, "Fetal Cells."

31. R. G. Edwards and Jean M. Purdy, eds., *Human Conception in Vitro: Proceedings of the First Bourn Hall Meeting* (London: Academic Press, 1982), p. 373.

32. According to Regina Morantz-Sanchez, medical historians have increasingly treated medicine "as an artifact of culture." "Good Guys in White Coats," review of *Doctors: The Biography of Medicine,* by Sherwin B. Nuland, *New York Times Book Review,* October 23, 1988, pp. 36–37.

33. See, for example, Eric J. Cassell, "The Principles of the Belmont Report Revisited: How Have Respect for Persons, Beneficence, and Justice Been Applied to Clinical Medicine?" *Hastings Center Report* 30, no. 4 (July–August 2000): 12–21.

34. Jacqueline A. Lutz and Hindy J. Shaman, "The Impact of Consumerism on Managed Health Care," in *Essentials of Managed Health Care,* ed. Peter R. Kongstvedt, 4th ed. (Gaithersburg, Md.: Aspen, 2001), pp. 573–74. Their characterization is based on a study by the Center for the Advancement of Health.

35. James R. Sorenson, "Biomedical Innovation, Uncertainty and Doctor-Patient Interaction," *Journal of Health and Social Behavior* 14, no. 4 (December

1974): 366–74; and Bernard Barber, *Informed Consent in Medical Therapy and Research* (New Brunswick, N.J.: Rutgers University Press, 1980), pp. 28–29.

36. Edward C. Hill, "Your Morality or Mine? An Inquiry into the Ethics of Human Reproduction," *American Journal of Obstetrics and Gynecology* 154, no. 6 (June 1986): 1180.

37. See, for example, the strong caveats expressed in Neil A. Holtzman, *Proceed with Caution: Predicting Genetic Risks in the Recombinant DNA Era* (Baltimore: Johns Hopkins University Press, 1989).

38. Susan R. Johnson and Thomas E. Elkins, "Ethical Issues in Prenatal Diagnosis," *Clinical Obstetrics and Gynecology* 31, no. 2 (June 1988): 408–17. At the time, Dr. Johnson was at the Department of Obstetrics and Gynecology at the University of Iowa Hospitals and Clinics, and Dr. Elkins at the University of Michigan College of Medicine. Five years later, however, Dr. Elkins, now at the Louisiana State University School of Medicine, strongly criticized extending prenatal diagnosis to "low risk" patients across the age spectrum. See below and chapter 9.

39. The word "forcing" is theirs. Does it imply that some circumstances might justify forcing a patient to be tested?

40. For a critique of this obstetric model, see Susan S. Mattingly, "The Maternal-Fetal Dyad: Exploring the Two-Patient Obstetric Model," *Hastings Center Report* 22, no. 1 (January–February 1992): 13–18. See chapter 10 for a feminist analysis of this adversarial mindset.

41. F. A. Chervenak, L. B. McCullough, and A. Kurjak, "An Essential Clinical Ethical Concept," in Chervenak and Kurjak, *Current Perspectives,* p. 2.

42. In an in-depth survey of ob/gyns, sociologist Jonathan Imber found "nearly unanimous avoidance of second trimester abortions." Jonathan B. Imber, *Abortion and the Private Practice of Medicine* (New Haven: Yale University Press, 1986), p. 115. See also Gina Kolata, "Under Pressures and Stigma, More Doctors Shun Abortion," *New York Times,* January 8, 1990, pp. A1, C8; and personal communication from Ruth Schwartz Cowan, who is researching a forthcoming study of the history of prenatal diagnosis.

43. Evans and Johnson, "Prenatal Diagnosis in the '90s," p. 388.

44. Council on Scientific Affairs, American Medical Association, "Genetic Counseling and Prevention of Birth Defects," *Journal of the American Medical Association* 248, no. 2 (July 9, 1982): 222.

45. Evans and Johnson, "Prenatal Diagnosis in the '90s," p. 388. A newspaper article at the time quoted physicians hailing this work as just the beginning and a major leap forward. See Gina Kolata, "Genetic Defects Detected in Embryos Just Days Old," *New York Times,* September 24, 1992, pp. A1, B10.

46. Joseph Schulman, "Prenatal Diagnosis of Rare Diseases," in *Frontiers in Rare Disease Research: Proceedings of a Symposium Held in Bethesda, MD, and Washington, DC, May 2 and 3, 1990,* publication 1992—621-953 (Washington, D.C.: U.S. Government Printing Office), pp. 116, 118.

47. Joseph D. Schulman, Andrew Dorfmann, and Mark I. Evans, "Genetic

Aspects of In Vitro Fertilization," *Annals of the New York Academy of Sciences* 442 (1985): 474. Britain's Dr. Robert Edwards had expressed support for gene modification in the human embryo as early as 1971. See Robert G. Edwards and David J. Sharpe, "Social Values and Research in Human Embryology," *Nature* 231, no. 5298 (May 14, 1971): 87–91. However, in the mid-1980s the leading specialist in IVF in France, Dr. Jacques Testart, declared his opposition to further research on human embryos for preimplantation diagnosis, fearing its manipulation for eugenic purposes. See Robert Walgate, "In Vitro Fertilization: French Scientist Makes a Stand," *Nature* 323, no. 6087 (October 2, 1986): 385; Gail Vines, "Test-Tube Pioneer Fears Rise of Eugenics," *New Scientist* (October 9, 1986): 17; and "French Researcher Says 'Non' to Egg Manipulation," *Hastings Center Report* 16, no. 6 (December 1986): 4. A decade later Dr. Testart restated his qualms. See Jacques Testart and B. Sele, "Towards an Efficient Medical Eugenics: Is the Desirable Always Feasible?" *Human Reproduction* 10, no. 12 (December 1995): 3086–90. See also Dr. Alan Handyside's response, calling "preposterous" Testart and Sele's contention that preimplantation diagnosis "could in future be used for eugenic selection of embryos with 'desirable' characteristics." Alan H. Handyside, "Commonsense as Applied to Eugenics—Response to Testart and Sèle," *Human Reproduction* 11, no. 4 (April 1996): 707.

48. Aubrey Milunsky, preface to *Genetic Disorders and the Fetus: Diagnosis, Prevention, and Treatment,* ed. Aubrey Milunsky, 2nd ed. (New York: Plenum, 1986), p. xi.

49. Aubrey Milunsky, *The Prevention of Genetic Disease and Mental Retardation* (Philadelphia: Saunders, 1975), pp. x, 87.

50. Aubrey Milunsky, *Choices Not Chances: An Essential Guide to Your Heredity and Health* (Boston: Little Brown, 1989); Aubrey Milunsky, *Choices Not Chances: How to Have the Healthiest Baby You Can* (New York: Simon & Schuster, 1986); and Aubrey Milunsky, *Know Your Genes* (Boston: Houghton Mifflin, 1977).

51. Aubrey Milunsky, ed., *Genetic Disorders and the Fetus: Diagnosis, Prevention, and Treatment,* 4th ed. (Baltimore: Johns Hopkins University Press, 1998), p. xi.

52. Margery Shaw, "Presidential Address: To Be or Not to Be? That Is the Question," *American Journal of Human Genetics* 36, no. 1 (January 1984): 9.

53. Margery Shaw, "Conditional Prospective Rights of the Fetus," *Journal of Legal Medicine* 5, no. 1 (March 1984): 63–116.

54. Jerome Yankowitz, Donald M. Howser, and John W. Ely, "Differences in Practice Patterns between Obstetricians and Family Physicians: Use of Serum Screening," *American Journal of Obstetrics and Gynecology* 174, no. 4 (April 1996): 1361–65.

55. See Maurice L. Druzin, Frank Chervenak, Laurence B. McCullogh, Robert N. Blatman, and Julie A. Neidich, "Should All Pregnant Patients Be Offered Prenatal Diagnosis Regardless of Age?" *Obstetrics and Gynecology* 81, no. 4 (April 1993): 615–18; the response letter by Marshall St. Amant, Thomas E. Elkins, Doug Brown, and Joseph G. Pastorek II, from the Louisiana State University School of

Medicine, and Dr. Druzin's response, *Obstetrics and Gynecology* 82, no. 2 (August 1993): 315–16.

56. See the thoughtful discussion in Jeffrey A. Kuller and Steven A. Laifer, "Contemporary Approaches to Prenatal Diagnosis," *American Family Physician* 52, no. 8 (December 1995): 2277–83. Kuller and Laifer call attention to the issue's editorial, which offers caveats on the subject: Mark A. Zamorski, "Prenatal Diagnosis: More Than Meets the Eye," ibid., 2173–74, 2177. Further responses and discussion appeared in letters under the heading "Issues Associated with Prenatal Testing for Fetal Abnormalities," *American Family Physician* 53, no. 8 (June 1996), 2435, 2439–40.

57. "Managed care is now by far the predominant form of health care coverage." Kongstvedt, *Essentials of Managed Health Care*, p. 1. The fourth edition of this managed care volume, at 884 pages, is double the size of the previous edition. Comprehensive in coverage, it is admittedly biased in its support for and promotion of the managed health care industry. According to *Physician Socioeconomic Statistics, 2000–2002 Edition* (Chicago: Center for Health Policy Research, American Medical Association, © 1999), p. 7, as of 1998, 94.1 percent of physicians in the U.S. had at least one contract with a managed care organization, with over half of physicians' revenue coming from such contracts, an "all-time high." In turn, the great majority of consumers with health care coverage receive medical services through such plans, including HMOs (health maintenance organizations), PPOs (preferred provider organizations), and POSs (point of service plans), usually through their place of employment or under Medicare or Medicaid. Dominated by large multi-state or national insurance companies, managed health care is a major industry. The largest firms are traded on the New York Stock Exchange, show high profits, and are headed by well-paid executives.

58. A series of articles appearing in the *New York Times* in the winter of 1990 described some of these changes for physicians. See Lawrence K. Altman and Elisabeth Rosenthal, "Changes in Medicine Bring Pain to Healing Profession," February 18, 1990, pp. l, 34–35; and Gina Kolata, "Wariness Is Replacing Trust between Healer and Patient," February 20, 1990, pp. A1, D15. See also S. J. O'Connor and J. A. Lanning, "The End of Autonomy? Reflections on the Postprofessional Physician," *Health Care Management Review* 17, no. 1 (Winter 1992): 1, 63–72; and J. W. Salmon, W. White, and J. Feinglass, "The Futures of Physicians: Agency and Autonomy Reconsidered," *Theoretical Medicine* 11, no. 4 (December 1990): 261–74.

59. John Ladd, "Physicians and Society: Tribulations of Power and Responsibility," in *The Law-Medicine Relation: A Philosophical Exploration*, ed. S. F. Spicker, J. M. Healey, and H. T. Engelhardt (Dordrecht: Reidel, 1981), pp. 33–52.

60. The Kaiser Family Foundation, *National Survey of Physicians, Part III: Doctors' Opinions about Their Profession*, March 2002, highlights and chart pack available on line at http://www.kff.org/kaiserpolls/20020426c-index.cfm, accessed September 20, 2004.

61. S. Daya, "Evidence-Based Reproductive Medicine," *Human Reproduction* 11: Abstract Book (June 1996): 1. On medicine's growing tendency to rely on

science, see Barbara Gutmann Rosenkrantz, "Damaged Goods: The Dilemmas of Responsibility for Risk," *Milbank Memorial Fund Quarterly/Health and Society* 57, no. 1 (Winter 1979): 1–37.

62. Obstetrics has been particularly hard hit by malpractice suits and costs. For a review of malpractice and related legal issues see Roger J. Bulger and Victoria P. Rostow, "Medical Professional Liability and the Delivery of Obstetrical Care," *Journal of Contemporary Health Law and Policy* 6, no. 8 (Spring 1990): 81–91. Among other issues, the authors note the breakdown of trust between physician and patient. See also Bulger and Rostow, eds., *An Interdisciplinary Review,* vol. 2 of *Medical Professional Liability and the Delivery of Obstetrical Care* (Washington, D.C.: National Academy of Sciences, 1989), a collection of papers from a symposium held at the Academy in 1988; and Institute of Medicine, *Professional Liability and the Delivery of Obstetrical Care,* ed. Victoria P. Rostow and Roger J. Bulger, vol. 1 (Washington, D.C.: National Academy of Sciences, 1989), a report of the results of a two-year study by the Institute. See also Ronni Sandroff, "When the Obstetrician Says 'No,'" *Health* 19, no. 11 (November 1987): 54.

63. Friedrich Vogel and Arno G. Motulsky, *Human Genetics: Problems and Approaches,* 2nd ed. (Heidelberg: Springer, 1986).

64. Perri Klass, "The Perfect Baby," *New York Times Magazine,* January 29, 1989, pp. 45–46.

65. Laurence E. Karp, "Genetic Drift toward the Perfect Child," *American Journal of Medical Genetics* 5, no. 2 (1980): 115–16.

6. THE PARENTS

1. Viviana A. Zelizer, *Pricing the Priceless Child: The Changing Social Value of Children* (1985; reprint, Princeton, N.J.: Princeton University Press, 1994), p. 11.

2. Ibid., p. 3, and introduction, passim. See also discussion in Regina H. Kenen, "A Look at Prenatal Diagnosis within the Context of Changing Parental and Reproductive Norms," in *The Custom-Made Child? Women's Perspectives,* ed. Helen B. Holmes, Betty B. Hoskins, and Michael Gross (Clifton, N.J.: Humana, 1981): 67–73.

3. Zelizer, *Pricing the Priceless Child,* p. 15.

4. Judith Walzer Leavitt, *Brought to Bed: Childbearing in America, 1750 to 1950* (New York: Oxford University Press, 1986). See also Janet Carlisle Bogdan, "Childbirth in America, 1650 to 1990," in *Women, Health and Medicine in America: A Historical Handbook,* ed. Rima D. Apple (1990; reprint, New Brunswick, N.J.: Rutgers University Press, 1992), chapter 4, especially pp. 117–20; and Philip K. Wilson, ed., *The Medicalization of Obstetrics: Personnel, Practice, and Instruments,* vol. 2 of *Childbirth: Changing Ideas and Practices in Britain and America, 1600 to the Present* (Hamden, Conn.: Garland, 1996), for further background. On infant mortality, see chart in Wertz and Wertz, *Lying-In,* p. 163. A further useful review of literature in this field is Charlotte G. Borst, "The Professionalization of Obstetrics: Childbirth Becomes a Medical Specialty," in Apple, *Women, Health and Medicine in America,* chapter 8, pp. 197–216.

5. On access, see Mary Ann Curry, "Nonfinancial Barriers to Prenatal Care," *Women & Health* 15, no. 3 (1989): 85–99; and Marilyn Poland, Joel Ager, and Jane Olson, "Barriers to Receiving Adequate Prenatal Care," *American Journal of Obstetrics and Gynecology* 157, no. 2 (August 1987): 297–303. On attitudinal factors affecting prenatal diagnosis usage, see Klaus J. Roghmann, Richard A. Doherty, Jennifer L. Robinson, Joel N. Nitzkin, and Ralph R. Sell, "The Selective Use of Prenatal Genetic Diagnosis: Experiences of a Regional Program in Upstate New York during the 1970s," *Medical Care* 21, no. 11 (November 1983): 1111–25; Rayna Rapp, "Moral Pioneers: Women, Men and Fetuses on a Frontier of Reproductive Technology," *Women & Health* 13, nos. 1–2 (1987): 101–16; Kate M. Brett, Kenneth C. Schoendorf, and John L. Kiely, "Differences between Black and White Women in the Use of Prenatal Care Technologies," *American Journal of Obstetrics and Gynecology* 170, no. 1 part 1 (January 1994): 41–46; and J. A. Gazmararian, K. S. Schwarz, L. B. Amacker, and C. L. Powell, "Barriers to Prenatal Care among Medicaid Managed Care Enrollees: Patient and Provider Perceptions," *HMO Practice* 11, no. 1 (March 1997): 18–24. See also Aliza Kolker and B. Meredith Burke, *Prenatal Diagnosis: A Sociological Perspective* (Westport, Conn.: Bergin & Garvey, 1994), chapter 6.

6. Even though expertise may separate them from the medical professionals with whom they come into contact, these women (and their partners) will frequently share class and cultural values with them. Imber, *Abortion,* pp. 112–13; and Rosenkrantz, "Damaged Goods," p. 5.

7. Robin Blatt notes that the term "maternal anxiety" is "the diagnosis necessary for the doctor to document in order to be reimbursed by third-party insurers for performing an amniocentesis on a woman under 35 years of age." Robin J. Blatt, "To Choose or Refuse Prenatal Testing," *GeneWatch* (January–February 1987): 5n.

8. Most of the studies of parental attitudes and decisions that I draw on have been of women, although some have looked at "couples" and a few specifically at men's attitudes. Genetic counselors also report that male partners are often at counseling sessions and do participate in decisions if a defect is found. I will distinguish between women and men where possible, while reviewing mainly women's responses.

9. Carole H. Browner, Mabel Preloran, and Nancy A. Press, "The Effects of Ethnicity, Education and an Informational Video on Pregnant Women's Knowledge and Decisions about a Prenatal Diagnostic Screening Test," *Patient Education and Counseling* 27, no. 2 (March 1996): 135–46.

10. Barbara Katz Rothman, *The Tentative Pregnancy: Prenatal Diagnosis and the Future of Motherhood* (New York: Viking, 1986).

11. G. Barsel-Bowers, D. N. Abuelo, M. R. Hopmann, and A. M. Goldstein, "Anxiety in Women with Low Maternal Serum Alpha-Fetoprotein Screening Tests," abstract, *American Journal of Human Genetics* 43, no. 3, supplement (September 1988): A225; K. Keenan, D. Basso, J. Goldkrand, and W. Butler, "The Effect of Genetic Counseling on Anxiety Associated with Low MSAFP," abstract, ibid., p.

A168; and D. M. Greene and A. P. Walker, "Maternal Anxiety and Perception of Benefit from the California Maternal Alpha Fetoprotein Screening Program," abstract, ibid., p. A167. The first two studies reported high anxiety among women less than 35 years old. Regina Kenen, questioning the concept of "at-risk health labeling" as developed in the previous two decades and the "'gift' of knowing," notes the anxiety experienced by the pregnant woman, especially when screening is thrust upon her without her knowledge. Regina H. Kenen, "The At-Risk Health Status and Technology: A Diagnostic Invitation and the 'Gift' of Knowing," *Social Science and Medicine* 42, no. 11 (June 1996): 1545–53. See also Randi Hutter Epstein, "Advances, and Angst, in a New Era of Ultrasound," *New York Times*, May 9, 2000, pp. F7, F12.

12. There is a considerable literature on the psychological aspects of fetal "loss" and prenatal diagnosis. See, for example, Natalie Rice, "Psychological Reaction to Prenatal Diagnosis and Loss," in Evans, *Reproductive Risks*, pp. 277–82; Rita Beck Black, "Prenatal Diagnosis and Fetal Loss: Psychosocial Consequences and Professional Responsibilities," *American Journal of Medical Genetics* 35, no. 4 (April 1990): 586–87; Jodi Rucquoi and M. J. Mahoney, "A Protocol to Address the Depressive Effects of Abortion for Fetal Abnormalities Discovered Prenatally via Amniocentesis," in *Psychosocial Aspects of Genetic Counseling*, ed. Gerry Evers-Kiebooms, Jean-Pierre Fryns, and Jean-Jacques Cassiman, Birth Defects Original Article Series 28, no. 1 (New York: John Wiley, 1992), 57–60; and Linda L. Layne, "Of Fetuses and Angels: Fragmentation and Integration in Narratives of Pregnancy Loss," *Knowledge and Society: The Anthropology of Science and Technology* 9 (1992): 29–58.

13. See, for example, discussions in *Genetic Risk, Risk Perception, and Decision Making*, ed. Gerry Evers-Kiebooms, Jean-Jacques Cassiman, Herman Vanden Berghe, and Gery d'Ydevalle, Birth Defects Original Article Series 23, no. 2 (New York: Alan R. Liss, 1987).

14. Gery d'Ydevalle, in ibid., p. 210.

15. Abby Lippman-Hand and F. Clarke Fraser, "Genetic Counseling: Provision and Perception of Information," *American Journal of Medical Genetics* 3, no. 2 (1979): 113–27; and Diane Beeson and Mitchell S. Golbus, "Decision-Making: Whether or Not to Have Prenatal Diagnosis and Abortion for X-Linked Conditions," *American Journal of Medical Genetics* 20, no. 1 (January 1985): 107–14.

16. Data are from National Opinion Research Center studies covering a 15-year period, 1972–1987, cited by Dorothy C. Wertz and John C. Fletcher, "Ethical Issues in Prenatal Diagnosis," *Pediatric Annals* 18, no. 11 (November 1989): 739, note 5. A *New York Times*/CBS News Poll conducted in early 1998 confirmed the consistency of support for legal abortion if "there is a strong chance of a serious defect in the baby," percentages fluctuating between 75 percent and just over 80 percent in the period from 1972 to 1998, even though other limitations appeared to gain ground. Carey Goldberg, with Janet Elder, "Public Still Backs Abortion, but Wants Limits, Poll Says," *New York Times*, January 16, 1998, pp. A1, A16.

17. Abby Lippman, "Prenatal Diagnosis: Reproductive Choice? Reproductive

Control?" in *The Future of Human Reproduction,* ed. Christine Overall (Toronto: Women's Press, 1989), p. 183. Lippman argues that possible reasons for physicians' developing the criterion included justifying the abortion of a clinically normal pregnancy and to provide justification in places where a serious defect was one of the few legal grounds for abortion.

18. Arie Drugan, Anne Greb, Mark Paul Johnson, Eric L. Krivchenia, Wendy R. Uhlmann, Kamran S. Moghissi, and Mark I. Evans, "Determinants of Parental Decisions to Abort for Chromosome Abnormalities," *Prenatal Diagnosis* 10, no. 8 (August 1990): 483–90.

19. Mark I. Evans, Michelle A. Sobiecki, Eric L. Krivchenia, Debra A. Duquette, Arie Drugan, Roderick F. Hume, Jr., and Mark P. Johnson, "Parental Decisions to Terminate/Continue following Abnormal Cytogenetic Prenatal Diagnosis: 'What' Is Still More Important Than 'When,'" *American Journal of Medical Genetics* 61, no. 4 (February 1996): 354. See also Peter G. Pryde, Arie Drugan, Mark P. Johnson, Nelson B. Isada, and Mark I. Evans, "Prenatal Diagnosis: Choices Women Make about Pursuing Testing and Acting on Abnormal Results," *Clinical Obstetrics and Gynecology* 36, no. 3 (September 1993): 496–509; this article, too, grouped trisomies 13, 18, and 21 together.

20. See Arthur Robinson, Bruce G. Bender, and Mary G. Linden, "Decisions following the Intrauterine Diagnosis of Sex Chromosome Aneuploidy," *American Journal of Medical Genetics* 34, no. 4 (December 1989): 552–54.

21. There is apparently greater concern over Klinefelter's and Turner's syndromes, even though the prognosis for the other conditions is mixed, especially for XXX females, who may have learning disabilities, physical problems, and low self-esteem. Ibid.

22. The termination rates for CVS-diagnosed conditions fell from 50 percent in 1986–88, to 39 percent in 1989–91, to 29 percent in 1992–94, with an average of 37 percent terminations, or slightly less than two out of every three women continuing their pregnancies; for amniocentesis diagnoses the termination rates were 22 percent, 24 percent, and 19 percent, with an average of 20 percent, or four out of five women keeping their pregnancies. Evans, Sobiecki, et al., "Parental Decisions to Terminate/Continue." An earlier report from Northwestern University Medical School covering the years 1977 to 1986 which did distinguish among chromosomal anomalies clearly showed parents choosing among severities, e.g., between Down syndrome and fatal conditions, and between sex chromosome discrepancies and others; further, researchers noted that with first-trimester diagnosis becoming available, termination rates could rise for all such pregnancies. Marion S. Verp, Allan T. Bombard, Joe Leigh Simpson, and Sherman Elias, "Parental Decision following Prenatal Diagnosis of Fetal Chromosome Abnormality," *American Journal of Medical Genetics* 29, no. 3 (March 1988): 613–22.

23. C. Grevengood, L. P. Shulman, J. S. Dungan, P. Martens, O. P. Phillips, D. S. Emerson, R. E. Felker, J. L. Simpson, and S. Elias, "Severity of Abnormality Influences Decision to Terminate Pregnancies Affected with Fetal Neural Tube

Defects," *Fetal Diagnosis and Therapy* 9, no. 4 (July–August 1994): 273–77. All 23 women carrying fetuses with anencephaly chose to terminate their pregnancies.

24. Kenneth B. Schechtman, Diana L. Gray, Jack D. Baty, and Steven M. Rothman, "Decision-Making for Termination of Pregnancies with Fetal Anomalies: Analysis of 53,000 Pregnancies," *Obstetrics and Gynecology* 99, no. 2 (February 2002): 217. The study, conducted at Washington University in St. Louis, covered pregnancies over a 15-year period, from 1984 to 1997.

25. As many as one out every 259 women in the general population may carry the premutation, which, if passed on to her daughters, can expand into a full mutation in the next generation. Finucane, "Should All Pregnant Women."

26. D. L. Meryash, "Genetic Counseling Needs of Women At-Risk for Bearing Children with the Fragile-X Syndrome," abstract, *American Journal of Human Genetics* 39, supplement (September 1986): A180.

27. J. Riordan, J. Rommens, B.-S. Kerem, N. Alon, R. Rozmahel, Z. Grzelczak, et al., "Identification of the Cystic Fibrosis Gene: Cloning and Characterization of Complementary DNA," *Science* 245, no. 4922 (September 8, 1989): 1066–73.

28. David M. Orenstein, Glenna B. Winnie, and Harold Altman, "Cystic Fibrosis: A 2002 Update," *Journal of Pediatrics* 140, no. 2 (February 2002): 156–64.

29. S. Loader, P. Caldwell, A. Kozyra, J. C. Levenkron, C. D. Boehm, H. H. Kazazian, Jr., and Peter T. Rowley, "Cystic Fibrosis Carrier Population Screening in the Primary Care Setting," *American Journal of Human Genetics* 59, no. 1 (July 1996): 234.

30. Orenstein, Winnie, and Altman, in "Cystic Fibrosis," note that early and aggressive treatment, using a variety of means to control airway and respiratory damage, plus careful attention to nutrition and other health measures, improves prognosis. The outcome for lung transplants, when respiratory failure is irreversible, is improving. Progress in gene therapy remains slow. On median age at death, see Cystic Fibrosis Foundation, *Patient Registry 1998 Annual Data Report* (Bethesda, Md.: Cystic Fibrosis Foundation, 1999), and a Foundation communication to me, 2002.

31. Dorothy C. Wertz, J. M. Rosenfield, S. R. Janes, and R. W. Erbe, "Psycho-Social Factors in Utilization of DNA-Based Prenatal Diagnosis for Cystic Fibrosis," abstract, *American Journal of Human Genetics* 45, no. 4, supplement (October 1989), p. A273. Most respondents, however, did not intend to have more children, so the sample was small.

32. J. S. Lee, R. Wallerstein, and S. R. Young, "Parental Attitudes toward Prenatal Diagnosis of Cystic Fibrosis," abstract, *American Journal of Human Genetics* 41, no. 3, supplement (September 1987): A198. Sixty-four percent of those who would not have prenatal diagnosis rejected abortion.

33. A study comparing the attitudes of consumers, with and without a family history of CF, and of genetics professionals toward severity, prenatal diagnosis, and abortion for eight diseases ranked "severe MR [mental retardation], death in childhood" as the most severe, and "facial disfigurement, normal IQ, normal

lifespan" as the least; consumers were more likely to want prenatal diagnosis but less likely to favor abortion than were professionals. See M. F. Myers, B. A. Bernhardt, E. S. Tambor, and N. A. Holtzman, "Consumer and Professional Perception of Disease Severity, Desire for Prenatal Diagnosis, and Willingness to Terminate a Pregnancy," abstract, *American Journal of Human Genetics* 51, no. 4, supplement (1992): A269.

34. Loader et al., "Cystic Fibrosis Carrier Population Screening," p. 234.

35. A. M. Vintzileos, C. V. Anath, J. C. Smulian, A. J. Fisher, D. Day-Salvatore, and T. Beazoglou, "A Cost-Effective Analysis of Prenatal Carrier Screening for Cystic Fibrosis," *Obstetrics and Gynecology* 91, no. 4 (April 1998): 529–34. The program was deemed to be cost-effective for Whites but not "for blacks, Asians, or Hispanics."

36. See R. White and P. O'Connell, "Identification and Characterization of the Gene for Neurofibromatosis Type 1," *Current Opinion in Genetic Development* 1, no. 1 (June 1991): 15–19; V. M. Riccardi, "The Prenatal Diagnosis of NF-1 and NF-2," *Journal of Dermatology* 19, no. 11 (November 1992): 885–91; and K. J. Hofman, "Diffusion of Information about Neurofibromatosis Type 1 DNA Testing," *American Journal of Medical Genetics* 49, no. 3 (February 1994): 299–301.

37. NF is frequently, but erroneously, referred to as "Elephant Man's Disease," named after the nineteenth-century Londoner Joseph Merrick. Merrick did not have NF, but a cranial disease, Proteus syndrome. Information on the symptoms and manifestations of NF is drawn from materials from Neurofibromatosis, Inc., a national support group for NF.

38. K. A. Crandall, J. G. Edwards, and V. M. Riccardi, "Attitudes of Individuals Affected with Neurofibromatosis toward Prenatal Diagnosis," *American Journal of Human Genetics* 43, no. 3, supplement (September 1988): A165.

39. Bracie Watson, Roswell Eldridge, Karen Stewart, Sandra Schlesinger, Dilys M. Parry, James Dambrosia, and John Mulvihill, "Neurofibromatosis 1: Attitudes toward Predictive Genetic Testing," draft, Neuroepidemiology Branch, National Institute of Neurological Disorders and Stroke, National Institutes of Health, Bethesda, Md., August 1990.

40. Watson et al., "Attitudes toward Predictive Genetic Testing," table 10, p. 22. Unlike NF-1, Huntington's does not manifest itself until early middle age—usually after childbearing has occurred. It is progressively debilitating, and eventually fatal.

41. J. B. Bernier, D. L. Meryash, and N. V. Ahmad, "Attitudes toward Prenatal Diagnosis among Mothers of Children with Spina Bifida (SB)," abstract, *American Journal of Human Genetics* 45, no. 4, supplement (October 1989): A119; and D. L. Meryash, J. B. Bernier, and N. V. Ahmad, "Perception of Burden among Mothers of Children with Spina Bifida (SB) of Raising an Affected Child," ibid., p. A123.

42. Denise M. Main and Michael T. Mennuti, "Neural Tube Defects: Issues in Prenatal Diagnosis and Counseling," *Obstetrics and Gynecology* 67, no. 1 (January 1986): 1–16.

43. In the study cited earlier in which 21 of 27 women chose to terminate SB

fetuses, only five of the fetuses had cranial lesions, indicating the most severe form of SB. Grevengood et al., "Severity of Abnormality."

44. Caroline Mansfield, Suellen Hopfer, and Theresa M. Marteau, "Termination Rates after Prenatal Diagnosis of Down Syndrome, Spina Bifida, Anencephaly, and Turner and Klinefelter Syndromes: A Systematic Literature Review," *Prenatal Diagnosis* 19, no. 9 (September 1999): 808–12.

45. Testing and selecting for sex retains its medical rationale for the rarer X-linked conditions whose causes have not been identified. In these cases it is done by preimplantation genetic diagnosis. See discussion below.

46. "New Chinese Law Prohibits Sex-Screening of Fetuses," *New York Times,* November 15, 1994, p. A5.

47. Philip Shenon, "A Chinese Bias against Girls Creates Surplus of Bachelors," *New York Times,* August 16, 1994, pp. A1, A8.

48. Edward A. Gargan, "Ultrasound Skews India's Birth Ratio," *New York Times,* December 13, 1991, p. A13.

49. See Nicholas D. Kristof, "Stark Data on Women: 100 Million Are Missing," *New York Times,* November 5, 1991, pp. C1, C12, which documents the birth rates in favor of boys in several Asian countries, as well as Egypt; Sheryl WuDunn, "Korean Women Still Feel Demands to Bear a Son," *New York Times,* January 14, 1997, p. A3; Celia W. Dugger, "Abortions in India Spurred by Sex Test Skew the Ratio against Girls," *New York Times,* April 22, 2001, p. 12; and Celia W. Dugger, "Modern Asia's Anomaly: The Girls Who Don't Get Born," *New York Times,* May 6, 2001, sec. 4, p. 4. See also David Rohde, "India Steps Up Effort to Halt Abortions of Female Fetuses," *New York Times,* October 26, 2003, p. 3.

50. Dorothy C. Wertz and John C. Fletcher, "Fatal Knowledge? Prenatal Diagnosis and Sex Selection," *Hastings Center Report* 19, no. 3 (May–June 1989): 21–27.

51. Ethics Committee, American Society for Reproductive Medicine, "Sex Selection and Preimplantation Genetic Diagnosis," *Fertility & Sterility* 72, no. 4 (October 1999): 595–98. The three cases disapproved were when the patient undergoing IVF asks that sex be added to the list of conditions to be diagnosed, when the IVF patient requests PGD solely for sex identification, and when the patient requests both IVF and PGD solely for sex identification. Among the committee's reasons for objecting is the unwarranted diversion of medical resources. Sex identification was allowable only if the information was obtained as part of or a by-product of PGD performed for medical reasons.

52. Ethics Committee, American Society for Reproductive Medicine, "Preconception Gender Selection for Nonmedical Reasons," *Fertility & Sterility* 75, no. 5 (May 2001): 861–64.

53. U.S. Congress, Office of Technology Assessment, *Artificial Insemination: Practice in the United States: Summary of a 1987 Survey.* Background Paper OTA-BP-BA-48 (Washington, D.C.: U.S. Government Printing Office, August 1988). No similarly comprehensive report seems to have been issued since. The OTA no longer exists.

54. American Fertility Society, "New Guidelines for the Use of Semen Donor Insemination: 1990," *Fertility & Sterility* 53, supplement 1 (March 1990): S1–S13.

55. American Society for Reproductive Medicine, "2002 Guidelines for Gamete and Embryo Donation," *Fertility & Sterility* 77, no. 6 (June 2002): S1–S16. Recommendations for minimal genetic screening are in appendix A, p. S15.

56. Mary E. Guinan, "Artificial Insemination by Donor: Safety and Secrecy," *Journal of the American Medical Association* 273, no. 11 (March 15, 1995): 890–91; E. A. Conrad, B. Fine, B. R. Hecht, and E. Pergament, "Current Practices of Commercial Cryobanks in Screening Prospective Donors for Genetic Disease and Reproductive Risk," *International Journal of Fertility and Menopausal Studies* 41, no. 3 (May–June 1996): 298–303; and J. K. Critser, "Current Status of Semen Banking in the USA," *Human Reproduction* 13, supplement 2 (May 1998): 55–67, 68–69. Critser anticipates that the Food and Drug Administration will require registration of all donor banks, to be followed by mandatory inspection and accreditation. See also D. B. Resnik, "Regulating the Market for Human Eggs," *Bioethics* 15, no. 1 (February 2001): 1–25.

57. U.S. Congress, Office of Technology Assessment, *Artificial Insemination,* pp. 40–41.

58. There is a bias for married couples with a male infertility problem as candidates for insemination performed by physicians. According to the OTA report, more than 90 percent of women seeking insemination "present themselves" to their physicians "as married or living with a man." Ibid., p. 23. Indeed, the major non-medical reason for rejecting an applicant is that she is unmarried. Ibid., p. 27.

59. See, for example, Judith N. Lasker and Susan Borg, *In Search of Parenthood: Coping with Infertility and High-Tech Conception* (Boston: Beacon, 1987), pp. 111, 189–90. My own telephone inquiries of sperm banks confirm this. One respondent (not a physician) who cited the importance of intelligence to me in a phone interview saw "no problem" because all of their donors were college or graduate students!

60. U.S. Congress, Office of Technology Assessment, *Artificial Insemination,* p. 40. Whether or not physicians believed that such abilities (in music or other creative arts, for example) were at all inheritable was not probed in the study, nor were their views about the degree of inheritability of intelligence. Their agreeing to match for such traits could be interpreted as a matter of pleasing their clients rather than necessarily sharing parents' acceptance of genetic determinism.

61. The Repository for Germinal Choice was established in 1979 by Robert Klark Graham, the developer of shatterproof plastic eyeglass lenses. He and the repository came under criticism for trying to foster a superior race. Embarrassment followed the news that one of the first women who became pregnant with sperm from this bank had a criminal record. Graham died in February 1997 at the age of 90. See obituary in *New York Times,* February 18, 1997, p. B7. The sperm bank closed its doors two years later.

62. So-called surrogate mothers are not "surrogates," but the real mothers

since their egg is used, they are impregnated, and they carry the child to term. *Surrogate* is only appropriate if a woman carries an embryo that is not her own, as in a case reported in California in 1990, for example.

63. Lasker and Borg, *In Search of Parenthood,* pp. 111–12.

64. Rene Almeling, "Gendering Commodification: How Egg Donation Agencies and Sperm Banks Structure Medical Markets in Genetic Material," M.A. thesis, Department of Sociology, UCLA, 2004.

65. Five years after the *New York Times* reported on egg-selling in 1991, the practice became widespread enough to raise ethical concerns. See Gina Kolata, "Young Women Offer to Sell Their Eggs to Infertile Couples," *New York Times,* November 10, 1991, pp. 1, 30; and Jan Hoffman, "Egg Donations Meet a Need and Raise Ethical Questions," *New York Times,* January 8, 1996, pp. 1, 10. By late 1997, embryos had entered the marketplace. Kolata's "Clinics Selling Embryos Made for 'Adoption'" (*New York Times,* November 23, 1997, pp. 1, 34) indicated that some selection for ancestry was possible. Web sites were the next step, such as the Options National Fertility Registry, which advertised sperm and egg donors meeting various physical specifications: Gina Kolata, "Infertile Foreigners See Opportunity in U.S.," *New York Times,* January 4, 1998, pp. 1, 15. In 1998 the American Society for Reproductive Medicine estimated that 6,000 women in the U.S. had given birth using donor eggs: Sheryl Gay Stolberg, "Quandary on Donor Eggs: What to Tell the Children," *New York Times,* January 18, 1998, pp. 1, 20. See also Gina Kolata, "$50,000 Offered to Tall, Smart Egg Donor," *New York Times,* March 3, 1999, p. A10; and Joseph Berger, "Yale Gene Pool Seen as Route to Better Baby," *New York Times,* January 10, 1999, p. 19.

66. A British survey in 1994 of almost 1,000 members of the general public of childbearing age found respondents more willing to test prenatally and terminate the pregnancy to eliminate certain diseases and characteristics, ranking them in the process, while less willing to enhance or prevent specific characteristics by gene therapy. Researchers pointed out, however, that the proportion supporting gene therapy for enhancement had doubled in the year since the public was last polled. Theresa Marteau, Susan Michie, Harriet Drake, and Martin Bobrow, "Public Attitudes towards the Selection of Desirable Characteristics in Children," *Journal of Medical Genetics* 32, no. 10 (October 1995): 796–98.

67. As evidence mounts that defective sperm can be a key cause of defects in the offspring, this fixing of blame becomes untenable on more than social and emotional grounds. Aging sperm, older fathers, and men's exposure to various toxins are cited. See Patricia A. Martin-DeLeon and Mary B. Williams, "Sexual Behavior and Down Syndrome: The Biological Mechanism," *American Journal of Medical Genetics* 27, no. 3 (July 1987): 693–700; Natalie Angier, "Genetic Mutations Tied to Father in Most Cases," *New York Times,* May 17, 1994, p. C12, which cites the continuing cell division for sperm and therefore faster mutation rate; Tamar Lewin, "Ask Not for Whom the Clock Ticks," *New York Times,* April 15, 2001, sec. 4, p. 4; and Sandra Blakeslee, "Research on Birth Defects Shifts to Flaws in Sperm," *New York Times,* January 1, 1991, pp. 1, 36, on exposure to toxins. A

French study of trisomy 21 (Down syndrome) found that the extra chromosome came from the father in 11 percent of the cases, significantly higher than the percentage found in previous studies: Muller et al., "Parental Origin of the Extra Chromosome."

68. Carol Levine, "Genetic Counseling: The Client's Viewpoint," in Capron et al., *Genetic Counseling*, 123–25.

69. Joan O. Weiss, "Genetic Counseling: A Social Worker's View," *Hospital Practice* 18, no. 3 (March 1983): 40H. A social worker when this was written, Weiss subsequently became coordinator of the Alliance of Genetic Support Groups (see discussion in chapter 9).

70. R. Neil Schimke, "Genetic Counseling: The Physician's Experience," *Hospital Practice* 18, no. 3 (March 1983): 38.

71. Regina Kenen and Robert Schmidt, "Stigmatization of Carrier Status: Implications of Screening Programs," *American Journal of Public Health* 68, no. 11 (July 1978): 1116–20.

72. Jessica G. Davis, "A Counselor's Viewpoint," in Capron et al., *Genetic Counseling*, 120.

73. Eleanor Gordon Applebaum and Stephen K. Firestein, *A Counseling Casebook* (New York: Free Press, 1983), p. 2.

74. Ray M. Antley and Lawrence C. Hartlage, "Psychological Responses to Genetic Counseling for Down's Syndrome," *Clinical Genetics* 9, no. 3 (March 1976): 257–65.

75. Beth Blodgett, Patricia Daugherty, Neita McClure, Karen J. Miller, Eileen Van Schaik, and Joseph Engelberg, "Spina Bifida: Family Therapy," *Hospital Practice* 23, no. 6 (June 15, 1988): 190.

7. DISCOURSES OF THE IMPERFECT

1. The *Eugenics Quarterly* appears to have introduced the term "Down's Syndrome" in the September 1963 issue in an article by Sheldon Reed on genetic counseling. See Sheldon Reed, "Down's Syndrome (Mongolism)," *Eugenics Quarterly* 10, no. 3 (September 1963): 139–42. "Down's" is used throughout the article. However, in the indexes to volumes 12 (1965) and 13 (1966), the entry "Down's Syndrome" is followed by "See Mongolism," (pp. 268 and 381 respectively). While the Down's entry in the index for volume 15 (1968) stands alone (p. 310), discussion of an abstract with "Down's" in the title uses the term "Mongolism" rather than "Down's Syndrome" (p. 218).

2. Kenneth Keniston, foreword to *The Unexpected Minority: Handicapped Children in America*, by John Gliedman and William Roth (New York: Harcourt Brace Jovanovich, 1980), p. iii.

3. Marsha Saxton, "Born and Unborn: The Implications of Reproductive Technologies for People with Disabilities," in *Test-Tube Women*, ed. Arditti, Klein, and Minden, pp. 299, 307.

4. Barbara M. Altman, "Studies of Attitudes toward the Handicapped: The Need for a New Direction," *Social Problems* 28, no. 3 (February 1981): 323.

5. Harlan Hahn, "Paternalism and Public Policy," *Society* 20, no. 3 (March–April 1983): 44.

6. Robert Funk, "Disability Rights: From Caste to Class in the Context of Civil Rights," in *Images of the Disabled, Disabling Images*, ed. Alan Gartner and Tom Joe (New York: Praeger, 1987), pp. 22–23.

7. Erving Goffman, *Stigma: Notes on the Management of Spoiled Identity* (Englewood Cliffs, N.J.: Prentice Hall, 1963), pp. 5, 9.

8. Stuart Oskamp, "The Editor's Page," in "Moving Disability beyond 'Stigma,'" ed. Adrienne Asch and Michelle Fine, special issue, *Journal of Social Issues* 44, no. 1 (1988). The Americans with Disabilities Act of 1990 defines a person with a disability as someone with "a physical or mental impairment that substantially limits one or more of the major life activities of such individual." Quoted in Mitchell P. LaPlante, "How Many Americans Have a Disability?" Disabilities Statistics Abstract 5 (San Francisco: Disability Statistics Rehabilitation Research and Training Center, June 1992), p. 1.

9. William Roth, "Handicap as a Social Construct," *Society* 20, no. 3 (March–April 1983): 56–61.

10. Funk, "Disability Rights," p. 14.

11. Ibid., p. 22.

12. Alan Gartner and Tom Joe, introduction to *Images of the Disabled*, p. 5.

13. Rosalyn Benjamin Darling and Jon Darling, *Children Who Are Different: Meeting the Challenge of Birth Defects in Society* (St. Louis: C. V. Mosby, 1982), pp. 43–44; see also pp. 214–19.

14. Douglas Biklen, "Framed: Print Journalism's Treatment of Disability Issues," in Gartner and Joe, *Images of the Disabled*, pp. 79–95.

15. Darling and Darling, *Children Who Are Different*, p. 45.

16. Lee Meyerson, "The Social Psychology of Physical Disability: 1948 and 1988," in Asch and Fine, "Moving Disability beyond 'Stigma,'" 186–87. A study in the early 1970s had found "essential equivalence in life satisfaction for handicapped, retarded, and normal persons," indicating that at least some clinical psychologists held a different view; evidently that view did not prevail. See Paul Cameron, Donna Gnadinger Titus, John Kostin, and Marilyn Kostin, "The Life Satisfaction of Nonnormal Persons," *Journal of Consulting and Clinical Psychology* 41, no. 2 (October 1973): 207–14.

17. Goffman, *Stigma*, pp. 3–5. For a useful summary of the literature on stigma see Lerita M. Coleman, "Stigma: An Enigma Demystified," in *The Disability Studies Reader*, ed. Lennard J. Davis (New York: Routledge, 1997), pp. 216–31.

18. Gliedman and Roth, *The Unexpected Minority*, pp. 374–75.

19. Leslie Fiedler, "The Tyranny of the Normal," in *Tyranny of the Normal: Essays on Bioethics, Theology & Myth* (Boston: David R. Godine, 1996), p. 152. This essay was originally published in 1984. See also his *Freaks: Myths and Images of the Secret Self* (1977; reprint, New York: Anchor, 1993).

20. Harlan Hahn, "The Politics of Physical Differences: Disability and Discrimination," in Asch and Fine, "Moving Disability beyond 'Stigma,'" 43.

21. Kaoru Yamamoto, "To Be Different," *Rehabilitation Counseling Bulletin* 14, no. 3 (March 1971): 182, 186.

22. Paul K. Longmore, "Screening Stereotypes: Images of Disabled People in Television and Motion Pictures," in Gartner and Joe, *Images of the Disabled*, p. 66. This paragraph and the next quote and paraphrase Longmore, pp. 66–70.

23. Interestingly enough, a musical play about Siamese twins, *Side Show*, which opened on Broadway in the 1997–98 season, flopped at the box office. It was based on the lives of the Hilton sisters, who performed in sideshows and films in the 1920s and '30s. Audiences, it seemed, could not accept the production's light musical approach, which treated their lives as near-normal, not dwelling on the difficulties of their "plight."

24. Leslie Fiedler, "Pity and Fear: Images of the Disabled in Literature and the Popular Arts," in Fiedler, *Tyranny of the Normal*, pp. 44, 46. The essay was originally published in 1982.

25. Bogdan, *Freak Show*, pp. x–xi, 280–81.

26. Robert Bogdan and Douglas Biklen, "Handicapism," *Social Policy* 7, no. 5 (March–April 1977): 16–17.

27. Longmore, "Screening Stereotypes," pp. 75–78.

28. Georgia Dullea, "Opening the World to a Generation," *New York Times*, October 12, 1989, pp. C1, C6.

29. Funk, "Disability Rights," pp. 23–24.

30. David Hevey, "The Enfreakment of Photography," in Davis, *Disability Studies Reader*, pp. 345, 346.

31. Hahn, "Politics of Physical Differences," p. 42.

32. Goffman, *Stigma*, p. 4.

33. Hanoch Livneh, "On the Origins of Negative Attitudes toward People with Disabilities," *Rehabilitation Literature* 43, nos. 11–12 (November–December 1982): 341.

34. Hahn, "Politics of Physical Differences," p. 44.

35. Roth, "Handicap as a Social Construct," p. 56.

36. Constantina Safilios-Rothschild, *The Sociology and Social Psychology of Disability and Rehabilitation* (New York: Random House, 1970), p. 5.

37. Stephen A. Richardson, Norman Goodman, Albert H. Hastorf, and Sanford M. Dornbusch, "Cultural Uniformity in Reaction to Physical Disabilities," *American Sociological Review* 26 (1961): 241–77; and Altman, "Studies of Attitudes," pp. 323–24.

38. Richardson et al., "Cultural Uniformity," pp. 246–47.

39. Stephen A. Richardson, "Age and Sex Differences in Values toward Physical Handicaps," *Journal of Health and Social Behavior* 11, no. 3 (September 1970): 207–14. Thirty years later obesity rates have climbed alarmingly; with at least one-quarter of all children in the U.S. now classified obese, such opinions may no longer hold.

40. Barbara Altman's careful review of studies of attitudes toward the handicapped cautions about certain limitations of these studies, such as their survey of

limited populations (mainly students), their use of stereotyped conditions as attitude objects, and their concentration on the more severe disabilities. Altman, "Studies of Attitudes."

41. Funk, "Disability Rights," p. 25.

42. The craze for fitness and perfect health, as noted in chapter 2, has a considerable history in American society. Harvey Green, pointing out how notions about gender, race, sex, and beauty evolved in the course of the nineteenth and twentieth centuries, explores why we remain obsessed by pursuing the perfect body today. See Harvey Green, *Fit for America: Health, Fitness, Sport, and American Society* (New York: Pantheon, 1986).

43. Rhoda Unger ascribes the first to K. K. Dion et al. 1972, the second to Gross and Crofton 1977. Rhoda Kesler Unger, "Personal Appearance and Social Control," in *Women's Worlds: From the New Scholarship*, ed. Marilyn Safir, Martha T. Mednick, Dafna Israeli, and Jessie Bernard (New York: Praeger, 1985): pp. 143, 148.

44. Ibid., pp. 143–46.

45. See Michelle Fine and Adrienne Asch, eds., *Women with Disabilities: Essays in Psychology, Culture, and Politics* (Philadelphia: Temple University Press, 1988), and further discussion in chapter 9.

46. Safilios-Rothschild, *Disability and Rehabilitation*, pp. 126–27.

47. Ibid., p. 127.

48. Lewis Anthony Dexter, "On the Politics and Sociology of Stupidity in Our Society," in *The Other Side: Perspectives on Deviance*, ed. Howard S. Becker (New York: Free Press, 1967), pp. 42–43. Becker's book has become a classic on deviance.

49. Robert Bogdan and Steven J. Taylor, *Inside Out: The Social Meaning of Mental Retardation* (Toronto; Buffalo, N.Y.: University of Toronto Press, 1982), pp. 6–8, 14, and passim.

50. Darwin, *The Descent of Man*, pp. 133–34, quoted in Greene, *Death of Adam*, p. 332; see also Greene, *Darwin and the Modern World View*.

51. See discussion in Greene, *Death of Adam*, pp. 332–34.

52. Dobzhansky, *Mankind Evolving*, p. 332.

53. Harlan Hahn, "Civil Rights for Disabled Americans: The Foundation of a Political Agenda," in Gartner and Joe, *Images of the Disabled*, p. 200.

54. Much of the material in this review comes from Reilly, *Surgical Solution*, as well as from Robitscher, *Powers of Psychiatry*, and from the legal sources cited below. See especially Reilly, *Surgical Solution*, pp. 94–95, for a summary of statistics.

55. Dunn, "Eugenic Sterilization Statutes," p. 280; and Richard K. Sherlock and Robert D. Sherlock, "Sterilizing the Retarded: Constitutional, Statutory and Policy Alternatives," *North Carolina Law Review* 60, no. 5 (June 1982): 946.

56. See discussion in "Appendix: American College of Obstetricians and Gynecologists Ethics Committee Statement: Sterilization of Women Who Are Mentally Handicapped," in Evans, Fletcher, et al., *Fetal Diagnosis and Therapy*, pp.

110–13. Designed "to provide background and guidance to the Fellows of ACOG," the statement points out in bold type, "Furthermore, the presence of a mental handicap alone does not, in itself, justify either sterilization or its denial" (p. 110), and sets out considerations that are "in the best interest of the patient" (p. 113).

Reports of government programs of forced sterilization for eugenic reasons in Scandinavia, which continued into the 1970s, surfaced in the mid-1990s. From 1935 to 1976 in Sweden, 60,000 women were sterilized as genetically or racially inferior, a category including the very poor, the learning-disabled, those of non-Nordic backgrounds. Finland sterilized 11,000 people with qualities such as poor eyesight and Gypsy features. "Swedish Scandal," editorial, *New York Times,* August 30, 1997, p. 22; Nicholas Wade, "Testing Genes to Save a Life without Costing You a Job," *New York Times,* September 14, 1997, sec. 4. p. 5. In France, it was alleged that 15,000 women "deemed mentally or physically inferior were sterilized without their consent." "15,000 Frenchwomen Reportedly Sterilized," *New York Times,* September 11, 1996, p. A4. Under a law passed in 1948 and revoked only in 1996 in Japan, doctors could "sterilize people with mental or physical handicaps or certain hereditary diseases without their consent"; from 1949 to 1995, 16,520 women were sterilized under this law. "Japan Says Forced Sterilizations Merit No Payments, No Apology," *New York Times,* September 18, 1997, p. A12. Since the late 1980s, China has had eugenics legislation in place to use sterilization to "improve the population quality" and "avoid new births of inferior quality." Nicholas D. Kristof, "Some Chinese Provinces Forcing Sterilization of Retarded Couples," *New York Times,* August 15, 1991, pp. A1, A8; and "Preventing 'Inferior' People in China," editorial, *New York Times,* December 27, 1993, p. A16, which called on the Clinton administration to respond. See also "Chinese Deal Sparks Eugenics Protests," *New Scientist,* November 16, 1996, p. 4, reprinted in *GeneWatch* 10, nos. 4–5 (February 1997): 2, 5, on protests against a French company's plans to research genetic diseases among the Chinese.

57. Kristin Luker, *Abortion and the Politics of Motherhood* (Berkeley: University of California Press, 1984), chapters 3 and 4 (from which much of the discussion in this section is drawn). Luker cites a small survey of physicians in the South in 1930 showed that one-third approved of aborting for a " 'dominant hereditary taint in both parents' " (p. 47).

58. Robert E. Hall, "Therapeutic Abortion, Sterilization, and Contraception," *American Journal of Obstetrics and Gynecology* 91 (February 15, 1965): 518–32; and J. J. Rovinsky and S. B. Gusberg, "Current Trends in Therapeutic Termination of Pregnancy," *American Journal of Obstetrics and Gynecology* 98, no. 1 (May 1, 1967): 11–17. Performing abortions for fetal indications was by no means uncontroversial.

59. Luker, *Politics of Motherhood,* pp. 69, 278 n. 7. As described by Luker, the American Law Institute was "a national nonprofit organization" composed of judges, lawyers, and law professors whose goal was "to 'modernize' American law."

60. Interestingly enough, the provision was deleted from the final version of

the law passed in California, the state that spearheaded reform efforts and which had extensive press coverage of the Finkbine case. The fetal deformity provision was removed at the request of then governor Ronald Reagan, in response to anti-abortionist demands.

61. Luker, *Politics of Motherhood*, pp. 89, 122. From extensive interviews conducted for her book, Luker concluded that the fetal indications provisions continued to be "the least ideologically tolerable," a virtual anathema, to activists opposing abortion. The issue cut to the deepest level of the personhood of the fetus, suggesting the "idea that humans can be ranked along some scale of perfection," excluding those that fall below a certain standard. She predicted that anti-choicers would remain intransigent on this, citing their strong opposition to amniocentesis as an example. Ibid., p. 236.

62. George Gallup, *The Gallup Poll* 1, no. 3 (1959–71): 1784, as cited in Luker, *Politics of Motherhood*, pp. 82, 280 n. 20.

63. Donald Granberg and Beth Wellman Granberg, "Abortion Attitudes, 1965–1980: Trends and Determinants," *Family Planning Perspectives* 12, no. 5 (September–October 1980): 252.

64. The *Webster* decision in 1989 returned some power to regulate abortion to the states. *Casey* in 1992 changed the standard of Roe from no restrictions to those not placing an "undue burden" on the woman. *Webster v. Reproductive Health Services,* 109 S.Ct. 3040, 3077–3079 (1989); and *Planned Parenthood of Southeastern Pennsylvania v. Casey* 112 S.Ct. 2791 (1992). In 2003, Congress passed and President Bush signed the so-called "Partial-Birth Abortion Law" placing restrictions on certain late-term abortions, in effect attempting to redefine the point of viability.

65. Gliedman and Roth, *The Unexpected Minority*, p. 376.

66. Michael J. Begab, "The Major Dilemma of Mental Retardation: Shall We Prevent It?" *American Journal of Mental Deficiency* 78, no. 5 (March 1974): 519, 524.

67. See Abby Lippman, "Prenatal Genetic Testing and Screening: Constructing Needs and Reinforcing Inequities," *American Journal of Law and Medicine* 17, nos. 1–2 (1991): 15–50. Lippman coined the term *geneticization.*

68. Gliedman and Roth, *The Unexpected Minority*, p. 302.

69. Infirmities of age, rather, increase the likelihood of having a disability, the person joining the one in five Americans with a disability, or the more than one in ten with a disability classed as severe. Using statistics from the 1996 Survey of Income and Program Participation (SIPP), the U.S. Census Bureau reports that in 1997, out of a "population of 267.7 million noninstitutionalized individuals" aged 15 and older, "52.6 million (or 19.7 percent) had some type of disability. Among those with a disability, 33.0 million (or 12.3 percent) had a severe disability." The Census Bureau follows the Americans with Disabilities Act of 1990 in defining disability as "a substantial limitation in a major life activity." U.S. Census Bureau, "Americans with Disabilities: 1997," March 1, 2001, available on line at http://www.census.gov/hhes/www/disable/sipp/disable97.html, accessed September 20, 2004.

This Census Bureau report, however, does not include children. According to the Disability Statistics Research and Training Center in San Francisco, four million children under 18, or 6.1 percent, have a disability. We might estimate that perhaps one million of these disabilities are due to birth defects. Barbara L. Wenger, H. Stephen Kaye, and Mitchell LaPlante, "Disabilities among Children," Disabilities Statistics Abstract 15 (San Francisco: Disability Statistics Rehabilitation Research and Training Center, September 1997).

70. National Center on Birth Defects and Developmental Disabilities, *Birth Defects: Frequently Asked Questions* (National Center on Birth Defects and Developmental Disabilities, Centers for Disease Control, 2002).

71. Birth Defects Prevention Act of 1998, Public Law 105-68. Among the programs are a campaign to educate the public on the benefits of folic acid (to prevent NTDs), projects in cooperation with the National Birth Defects Prevention Network, including a national program for birth defects surveillance, and informational campaigns on the detrimental effects of alcohol and smoking.

72. Deborah Kaplan, "Prenatal Screening and Its Impact on Persons with Disabilities," *Clinical Obstetrics and Gynecology* 36, no. 3 (September 1993): 610.

73. Dana Canedy, "More Toys Are Reflecting Disabled Children's Needs," *New York Times*, December 25, 1997, pp. A1, D4; and Tamar Lewin, "Where All Doors Are Open for Disabled Students," *New York Times*, December 28, 1997, pp. 1, 20.

74. Steven A. Holmes, "In 4 Years, Disabilities Act Hasn't Improved Jobs Rate," *New York Times*, October 23, 1994, p. 22.

75. "Acceptance of Disability and Its Correlates," session 130, American Sociological Association Annual Meeting, New York City, August 17, 1996. I attended the session.

76. "A Disabled Child Is Seen More Likely to Be Abused," *New York Times*, October 7, 1993, p. A21.

77. Theresa M. Marteau, "Psychological Implications of Genetic Screening," in Evers-Kiebooms, Fryns, and Cassiman, *Psychosocial Aspects of Genetic Counseling*, 189.

78. Eleanor Singer, "Public Attitudes toward Genetic Testing," *Population Research and Policy Review* 10 (1991): 251. Singer's first conclusion was that "attitudes toward prenatal testing for genetic defects are overwhelmingly favorable at this time" (p. 250).

79. Shoshana Shiloh and Michael Berkenstadt, "Lay Conceptions of Genetic Disorders," in Evers-Kiebooms, Fryns, and Cassiman, *Psychosocial Aspects of Genetic Counseling*, 191–200.

80. Sociologist Troy Duster is especially concerned that eugenics might enter via the "back door," through government-mandated mass screenings aimed at various racially and ethnically designated target populations. See Troy Duster, *Backdoor to Eugenics* (New York: Routledge, 1990).

81. Lennard J. Davis, "Introduction: The Need for Disability Studies," in Davis, *Disability Studies Reader*, p. 5.

8. BIOETHICS DISCOURSE AND REPRODUCTIVE PRACTICE

1. LeRoy Walters and Tamar Joy Kahn, introduction to *Bibliography of Bioethics*, vol. 24 (Washington, D.C.: Kennedy Institute of Ethics, 1998), p. 3.

2. Joseph Fletcher, "Ethical Aspects of Genetic Controls: Designed Genetic Changes in Man," *New England Journal of Medicine* 285, no. 14 (September 30, 1971): 780–82. For a telling critique of this argument, see Richard A. McCormick, *How Brave a New World? Dilemmas in Bioethics* (Garden City, N.Y.: Doubleday, 1981).

3. Joseph Fletcher, "Ethics and Genetic Control," in *Medical Ethics: A Guide for Health Professionals,* ed. John F. Monagle and David C. Thomasma (Rockville, Md.: Aspen, 1988), p. 6.

4. Bentley Glass, "Human Heredity and Ethical Problems," *Perspectives in Biology and Medicine* 15, no. 2 (Winter 1972): 246–47.

5. Ibid., 252.

6. Bentley Glass, *Progress or Catastrophe: The Nature of Biological Science and Its Impact on Human Society* (New York: Praeger, 1985).

7. The symposium was held in Warrenton, Virginia, under the joint sponsorship of the John E. Fogarty International Center for Advanced Study at the National Institutes of Health and the Institute of Society, Ethics and the Life Sciences (later the Hastings Center). Following up an NIH-sponsored conference a year earlier on the impact of amniocentesis, symposium organizers sought to expand on that conference's largely medical orientation to produce a broad-based gathering of scholars and professionals from a wide range of fields. But participants were predominantly White, Western, and male—only eight women—and represented prestigious academic, medical, and research institutions, mostly in the United States. A professional gathering, no members of the general public attended. Bruce Hilton et al., eds., *Ethical Issues in Human Genetics: Genetic Counseling and the Use of Genetic Knowledge* (New York: Plenum, 1973). On the earlier conference, see Maureen Harris, ed., *Early Diagnosis of Human Genetic Defects: Scientific and Ethical Considerations* (Washington, D.C.: U.S. Government Printing Office, 1972).

8. Robert L. Sinsheimer, "Prospects for Future Scientific Developments: Ambush or Opportunity," in Hilton et al., *Ethical Issues in Human Genetics,* pp. 348–50. The Darwin Centennial was held in 1959. See chapter 3.

9. While not expressly ruling out genetic engineering, Sinsheimer questioned its ultimate application to redesigning human beings and human nature. He speculated whether, like splitting the atom, genetic engineering might not turn out to be "another Faustian bargain." Robert L. Sinsheimer, "Genetic Engineering and Gene Therapy: Some Implications," in *Genetic Issues in Public Health and Medicine,* ed. Bernice H. Cohen, Abraham M. Lilienfeld, and P. C. Huang (Springfield, Ill.: Charles C. Thomas, 1978), pp. 439, 456, and passim.

10. Robert L. Sinsheimer, "The Prospect of Designed Genetic Change," *American Scientist* 57, no. 1 (Spring 1969): 134–42; reprinted in *Ethics, Reproduction and Genetic Control,* ed. Ruth F. Chadwick (London: Croom Helm, 1987).

11. James V. Neel, "Social and Scientific Priorities in the Use of Genetic Knowledge," in Hilton et al., *Ethical Issues in Human Genetics,* pp. 353, 364, 361. The *New York Times* obituary for Dr. Neel, who died in 2000, quotes a colleague's appraisal that he "can be said to have birthed the field of human genetics." *New York Times,* February 3, 2000, p. C27.

12. Peter Condliffe and Daniel Callahan, preface to Hilton et al., *Ethical Issues in Human Genetics,* pp. x–xi.

13. Paul Ramsey, "Screening: An Ethicist's View," in Hilton et al., *Ethical Issues in Human Genetics,* p. 159.

14. Leon R. Kass, "Implications of Prenatal Diagnosis for the Human Right to Life," in Hilton et al., *Ethical Issues in Human Genetics,* pp. 191, 192, 198.

15. See Nicholas Wade, "Moralist of Science Ponders Its Power," *New York Times,* March 19, 2002, pp. F1, F2.

16. Judith Hall, "The Concerns of Doctors and Patients," in Hilton et al., *Ethical Issues in Human Genetics,* pp. 30, 31.

17. Jerome Lejeune, general discussion of "Survey of Counseling Practices," in Hilton et al., *Ethical Issues in Human Genetics,* pp. 17–22.

18. Ibid., p. 100.

19. Dr. Murray's remarks followed those of Sinsheimer and Neel. Robert Murray, "Screening: A Practitioner's View," in Hilton et al., *Ethical Issues in Human Genetics,* pp. 121–30.

20. David Eaton, discussion of presentations by Sinsheimer, Neel, and NIH representatives, in Hilton et al., *Ethical Issues in Human Genetics,* pp. 378–84.

21. David Eaton, "Decision-Making and the Interests of Minority Groups," and discussion following, in Hilton et al., *Ethical Issues in Human Genetics,* pp. 329–32.

22. The conference was co-sponsored by the Institute of Society, Ethics and the Life Sciences, the future Hastings Center. Research scientists were heavily represented, with many participants drawn from Harvard University or Harvard Medical School. Marc Lappé and Robert S. Morison, eds., *Ethical and Scientific Issues Posed by Human Uses of Molecular Genetics* (New York: New York Academy of Sciences, 1976).

23. Jon Beckwith, "Social and Political Uses of Genetics in the United States: Past and Present," in Lappé and Morison, *Ethical and Scientific Issues,* p. 53. Such decisions, he continued, "are a natural result of a series of distorted values influencing the situation." The "criminal chromosome" later resurfaced as the "criminal gene," when in 1992 NIH withdrew funds from a planned conference at the University of Maryland entitled "Genetic Factors in Crime: Findings, Uses and Implications." Daniel Goleman, "New Storm Brews on Whether Crime Has Roots in Genes," *New York Times,* September 15, 1992, pp. C1, C7. But in 1995, another such conference, "The Meaning and Significance of Research on Genetics and Criminal Behavior," did take place at the university; see criticism by Dorothy Nelkin, "Biology Is Not Destiny," *New York Times,* September 28, 1995, p. A27.

24. Beckwith, "Social and Political Uses of Genetics," in Lappé and Morison, *Ethical and Scientific Issues,* pp. 53–54.

25. A 1974 publication resulting from two years of deliberations by the Genetics Group of the Institute of Society, Ethics and the Life Sciences did pay more attention to reproductive issues. More tightly focused than other symposia in which many of these physicians, varied health professionals, research scientists, ethicists, lawyers, and philosophers also participated, the ethical discussions concentrated on mass and carrier screening, signaling the kind of bioethics specialization that would occur in the next decade. Daniel Bergsma, with Marc Lappé, Richard Roblin, and James M. Gustafson, eds., *Ethical, Social and Legal Dimensions of Screening for Human Genetic Disease,* Birth Defects Original Article Series 10, no. 6 (New York: Stratton Intercontinental Medical Book Corp., 1974).

26. Ramsey, "Screening," in Hilton et al., *Ethical Issues in Human Genetics,* p. 159.

27. Daniel Callahan, "The Meaning and Significance of Genetic Disease: Philosophical Perspectives," in Hilton et al., *Ethical Issues in Human Genetics,* pp. 86–87. Yet, despite the language of concern, Ramsey and Callahan used stigmatizing labels such as "defectives" and "abnormals." The terms "mongolism" and "mongoloid" were still used by conference participants rather than "Down syndrome." While there was less sensitivity to such language at the time, the tenor of symposium discussions remained that of "us" and "them."

28. Ramsey found that "aversion to abnormality" and "society's repulsion to disease" were reflected in the labeling of some persons as unacceptable. Ramsey, "Screening," in Hilton et al., *Ethical Issues in Human Genetics,* p. 159.

29. Callahan, "Meaning and Significance of Genetic Disease," in Hilton et al., *Ethical Issues in Human Genetics,* pp. 86, 88, 89.

30. At a panel discussing the implications of prenatal diagnosis for the right to human life, Peter Condliffe, one of the symposium planners, remarked how few women were participating there and at similar conferences. "Here we are discussing abortion without a single woman on the panel." He called on the panel to remember this, since especially "when it comes to abortion," women "have the star role." Peter Condliffe, "Discussion," in Hilton et al., *Ethical Issues in Human Genetics,* p. 214. He also noted the lack of practicing obstetricians at the symposium. Theologian and ethicist John Fletcher was alone among the ethicists in drawing on the actual experiences of patients, basing his talk on interviews with women undergoing amniocentesis and with their partners. John Fletcher, "Parents in Genetic Counseling: The Moral Shape of Decision-Making," ibid., pp. 301–27.

31. The conference proceedings were published as *Genetic Responsibility: On Choosing Our Children's Genes,* ed. Mack Lipkin, Jr., and Peter T. Rowley (New York: Plenum, 1974). The symposium, sponsored by the Task Force on Genetics and Reproduction at Yale and the Youth Council of the AAAS, consisted of four panels on the theme "On Choosing Our Children's Genes." The range of topics included a review of progress and problems in medical genetics, genetic counsel-

ing and screening, the impact on society, and how decision-making institutions could be made to face long-term consequences of individual genetic choices. In addition to the physicians, scientists, social scientists, theologians, lawyers, and policy makers participating on the panels, attending academics from a number of different fields brought lively, often radical critique to the proceedings.

32. John Fletcher, "Genetics, Choice and Society," in Lipkin and Rowley, *Genetic Responsibility*, pp. 95, 98. At this early stage, Fletcher was more willing than other moderates to take a position on prenatal diagnosis, stating he could not approve of social policy "promoting abortion" as a "long-range strategy" for "genetically defective fetuses. . . . The healing and not the elimination of handicapped human life should be our goal" (p. 96). Fletcher was specifically opposing the views that biologist Garrett Hardin and economist Thomas Schelling expressed at the symposium.

33. James R. Sorenson, "Sociological and Psychological Factors in Applied Human Genetics," in Hilton et al., *Ethical Issues in Human Genetics*, p. 298.

34. President's Commission for the Study of Ethical Problems in Medicine and Biomedical and Behavioral Research, *Screening and Counseling for Genetic Conditions: A Report on the Ethical, Social and Legal Implications of Genetic Screening, Counseling, and Educational Programs* (Washington, D.C.: U.S. Government Printing Office, 1983).

35. Capron et al., *Genetic Counseling*.

36. The first volume was published in 1976, presenting the proceedings of a national "Genetics and the Law" symposium in Boston in 1975. Aubrey Milunsky and George J. Annas, eds., *Genetics and the Law* (New York: Plenum, 1976). Authors included physicians and research scientists as well as lawyers.

37. Sherman Elias and George J. Annas, *Reproductive Genetics and the Law* (Chicago: Year Book Medical Publishers, 1987).

38. John C. Fletcher, "What Are Society's Interests in Human Genetics and Reproductive Technologies?" *Law, Medicine and Health Care* 16, nos. 1–2 (Spring–Summer 1988): 131–37.

39. See, for example, John Robertson, "Embryo Research," *University of Western Ontario Law Review* 24, no. 1 (June 1986): 15–37. In the 1990s, see his *Children of Choice: Freedom and the New Reproductive Technologies* (Princeton, N.J.: Princeton University Press, 1994). Robertson is a professor in the School of Law at the University of Texas.

40. Karen Lebacqz, "The Ghosts Are on the Wall: A Parable for Manipulating Life," in *The Manipulation of Life*, ed. Robert Esbjornson (New York: Harper & Row, 1984), pp. 22–41.

41. The international Human Genome Organization was founded in 1988 in Switzerland; the U.S. portion, the Human Genome Project (HGP), was established in 1990. See below.

42. Edward M. Berger and Bernard M. Gert, "Genetic Disorders and the Ethical Status of Germ-Line Gene Therapy," *Journal of Medicine and Philosophy*

16, no. 6 (December 1991): 667. The issue was guest-edited by Eric T. Juengst, then the director of ELSI, the ethics program of the Human Genome Project.

43. John Fletcher, "Ethical Issues in and beyond Prospective Clinical Trials of Human Gene Therapy," *Journal of Medicine and Philosophy* 10, no. 3 (August 1985): 306–309. The journal issue was devoted to the theme "Genetic and Reproductive Engineering," the articles including technical information about early human development, policy recommendations, a philosophical analysis of embryo and fetal personhood, and two on human gene therapy, one by Fletcher, the other by W. French Anderson. Dr. Anderson, chief of the Laboratory of Molecular Hematology at the National Heart, Lung, and Blood Institute of NIH, led the team that made the first successful trial of gene therapy in a human being. See chapter 4.

44. W. French Anderson, "Human Gene Therapy: Why Draw a Line?" *Journal of Medicine and Philosophy* 14, no. 6 (December 1989): 681–93.

45. Fletcher and Anderson suggested that the distinction be drawn between "corrective" and "enhancement" gene therapy rather than between somatic and germ-line therapy. Following the ethical principle of "beneficence," the criterion is, Will the use of gene therapy relieve "severe suffering," will it benefit the recipient, will it cure or prevent serious disease? (Anderson, "Why Draw a Line?"; John Fletcher, "Ethical Issues," 303–309). Anderson found somatic enhancement so medically hazardous and morally precarious as to be unacceptable. W. French Anderson, "Human Gene Therapy: Scientific and Ethical Considerations," *Journal of Medicine and Philosophy* 10, no. 3 (August 1985): 275–91.

46. "Germline Gene Therapy 'Must Be Spared Excessive Regulation,'" *Nature* 392, no. 6674 (March 26, 1998): 317. For further discussion of this symposium, see Gina Kolata, "Scientists Brace for Changes in Path of Human Evolution," *New York Times*, March 21, 1998, pp. A1, A12.

47. Burke K. Zimmerman, "Human Germ-Line Therapy: The Case for Its Development and Use," *Journal of Medicine and Philosophy* 16, no. 6 (December 1991): 593.

48. Ibid., p. 609.

49. Arthur L. Caplan, *Am I My Brother's Keeper? The Ethical Frontiers of Biomedicine* (Bloomington: Indiana University Press, 1997), pp. 190–91.

50. For a useful political analysis, showing the need for public inquiry, see Andrea L. Bonnicksen, "The Politics of Germline Therapy," *Nature Genetics* 19, no. 1 (May 1998): 10–11. See also a many-sided discussion in Audrey R. Chapman and Mark S. Frankel, eds., *Designing Our Descendants: The Promises and Perils of Genetic Modifications* (Baltimore: Johns Hopkins University Press, 2003).

51. Marc Lappé, "Ethical Issues in Manipulating the Human Germ Line," *Journal of Medicine and Philosophy* 16, no. 6 (December 1991): 638–39.

52. Berger and Gert, "Genetic Disorders," pp. 679–80.

53. David Resnik, "Debunking the Slippery Slope Argument against Human Germ-Line Gene Therapy," *Journal of Medicine and Philosophy* 19, no. 1 (February 1994): 38.

54. William Gardner, "Can Human Genetic Enhancement Be Prohibited?" *Journal of Medicine and Philosophy* 20, no. 1 (February 1995): 76.

55. Ibid., p. 80.

56. John C. Fletcher and Gerd Richter, "Human Fetal Gene Therapy: Moral and Ethical Questions," *Human Gene Therapy* 7, no. 13 (August 20, 1996): 1609. Edited by W. French Anderson, the journal *Human Gene Therapy* was established in 1990, marking the stepped-up pace of research and increasing interest in the field.

57. Caplan, *Am I My Brother's Keeper?* p. 210. In the preceding chapter Caplan had noted that the "greatest challenge to securing continued funding for the genome project does not originate from concerns about privacy, confidentiality, or coercive genetic testing. It is eugenics, manipulating the human genome in order to improve or enhance the human species" (p. 190).

58. When first proposed, the project to map and sequence the human genome evoked enthusiasm, as well as questions and cautions, from within and outside the bioethics mainstream. Alexander Morgan Capron, "The Rome Bioethics Summit," *Hastings Center Report* 18, no. 4 (August–September 1988): 11–13; and Santiago Grisola, "Mapping the Human Genome," *Hastings Center Report* 19, no. 4 (July–August 1989): S18–S19, report on a meeting in Valencia. Both accounts note endorsements from scientists at international meetings. Concerning the U.S., see Victor A. McKusick, "Mapping and Sequencing the Human Genome," *New England Journal of Medicine* 320, no. 14 (April 6, 1989): 910–15, which summarizes reports of the National Research Council and the Office of Technology Assessment (OTA) in 1988. The OTA, stating that the "humanitarian and scientific benefits will be great," encouraged more international exchange. U.S. Congress, Office of Technology Assessment, *Mapping Our Genes* (Washington, D.C.: Government Printing Office, 1988), p. 173. McKusick, along with Dr. Theodore Friedmann, pointed to scientists' support of the project for diagnosing, screening, and treating through gene therapy, plus benefits for cancer research. Friedmann, "The Human Genome Project."

Among the questioners, the Council for Responsible Genetics asked how the "normal" and "abnormal" would be redefined. "Position Paper on Human Genome Initiative" (Boston, Mass.: Council for Responsible Genetics, 1989). Lawyer George Annas, stating that the "genome project has been overhyped and oversold," called on those evaluating it "to insure that the dangers, as well as the opportunities, are rigorously and publicly explored." George Annas, "Who's Afraid of the Human Genome?" *Hastings Center Report* 19, no. 4 (July–August 1989): 21. Elsewhere he raised the issue of how possible recommendations, such as to restrict germ-line experiments or use of genetic information, could be enforced.

59. See the chronology in National Center for Human Genome Research, *Progress Report: Fiscal Years 1991 and 1992,* NIH Publication No. 93-3550 (Washington, D.C.: National Institutes of Health, March 1993), pp. 6–7. The NCHGR was subsequently renamed the National Human Genome Research Institute (NHGRI).

60. Lori B. Andrews, Jane E. Fullarton, Neil A. Holtzman, and Arno Motul-sky, eds., *Assessing Genetic Risks: Implications for Health and Social Policy* (Washington, D.C.: National Academy Press, 1994), executive summary, p. 2.

61. National Human Genome Research Institute, National Institutes of Health, "Ethical, Legal and Social Implications of the Human Genome Project," fact sheet summarizing the final report of ELSI, December 19, 1996.

62. George J. Annas and Sherman Elias, *Gene Mapping: Using Law and Ethics as Guides* (New York: Oxford University Press, 1992), pp. 272–75. Workshop chairs Annas and Elias noted that the four priorities identified by the NIH workshop were "substantially similar to the three priority areas identified by the Project's own Working Group . . . (ELSI) in late 1990," concluding that at the outset there was "a professional consensus on research priorities" for social policy of the HGP. They also noted in their preface that the memberships of the working group and the workshop overlapped somewhat.

63. Ibid., pp. 274, 275. They could find no mechanism within ELSI to take on the "should" issue, finding this "unremarkable" in that the project itself was not the "appropriate funder" for "an 'independent' or 'objective' assessment of its own priority in scientific research."

64. *ELSI Project Descriptions*, NHGRI ELSI Program—1990 to the Present (Bethesda, Md.: Ethical, Legal, and Social Implications Program, Division of Extramural Research, NHGRI, NIH/DOE, 1999).

65. Elizabeth J. Thomson and Karen Rothenberg, eds., "Reproductive Genetic Testing: Impact on Women," supplement to *Fetal Diagnosis and Therapy* 8 (April 1993). A book based in part on a lecture series at the California Institute of Technology in 1989–90 which received grants from ELSI and the National Science Foundation included only one article specifically devoted to prenatal diagnosis, although testing and abortion in relation to genetic knowledge and diagnosis did figure in a few of the other articles. Daniel J. Kevles and Leroy Hood, eds., *The Code of Codes: Scientific and Social Issues in the Human Genome Project* (Cambridge, Mass.: Harvard University Press, 1992).

66. ELSI's Committee on Genetic Risks found "significant gaps in data, research, and policy analysis that impede informed policy making for the future." Andrews et al., *Assessing Genetic Risks*, "Research and Policy Agenda" section, pp. 20, 21. The 15-member task force, chaired by Neil A. Holtzman and Michael Watson, was set up to fill some of these gaps. See Neil A. Holtzman and Michael S. Watson, eds., *Promoting Safe and Effective Genetic Testing in the United States: Final Report of the Task Force on Genetic Testing* (Bethesda, Md.: NIH-DOE Working Group on Ethical, Legal, and Social Implications of Human Genome Research, National Human Genome Research Institute, National Institutes of Health, 1997), executive summary, p. 18.

67. *Report of the Joint NIH/DOE Committee to Evaluate the Ethical, Legal, and Social Implications of the Human Genome Project* (Bethesda, Md.: National Human Genome Research Institute, National Institutes of Health, December 19, 1996); and Francis S. Collins, Ari Patrinos, Elke Jordan, Aravinda Chakravarti, Raymond

Gestelend, and LeRoy Walters, "New Goals for the U.S. Human Genome Project: 1998–2003," *Science* 282, no. 5389 (October 23, 1998): 682–89. See also the NHGRI's Web site at http://www.genome.gov.

68. National Human Genome Research Institute, National Institutes of Health, *A Review and Analysis of the ELSI Research Programs at the National Institutes of Health and the Department of Energy* (ERPEG Final Report), February 10, 2000.

69. These four revised program areas are "(1) privacy and fair use of genetic information; (2) clinical integration of genetic technologies; (3) ethical issues surrounding genetic research; and (4) education and resources." Ibid., executive summary, p. i.

70. Goals one, two, and three are: 1. "Examine the issues surrounding the completion of the human DNA sequence and the study of human genetic variation"; 2. "Examine issues raised by the integration of genetic technologies and information into health care and public health activities"; 3. "Examine issues raised by the integration of knowledge about genomics and gene-environment interactions into nonclinical settings." Collins et al., "New Goals." A pyramid rendering of the five goals shows how the HGP discoveries placed at the top are set within the other goals of integration of the knowledge, interdisciplinary and world view perspectives, and finally at the broad base the impact of socioeconomic, racial, and ethnic concepts.

71. Ibid., executive summary, p. ii.

72. The American medical profession's first code of ethics was drawn up in 1847, to be followed by "principles of ethics" at various intervals in the twentieth century. See Robert B. Baker, Arthur L. Caplan, Linda L. Emanuel, and Stephen R. Latham, eds., *The American Medical Ethics Revolution: How the AMA's Code of Ethics Has Transformed Physicians' Relationships to Patients, Professionals, and Society* (Baltimore: Johns Hopkins University Press, 1999).

73. Theodore Friedmann, "Prenatal Diagnosis of Genetic Disease," *Scientific American* 225, no. 5 (November 1971): 41.

74. Evans, Fletcher, et al., *Fetal Diagnosis and Therapy.* Dr. Mark I. Evans, as previously noted, is among the leading experts in prenatal diagnosis. Of the other co- editors, Alan O. Dixler is a practicing lawyer, John C. Fletcher was a theologian and bioethicist, and Dr. Joseph D. Schulman, as discussed in chapter 5, is a foremost exponent of IVF and advanced uses of reproductive genetics. There were 68 contributors to the volume in addition to the editors.

75. John Fletcher, "Ethical Issues," in ibid., p. 7.

76. Dorothy C. Wertz and James R. Sorenson, "Sociologic Implications," in ibid., p. 563. Wertz was then at the Boston University School of Public Health, and Sorenson at the School of Public Health of North Carolina. Their article appeared in the final section, "Nonmedical Issues."

77. See also Evans, *Reproductive Risks;* and Simpson and Elias, *Essentials of Prenatal Diagnosis.*

78. Michael M. Kaback, "Screening for Reproductive Counseling: Social, Ethical, and Medicolegal Issues in the Tay-Sachs Disease Experience," in *Medical*

Aspects, vol. 2 of *Human Genetics: Proceedings of the Sixth International Congress of Human Genetics,* ed. Batsheva Bonné-Tamir with Tirza Cohen and Richard M. Goodman (New York: Alan R. Liss, 1982), p. 455.

79. The issue of therapy vs. abortion goes back to the 1970s. At a symposium at the New York Academy of Sciences in 1975, Cynthia Tiff of the Genetics Program at Rutgers University, recalling that prenatal diagnosis was originally "envisioned as temporary," asked when, "if at all," prenatal diagnosis and selective abortion would be replaced by therapy. Dr. Theodore Friedmann suspected that prenatal diagnosis would be "around for a long time," given how long it would take for gene therapy to be available for diseases of very early onset. He observed that methods for detecting conditions and subsequent pressure to abort will "remain a stronger imperative" than for treatment "for a long period of time." Lappé and Morison, *Ethical and Scientific Issues,* "Discussion," p. 152. Referring to the issue again in 1990, Friedmann noted, "the obvious application to prenatal diagnosis of genetic disease predicts increasing use of medically indicated abortion." Friedmann, "The Human Genome Project," p. 412.

80. Theodore Friedmann, "Experiment or Treatment? A Personal View," in *Gene Therapy: Fact and Fiction in Biology's New Approach to Disease* (Cold Spring Harbor, N.Y.: Cold Spring Harbor Laboratory, 1983), p. 123. This was the final chapter of the edited transcripts of a conference on gene therapy at the Banbury Center in Cold Spring Harbor in 1982. Attendees were a notable group of molecular biologists and geneticists, many of whom were also physicians.

81. Theodore Friedmann, "Progress toward Human Gene Therapy," *Science* 244, no. 4910 (June 16, 1989): 1275–81.

82. Edmond A. Murphy, Gary A. Chase, and Alejandro Rodriguez, "Genetic Intervention: Some Social, Psychological, and Philosophical Aspects," in *Genetic Issues in Public Health and Medicine,* ed. Bernice H. Cohen, Abraham M. Lilienfeld, and P. C. Huang (Springfield, Ill.: Charles C. Thomas, 1978), p. 363. The book was aimed at health practitioners.

83. Kaback, "Screening for Reproductive Counseling," p. 454.

84. Klass, "The Perfect Baby," pp. 45–46.

85. See also Karp, "Genetic Drift toward the Perfect Child," discussed in chapter 5.

86. William Ruddick, "Can Doctors and Philosophers Work Together?" *Hastings Center Report* 11, no. 2 (April 1981): 12–17. The Philosophers in Medical Centers Project ran from 1976 to 1980. By involving ethicists in the clinical setting, the project sought to develop a more practical and useful ethics, what philosopher Richard Zaner has called "clinical ethics." Richard M. Zaner, *Ethics and the Clinical Encounter* (Englewood Cliffs, N.J.: Prentice Hall, 1988). A professor of medical ethics at Vanderbilt University, Zaner, like Ruddick, has criticized the bioethicist for being too remote from the practice of medicine to be useful, urging philosophers to get into the "marketplace."

87. See Alan R. Fleischman, "A Physician's View," *Hastings Center Report* 11, no. 2 (April 1981): 18–19.

88. Hill, "Your Morality or Mine?" pp. 1173–74.

89. Mark Siegler, "Clinical Ethics and Clinical Medicine," *Archives of Internal Medicine* 139, no. 8 (August 1979): 914–15.

90. Edmund G. Howe, the journal's editor in chief, stated in the first issue, "Future articles will generally be written for and by physicians, nurses, members of the clergy, philosophers, attorneys, and others whose decisions directly affect patients." Edmund G. Howe, "*The Journal of Clinical Ethics:* Genesis, Purposes, and Scope," *Journal of Clinical Ethics* 1, no. 1 (Spring 1990): 3.

91. Council on Ethical and Judicial Affairs, American Medical Association, "Ethical Issues Related to Prenatal Genetic Testing," *Archives of Family Medicine* 3, no. 7 (July 1994): 633.

92. Pergament and Fiddler, "Prenatal Gene Therapy," 1303–11. See chapter 4.

93. Kenneth L. Garver and Bettylee Garver, "The Human Genome Project and Eugenic Concerns," *American Journal of Human Genetics* 54, no. 1 (January 1994): 155.

94. Allan J. Jacobs, "Liberty, Equality, and Genetic Selection," *The Pharos* 64, no. 1 (Winter 2001): 15–20. See further discussion in chapter 9.

95. Kenneth L. Garver, Nadene Henderson, and Kay A. LeChien, "New Genetic Technologies: Our Added Responsibilities," *American Journal of Human Genetics* 54, no. 1 (January 1994): 120.

96. Lisa S. Parker, "Bioethics for Human Geneticists: Models for Reasoning and Methods for Teaching," *American Journal of Human Genetics* 54, no. 1 (January 1994): 146.

97. John La Puma, Cheryl M. Darling, Carol B. Stocking, and Katy Schiller, "A Perinatal Ethics Committee on Abortion: Process and Outcome in Thirty-One Cases," *Journal of Clinical Ethics* 3, no. 3 (Fall 1992): 196–203. An international survey of pediatric neurosurgeons that included religious perspectives showed general approval of abortion for prenatally detected neural tube malformations, if there was no other remedy. J. F. Hirsch, "Medical Abortion: Ethics, Laws and Religious Points of View—A Study by the 1994–1995 Ethics and Morals Committee of the ISPN," *Child's Nervous System* 12, no. 9 (September 1996): 507–14. (The ISPN is the International Society for Pediatric Neurosurgery.) Hirsch preferred the term "medical abortion" to "therapeutic abortion" because abortion is not a treatment.

98. See, for example, Bernard Lo, "Testing for Genetic Conditions," chapter 47 of *Resolving Ethical Dilemmas: A Guide for Clinicians* (Baltimore: Williams & Wilkins, 1995), pp. 353–62; Dan C. English, *Bioethics: A Clinical Guide for Medical Students* (New York: W. W. Norton, 1994), chapter 7, pp. 108–24; and Tom L. Beauchamp and LeRoy Walters, eds., *Contemporary Issues in Bioethics,* 6th ed. (Belmont, Calif.: Wadsworth-Thompson Learning, 2003), part 4.

99. *Journal of Clinical Ethics* 3, no. 1 (Spring 1992): 3–20; and "Review of the Literature: Feminist Approaches to Medical Ethics," *Journal of Clinical Ethics* 5, no. 1 (Spring 1994): 65–85.

100. Rosemary Tong, ed., "Feminist Approaches to Bioethics," special section, *Journal of Clinical Ethics* 7, no. 1 (Spring 1996): 13–47; *Journal of Clinical Ethics* 7,

no. 2 (Summer 1996): 150–76; *Journal of Clinical Ethics* 7, no. 3 (Fall 1996): 228–42; *Journal of Clinical Ethics* 7, no. 4 (Winter 1996): 315–40.

101. In his introduction, Howe fastened on the patient's "subjective experience" to characterize how feminist perspectives "profoundly challenge the way we now approach medical care." Edmund Howe, "Implementing Feminist Perspectives in Clinical Care," *Journal of Clinical Ethics* 7, no. 1 (Spring 1996): 8. Guest editor Tong amplified that perspective: "By becoming attentive to issues of power and care in the clinic," she wrote, "by asking who has the power and who delivers the care, we will become better able to share the privileges of power and the responsibilities of care with each other. Feminist approaches . . . provide bioethics with some powerful lenses capable of broadening and deepening everyone's line of moral vision." Rosemary Tong, "An Introduction to Feminist Approaches to Bioethics: Unity in Diversity," *Journal of Clinical Ethics* 7, no. 1 (Spring 1996): 19; and Edmund Howe, "The Need for Original Ethical Analysis for Women," *Journal of Clinical Ethics* 10, no. 4 (Winter 1999): 333–40, which followed an article on IVF.

102. See Michael Burgess and Lori d'Agincourt-Canning, "Genetic Testing for Hereditary Disease: Attending to Relational Responsibility," *Journal of Clinical Ethics* 12, no. 4 (Winter 2001): 361–72; and further discussion in chapter 10.

103. *Report of the Joint NIH/DOE Committee*, executive summary, p. 3.

104. Daniel Callahan, "Bioethics, Our Crowd, and Ideology," part of a symposium: "In Search of the Good Society: The Work of Daniel Callahan," *Hastings Center Report* 26, no. 6 (November–December 1996): 3–4. In his criticism of ELSI, Callahan might also have mentioned that much of the Hastings Center's research, as well as that of other centers and institutions, has been funded either by ELSI or by the HGP itself.

105. See Tod Chambers, *The Fiction of Bioethics: Cases as Literary Texts* (New York: Routledge, 1999) for a critique of "stories as data."

106. Glenn C. Graber, "Basic Theories in Medical Ethics," in Monagle and Thomasma, *Medical Ethics*, pp. 464–65.

107. A more detailed critique of the rights theory of moral obligation is developed in chapter 10.

108. For example, the Kennedy Institute of Ethics maintains an extensive library, bibliographic files, archives, and other resources.

109. In so doing, ELSI's focus recalls the conceptual questions and concerns about the consequences of advanced genetic research raised at its 1992 conference, "The Genetic Prism." The conference was funded by the National Human Genome Initiative, which was later renamed the Human Genome Project. See "Genetic Grammar: 'Health,' 'Illness,' and the Human Genome Project," *Hastings Center Report*, special supplement 22, no. 4 (July–August 1992): S1–S20.

110. "Eugenic Artificial Insemination: A Cure for Mediocrity?" *Harvard Law Review* 94, no. 8 (June 1981): 1863. This is a "Notes" article and does not list authors. Hans Jurgen Eysenck, Arthur R. Jensen, and Richard J. Herrnstein were three Harvard psychologists associated with genetic determinist views, especially concerning intelligence and IQ. See discussion below of *The Bell Curve*.

111. George P. Smith, "Genetics, Eugenics, and Public Policy," *Southern Illinois University Law Journal,* 1985, no. 3 (Summer), p. 453. Smith was cautious, however, about endorsing positive eugenics. Concerned more about population growth than a deteriorating gene pool, he held that "[g]enetic planning and screening as well as eugenic programming are more rational and humane alternatives to regulation of the population than premature death, famine and war." Among other things, he misinterpreted the ways genetic knowledge was to be used.

Somewhat surprisingly, given the Vatican's strong opposition to almost all manner of procreative technology, a good deal of the legal support for eugenic uses of genetic engineering can be found among law professors at Catholic institutions, as well as in journals sponsored by such law schools.

112. George P. Smith, *The New Biology: Law, Ethics, and Biotechnology* (New York: Plenum, 1989), p. vii.

113. Richard J. Herrnstein and Charles A. Murray, *The Bell Curve: Intelligence and Class Structure in American Life* (New York: Free Press, 1994).

114. "The IQ Gene," *Time,* September 13, 1999, pp. 54–62. Stephen Jay Gould debunked the notion that there is a single gene for anything, much less memory or intelligence, in the same issue: "Message from a Mouse: It Takes More Than Genes to Make a Smart Rodent, or High-IQ Humans," p. 62.

115. A sampling: June Goodfield, *Playing God: Genetic Engineering and the Manipulation of Life* (New York: Random House, 1977); Ted Howard and Jeremy Rifkin, *Who Should Play God? The Artificial Creation of Life and What It Means for the Future of the Human Race* (New York: Dell, 1977); and Ted Peters, *Playing God? Genetic Determinism and Human Freedom* (New York: Routledge, 1997). More balanced than others of the time is Yvonne Baskin, *The Gene Doctors: Medical Genetics at the Frontier* (New York: William Morrow, 1984).

116. Jeremy Rifkin, *The Biotech Century: Harnessing the Gene and Remaking the World* (New York: Jeremy P. Tarcher/Putnam, 1998); Jeremy Rifkin, with Nicanor Perlas, *Algeny: A New Word, a New World* (New York: Penguin, 1984); and Howard and Rifkin, *Who Should Play God?*

117. Two years later the press was headlining "Search for a Gay Gene." See Richard Horton, "Is Homosexuality Inherited?" review of *The Sexual Brain,* by Simon LeVay, and *The Science of Desire: The Search for the Gay Gene and the Biology of Behavior,* by Dean Hamer and Peter Copeland, *New York Review of Books,* July 13, 1995, pp. 36–41.

118. Bryan Appleyard, *Brave New Worlds: Staying Human in the Genetic Future* (New York: Viking, 1998), pp. 134, 172.

119. Gina Maranto, *Quest for Perfection: The Drive to Breed Better Human Beings* (New York: Scribner, 1996).

120. Lee M. Silver, *Remaking Eden: Cloning and Beyond in a Brave New World* (New York: Avon, 1997), p. 15. His argument is much like William Gardner's: that parents will demand enhancement.

121. In a way, his warnings accept a form of genetic reductionism: the prem-

ise that we can be reduced to our genes and that medicine will become able to fine-tune them.

122. Allen E. Buchanan, Dan W. Brock, Norman Daniels, and Daniel Wickler, *From Chance to Choice: Genetics and Justice* (Cambridge: Cambridge University Press, 2000), chapter 1.

123. One of the best of these was "Curveball" by Stephen Jay Gould in the *New Yorker*, November 28, 1994, pp. 139–49. Others include Russell Jacoby and Naomi Glauberman, eds., *The Bell Curve Debate: History, Documents, Opinions* (New York: Times Books, 1995); Steven Fraser, ed., *The Bell Curve Wars: Race, Intelligence, and the Future of America* (New York: Basic, 1995); Claude S. Fischer, Michael Hout, Martin Sanchez Jankowski, Samuel R. Lucas, Ann Swidler, and Kim Voss, *Inequality by Design: Cracking the Bell Curve Myth* (Princeton, N.J.: Princeton University Press, 1996); and Joe L. Kincheloe, Shirley R. Steinberg, and Aaron D. Gresson III, eds., *Measured Lies: The Bell Curve Examined* (New York: St. Martin's, 1996).

124. See, for example, "Public and Private Eugenics," special issue, *Gene Watch* 12, no. 3 (June 1999). *Gene Watch* is published by the Council for Responsible Genetics.

125. R. C. Lewontin, Steven Rose, and Leon J. Kamin, *Not in Our Genes: Biology, Ideology, and Human Nature* (New York: Pantheon, 1984). See also Steven Rose, "DNA and the Goal of Human Perfectibility," *Monthly Review* 38, no. 3 (July–August 1986): 48–60.

126. Ruth Hubbard and Elijah Wald, *Exploding the Gene Myth: How Genetic Information Is Produced and Manipulated by Scientists, Physicians, Employers, Insurance Companies, Educators, and Law Enforcers* (Boston: Beacon, 1993); and Philip Kitcher, *The Lives to Come: The Genetic Revolution and Human Possibilities* (New York: Simon & Schuster, 1996). For a particularly insightful historical analysis, see Evelyn Fox Keller, *The Century of the Gene* (Cambridge, Mass.: Harvard University Press, 2000).

127. Barbara Katz Rothman, *Genetic Maps and Human Imaginations: The Limits of Science in Understanding Who We Are* (New York: W. W. Norton, 1998), p. 222.

128. The Hubbard and Wald book was favorably reviewed in the *New York Times* by Daniel Callahan, then head of the Hastings Center. "They Dream of Genes," *New York Times Book Review*, September 12, 1993, p. 26.

9. SITES OF RESISTANCE

1. David A. Grimes, "Technology Follies: The Uncritical Acceptance of Medical Innovation," Commentary, *Journal of the American Medical Association* 269, no. 23 (June 16, 1993): 3030–33. Dr. Grimes is a member of the Department of Obstetrics, Gynecology and Reproductive Sciences at San Francisco General Hospital. A more sweeping condemnation of technology's hold on medicine came that same year from a professor of public health at Cornell Medical College who likened technologies to the brooms in *The Sorcerer's Apprentice:* they take on a life

of their own and doctors must bring them under control. Eric J. Cassell, "The Sorcerer's Broom: Medicine's Rampant Technology," *Hastings Center Report* 23, no. 6 (November–December 1993): 32–39.

2. "Study Questions Monitoring of Fetus at Birth," *New York Times*, March 10, 1996, p. 25.

3. See chapter 5, note 47.

4. Thomas E. Elkins and Douglas Brown, "The Cost of Choice: A Price Too High in the Triple Screen for Down Syndrome," *Clinical Obstetrics and Gynecology* 36, no. 3 (September 1993): 532–40.

5. Ibid., p. 537.

6. Weaver, with Brandt, *Catalog of Prenatally Diagnosed Conditions*, p. xiv.

7. Elkins and Brown, "The Cost of Choice," p. 538.

8. Margarete Sandelowski and Linda Corson Jones, "'Healing Fictions': Stories of Choosing in the Aftermath of the Detection of Fetal Anomalies," *Social Science and Medicine* 42, no. 3 (February 1996): 353–61.

9. Miriam Kuppermann, James D. Goldberg, Robert F. Nease, Jr., and A. Eugene Washington, "Who Should Be Offered Prenatal Diagnosis? The 35-Year-Old Question," *American Journal of Public Health* 89, no. 2 (February 1999): 163.

10. Bernard G. Ewigman, James P. Crane, Frederic D. Frigoletto, Michael L. LeFevre, Raymond P. Bain, Donald McNellis, and the RADIUS Study Group, "Effect of Prenatal Ultrasound Screening on Perinatal Outcome," *New England Journal of Medicine* 329, no. 12 (September 16, 1993): 821–27; and M. L. LeFevre et al., "A Randomized Trial of Prenatal Ultrasonographic Screening: Impact on Maternal Management and Outcome," *American Journal of Obstetrics and Gynecology* 169, no. 3 (September 1993): 483–89. See also Warren E. Leary, "Study Finds Waste in Ultrasound Use," *New York Times*, September 16, 1993, p. A17. Ultrasound is second only to MSAFP screening in frequency of use.

11. Richard L. Berkowitz, "Should Every Pregnant Woman Undergo Ultrasonography?" *New England Journal of Medicine* 329, no. 12 (September 16, 1993): 874–75.

12. Natalie Angier, "Doctors Favor Ultrasound Use in Right Hands," *New York Times*, July 15, 1997, pp. C1, C10. Accuracy rate for Eurofetus was 61.4% as against 34.8% for RADIUS.

13. Neil A. Holtzman, *Proceed with Caution: Predicting Genetic Risks in the Recombinant DNA Era* (Baltimore: Johns Hopkins University Press, 1989). He had earlier criticized the delivery of genetic services, citing the lack of national health care, and competition between private laboratories that does not always result in quality service: Holtzman, "Delivery of Genetic Services," in *Medical Aspects*, vol. 2 of *Human Genetics: Proceedings of the Sixth International Congress of Human Genetics*, ed. Batsheva Bonné-Tamir with Tirza Cohen and Richard M. Goodman (New York: Alan R. Liss, 1982), pp. 413–19.

14. Neil A. Holtzman, "Genetics," *Journal of the American Medical Association* 273, no. 16 (April 26, 1995): 1304–1306.

15. Jessica Davis, comments in a panel discussion, "Ethical and Scientific Issues Posed by Human Uses of Molecular Genetics," *Annals of the New York Academy of Sciences* 265 (January 23, 1976): 162, 163.

16. Barbara A. Bernhardt, Gail Geller, Theresa Doksum, S. M. Larson, D. Roter, and Neil A. Holtzman, "Prenatal Genetic Testing: Content of Discussions between Obstetric Providers and Pregnant Women," *Obstetrics and Gynecology* 91, no. 5, pt. 1 (May 1998): 648–55.

17. Seymour Kessler, "Process Issues in Genetic Counseling," in Evers-Kiebooms, Fryns, and Cassiman, *Psychosocial Aspects of Genetic Counseling*, 1–10.

18. Maria O. Vargas, "Tradition of Nontradition—Our Cultural Blindspot," in *Religious, Cultural and Ethnic Influences on the Counseling Process*, part 2 of *Strategies in Genetic Counseling*, Birth Defects Original Article Series 23, no. 6, ed. Barbara Biesecker, Patricia A. Magyari, and Natalie W. Paul (White Plains, N.Y.: March of Dimes Birth Defects Foundation, 1987), p. 130. This volume contains the proceedings of the Fifth Annual Education Conference of the National Society of Genetic Counselors, Salt Lake City, October 1985.

19. Juliet Yuen, "Asian Americans" in workshop "Defining Our Cultures—Bridging the Gap," in Biesecker, Magyari, and Paul, *Religious, Cultural and Ethnic Influences*, p. 164.

20. Rodger G. Lum, "The Patient-Counselor Relationship in a Cross-Cultural Context," in Biesecker, Magyari, and Paul, *Religious, Cultural and Ethnic Influences*, p. 137.

21. Diana Punales-Morejon and Victor B. Penchaszadeh, "Psychosocial Aspects of Genetic Counseling: Cross-Cultural Issues," in Evers-Kiebooms, Fryns, and Cassiman, *Psychosocial Aspects of Genetic Counseling*, 11–15.

22. K. Watson and Mary B. Mahowald, "Honoring Gender-Based Patient Requests for Obstetricians: Ethical Imperative or Employment Discrimination?" *Journal of Women's Health & Gender-Based Medicine* 8, no. 8 (October 1999): 1031–41; and D. L. Roter, G. Geller, B. A. Bernhardt, S. M. Larson, and T. Doksum, "Effects of Obstetrician Gender on Communication and Patient Satisfaction," *Obstetrics and Gynecology* 93, no. 5, pt. 1 (May 1999): 635–41.

23. See A. Paul Williams, Karin Dominick Pierre, and Eugene Vayda, "Women in Medicine: Toward a Conceptual Understanding of the Potential for Change," *Journal of the American Medical Women's Association* 48, no. 8 (July–August 1993): 115–21.

24. R. C. Juberg, A. E. Katz, and J. R. Nelson, "Reasons for Refusing Amniocentesis," abstract, *American Journal of Human Genetics* 43, no. 3, supplement (September 1988): A167. For a roundup of literature on this issue, see Brenda F. Seals, Edem E. Ekwo, Roger A. Williamson, and James W. Hanson, "Moral and Religious Influences on the Amniocentesis Decision," *Social Biology* 32, nos. 1–2 (Spring–Summer 1985): 13.

25. Complicating the picture, however, as discussed in chapter 7, is the way that anti-abortion attitudes, views about birth defects, and abortion policy may

intersect. Some abortion opponents make an exception for fetal defects and support legislation allowing such exceptions, thus putting them at odds with women personally opposed to abortion, and therefore testing, for any reason.

26. Anna Quindlen, "This Child I Carry, Like My Other Two, Is Wanted. Healthy or Not," Life in the '30s, *New York Times,* May 12, 1988, p. C2; and "Readers React to Anna Quindlen's Decision Not to Have Amniocentesis," *New York Times,* June 9, 1988, p. C12.

27. Except as otherwise noted, the responses referred to are drawn from my conversations over time with women who belong to this class of testing candidates.

28. See Nancy E. Adler, Susan Keyes, and Patricia Robertson, "Psychological Issues in New Reproductive Technologies: Pregnancy-Inducing Technology and Diagnostic Screening," in *Women and New Reproductive Technologies: Medical, Psychosocial, Legal, and Ethical Dilemmas,* ed. Judith Rodin and Aila Collins (Hillsdale, N.J.: Lawrence Erlbaum, 1991): 117ff.

29. Susan Markens, Carole H. Browner, and Nancy Press, " 'Because of the Risks': How U.S. Pregnant Women Account for Refusing Prenatal Screening," *Social Science & Medicine* 49, no. 3 (August 1999): 359–69.

30. Adler, Keyes, and Robertson, "Psychological Issues," p. 119.

31. Nancy Press, Carole H. Browner, Diem Tran, Christine Morton, and Barbara Le Master, "Provisional Normalcy and 'Perfect Babies': Pregnant Women's Attitudes toward Disability in the Context of Prenatal Testing," in *Reproducing Reproduction: Kinship, Power and Technological Innovation,* ed. Sarah Franklin and Helena Ragoné (Philadelphia: University of Pennsylvania Press, 1998), pp. 50–52.

32. See Peter A. Benn, Lillian Y. F. Hsu, Ann Carlson, and Hody L. Tannenbaum, "The Centralized Prenatal Genetics Screening Program of New York City III: The First 7,000 Cases," *American Journal of Medical Genetics* 20, no. 2 (February 1985): 369–84. A 1988 report, assessing these services at the Prenatal Diagnosis Laboratory, showed steady yearly growth in the number of women coming in for counseling and accepting amniocentesis when indicated. See E. Lieber, H. Tannenbaum, E. Kahn, P. Nelson, T. Perlis, and L. Y. F. Hsu, "Prenatal Genetic Services to an Inner-City Community Hospital: Problems of Health Care Delivery," abstract, *American Journal of Human Genetics* 43, no. 3, supplement (September 1988): A168.

33. For a description of Rapp's methodology, see Rayna Rapp, *Testing Women, Testing the Fetus: The Social Impact of Amniocentesis in America* (New York: Routledge, 2000), chapter 1.

34. Ibid., especially discussion in chapters 3, 4, and 5.

35. Rayna Rapp, "Chromosomes and Communication: The Discourse of Genetic Counseling," *Medical Anthropology Quarterly,* n.s. 2, no. 2 (June 1988): 143–57. See also Rayna Rapp, "Communicating about the New Reproductive Technologies: Cultural, Interpersonal, and Linguistic Determinants of Understanding," in Rodin and Collins, *Women and New Reproductive Technologies,* pp. 135–52.

36. Rapp, "Chromosomes and Communication." Rapp notes in a footnote that religious reasons were more Evangelical than Catholic, at least among Hispanics and Caribbean Blacks. In *Testing Women, Testing the Fetus,* especially in chapter 4, Rapp is at great care to point out that the diversity of Spanish-speaking cultures in New York City, and in other large U.S. cities, is "quite profound," including, for example, Puerto Rican, Dominican, Central American, middle-class as well as poor, and crossing race classifications. This diversity, of course, contributes to the diversity of responses to prenatal testing.

37. Susan Klein, quoted in Rapp, "Chromosomes and Communication."

38. Lieber et al., "Prenatal Genetic Services to an Inner-City Community Hospital," A168.

39. A study in Washington state showed high correlations between use of amniocentesis and race: use was highest among Chinese, Japanese, and Whites; Native Americans, other Asians, and Filipinas had the lowest use; and African Americans and Latinas were in the middle. Use correlated with socioeconomic status as well: the higher their status, the more likely women were to use amniocentesis, and the lower, the less. W. Burke and C. D. Dugowson, "Race and Socioeconomic Status in the Utilization of Amniocentesis," abstract #1084, *American Journal of Human Genetics* 45, no. 4, supplement (October 1989): A275.

40. Interestingly enough, contrary to expectations (and unlike the pattern among some middle-class couples), male partners of women of Mexican origin were generally supportive of the women's amniocentesis decisions. See Carole H. Browner and H. Mabel Preloran, "Male Partners' Role in Latinas' Amniocentesis Decisions," *Journal of Genetic Counseling* 8, no. 2 (April 1999): 85–108.

41. Carole H. Browner, H. Mabel Preloran, and Simon J. Cox, "Ethnicity, Bioethics, and Prenatal Diagnosis: The Amniocentesis Decisions of Mexican-Origin Women and Their Partners," *American Journal of Public Health* 89, no. 11 (November 1999): 1665.

42. Carole H. Browner and H. Mabel Preloran, "*Para Sacarse la Espina* (To Get Rid of the Doubt): Mexican Immigrant Women's Amniocentesis Decisions," in *Bodies of Technology: Women's Involvement in Reproductive Medicine,* ed. Ann Rudinow Saetnan, Nelly Oudshoorn, and Marta Kirejczyk (Columbus: Ohio State University Press, 2000), p. 380.

43. Natalie Angier, "Ultrasound and Fury: One Mother's Ordeal," *New York Times,* November 26, 1996, pp. C1, C8.

44. "Account of Sonogram Dilemma Prompts Letters of Joy and Grief," *New York Times,* July 15, 1997, p. C10.

45. Kathleen McAuliffe, "A Little Knowledge, a Lot of Agony," *Women's Health, New York Times,* June 21, 1998, p. 22.

46. Rapp, "Chromosomes and Communication."

47. E. Q. Wooldridge and R. F. Murray, Jr., "The Health Orientation Scale: A Measure of Feelings about Sickle Cell Trait," *Social Biology* 35, nos. 1–2 (Spring–Summer 1988): 123–33.

48. C. C. Kocun, J. T. Harrigan, J. C. Canterino, S. M. Feld, and C. O.

Fernandez, "Changing Trends in Patient Decisions concerning Genetic Amnio-centesis," *American Journal of Obstetrics and Gynecology* 182, no. 5 (May 2000): 1018–20.

49. Erik Parens and Adrienne Asch, eds., *Prenatal Testing and Disability Rights* (Washington, D.C.: Georgetown University Press, 2000).

50. National Down Syndrome Society, "The National Down Syndrome Society's Recommendations for Accountability under IDEA," http://www.ndss.org/content.cfm?fuseaction=NwsEvt.Article&article=531, accessed September 20, 2004.

51. Spina Bifida Association of America, http://www.sbaa.org, under links "About SBAA/SBF" and then "About SBAA."

52. "History," a timeline furnished by the Genetic Alliance, Washington, D.C., p. 6.

53. Ibid., p. 1. Major funding for the Alliance comes from the Genetic Services Branch of the Bureau of Maternal and Child Health, a federal agency. Additional funds are from the March of Dimes, membership dues, and various private, foundation, and corporate grants, plus the National Center for Human Genome Research. The Alliance describes itself as "an international coalition of all the stakeholders in genetics—families, professionals, genetic lay advocacy organizations, government and industry, working to promote healthy lives for everyone impacted by genetic conditions" (Genetic Alliance, "Genetic Alliance Strategic Plan," http://geneticalliance.org/aboutus/strategicplan.html, accessed September 20, 2004).

54. E-mail from Janine Lewis, director, Information Resource Network, Genetic Alliance, December 14, 2000. My question used the term "prenatal diagnosis" rather than "prenatal testing."

55. E-mail from Marybeth Leongini, public relations manager, Spina Bifida Association of America, December 18, 2000.

56. The NDSS statement says, "prenatal testing for Down syndrome should be made available to any pregnant woman who wishes to receive the tests, regardless of the woman's age, reproductive history or disability status. Knowing in advance either the risk or diagnosis of Down syndrome can help parents educate, inform and prepare themselves for all issues regarding this genetic condition. However, the decision whether to undergo prenatal testing must be solely that of the pregnant woman. All forms of prenatal testing for Down syndrome should remain strictly confidential and voluntary." NDSS Position Statement on Prenatal Testing, April 19, 2004, http://www.ndss.org/content.cfm?fuseaction=NwsEvt.PressPSArticle&article=700, accessed September 20, 2004.

57. Marsha Saxton, "Why Members of the Disability Community Oppose Prenatal Diagnosis and Selective Abortion," in Parens and Asch, *Prenatal Testing and Disability Rights*, pp. 147–64.

58. Americans with Disabilities Act (Public Law No. 101-336, 1990).

59. Steven A. Holmes, "Sweeping U.S. Law to Help Disabled Goes into Effect," *New York Times*, January 27, 1992, pp. A1, A12.

60. Adrienne Asch, "Prenatal Diagnosis and Selective Abortion: A Challenge to Practice and Policy," *American Journal of Public Health* 89, no. 11 (November 1999): 1651.

61. Erik Parens and Adrienne Asch, "The Disability Rights Critique of Prenatal Genetic Testing: Reflections and Recommendations," in Parens and Asch, *Prenatal Testing and Disability Rights*, pp. 12–13.

62. Nancy Press, "Assessing the Expressive Character of Prenatal Testing: The Choices Made or the Choices Made Available?" in Parens and Asch, *Prenatal Testing and Disability Rights*, pp. 214–33. See also Nancy Press and Carole H. Browner, "Collective Silences and Collective Fictions: How Prenatal Diagnostic Testing Became Part of Routine Prenatal Care," in *Women and Prenatal Testing: Facing the Challenges of Genetic Technology*, ed. Karen H. Rothenberg and Elizabeth J. Thomson (Columbus: Ohio State University Press, 1994), pp. 201–18.

63. Philip M. Ferguson, Alan Gartner, and Dorothy K. Lipsky, "The Experience of Disability in Families: A Synthesis of Research and Parent Narratives," in Parens and Asch, *Prenatal Testing and Disability Rights*, p, 85.

64. Barbara Bowles Biesecker and Lori Hamby, "What Difference the Disability Community Arguments Should Make for the Delivery of Genetic Services," in Parens and Asch, *Prenatal Testing and Disability Rights*, pp. 340–57.

65. Asch, "Prenatal Diagnosis and Selective Abortion," 1654, 1655.

66. Adrienne Asch and Michelle Fine, "Shared Dreams: A Left Perspective on Disability Rights and Reproductive Rights," in Fine and Asch, *Women with Disabilities*, p. 302.

67. Adrienne Asch, "Why I Haven't Changed My Mind about Prenatal Diagnosis: Reflections and Refinements," in Parens and Asch, *Prenatal Testing and Disability Rights*, pp. 234–58.

68. Asch and Fine, "Shared Dreams," pp. 298–99.

69. Ibid., p. 298. For a useful appraisal of feminist work on disability, see the review essay by Barbara Hillyer, "Women and Disabilities," *NWSA Journal* 4, no. 1 (Spring 1992): 106–14.

70. Murphy, Chase, and Rodriguez, "Genetic Intervention," pp. 365, 369. See chapter 8.

71. Steven J. Ralston, "Reflections from the Trenches: One Doctor's Encounter with Disability Rights Arguments," in Parens and Asch, *Prenatal Testing and Disability Rights*, pp. 335, 337.

72. Jacobs, "Liberty, Equality, and Genetic Selection," p. 19.

73. Interview with Dr. Davis, June 20, 1990.

74. Ralston, "Reflections from the Trenches," p. 338.

10. TRANSFORMING THE DREAM OF THE PERFECT CHILD

1. FINNRET, the Feminist International Network on New Reproductive Technologies, was founded at the Second International Interdisciplinary Congress on Women in Gronigen, The Netherlands, in April 1984. The core "author-activists" were Gena Corea, Renate D. Klein, Janice Raymond, and Robyn Row-

land. At an "emergency" conference in Vallinge, Sweden, in July 1985, the name was changed to FINRRAGE, Feminist International Network of Resistance to Reproductive and Genetic Engineering. See Nancy Lublin, *Pandora's Box: Feminism Confronts Reproductive Technology* (Lanham, Md.: Rowman & Littlefield, 1998), pp. 63ff. Jana Sawicki, critiquing the radical feminist position, holds that viewing the technologies as all-powerful and women as hapless victims precludes their being able to join as sites of resistance to the dominant discourse. Jana Sawicki, *Disciplining Foucault: Feminism, Power, and the Body* (New York: Routledge, 1991), chapter 4.

2. Lorraine Code, Sheila Mullett, and Christine Overall, introduction to *Feminist Perspectives: Philosophical Essays on Method and Morals* (Toronto: University of Toronto Press, 1988), p. 8.

3. Carol Gilligan, *In a Different Voice: Psychological Theory and Women's Development* (Cambridge, Mass.: Harvard University Press, 1982). See, for example, the recent critique of Joy Kroeger-Mappes, "The Ethic of Care vis-à-vis the Ethic of Rights: A Problem for Contemporary Moral Theory," *Hypatia* 9, no. 3 (Summer 1994): 108–31.

4. See the useful discussion in Joan C. Callahan, introduction to *Reproduction, Ethics, and the Law: Feminist Perspectives,* ed. Joan C. Callahan (Bloomington: Indiana University Press, 1995).

5. Patrice DiQuinzio and Iris Marion Young, introduction to "Feminist Ethics and Social Policy, Part 1," special issue, *Hypatia* 10, no. 1 (Winter 1995): 1. See also rest of introduction and articles in this issue further articulating the arguments in this section.

6. Caroline Whitbeck, "A Different Reality: Feminist Ontology," in *Beyond Domination: New Perspectives on Women and Philosophy,* ed. Carol C. Gould (Totowa, N.J.: Rowman & Allanheld, 1983), p. 79.

7. Ibid., p. 64. In a comprehensive footnote, Whitbeck discusses the early development of the feminist critique of dualism. See p. 82 n. 1.

8. See Alison M. Jaggar, *Feminist Politics and Human Nature* (Totowa, N.J.: Rowman & Allanheld, 1983), chapter 3, "Liberal Feminism and Human Nature," pp. 27–50; and Macpherson, *Political Theory of Possessive Individualism.*

9. Beverly Wildung Harrison, "Feminism and Ethics," introduction to *Making the Connections: Essays in Feminist Social Ethics* (Boston: Beacon, 1985), p. 1.

10. Christine Overall, *Ethics and Human Reproduction: A Feminist Analysis* (Boston: Allen & Unwin, 1987), p. 6.

11. Caroline Whitbeck, "The Moral Implications of Regarding Women as People: New Perspectives on Pregnancy and Personhood," in *Abortion and the Status of the Fetus,* ed. William B. Bondeson, H. Tristram Englehardt, Jr., Stuart F. Spicker, and Daniel Winship (Dordrecht: D. Reidel, 1983), p. 254.

12. Iris Marion Young, "Pregnant Embodiment: Subjectivity and Alienation," *Journal of Medicine and Philosophy* 9, no. 1 (February 1984): 45–62. This article was reprinted in Young's collection *Throwing Like a Girl and Other Essays in Feminist Philosophy and Social Theory* (Bloomington: Indiana University Press,

1990), pp. 160–74. Citations are to the 1984 publication. Young cautions that her analysis is limited "to the specific experience of women in technologically sophisticated Western societies" and to pregnancies that are chosen or at least positively accepted, adding that this is not so for most women in the world. Whether or not her experience does transcend these limits, and it may well do so, I find her analysis especially relevant since it is such privileged women who are caught up in the "perfect child" discourse. It also may be that the dialectical consciousness she describes is more widely applicable to the pregnancy experience than she is willing to project.

13. Ibid., pp. 48, 49, 52, 54.

14. Sheila Mullett, "Shifting Perspective: A New Approach to Ethics," in Code, Mullett, and Overall, *Feminist Perspectives*, 122–23.

15. Carol Gilligan, "Hearing the Difference: Theorizing the Connection," in "Feminist Ethics and Social Policy, Part II," special issue, *Hypatia* 10, no. 2 (Spring 1995): 122. Her remarks were part of a "Symposium on Care and Justice" at the September 1994 meeting of the American Political Science Association in New York City.

16. Christine Overall, "Feminism, Ontology, and 'Other Minds,'" in Code, Mullett, and Overall, *Feminist Perspectives*, pp. 98, 99.

17. Whitbeck, "Regarding Women as People," p. 256.

18. Ibid., p. 250.

19. Overall, *Ethics and Human Reproduction*, p. 28.

20. Mary Mahowald's relational model is a "parentalist" ethical model for reproductive medicine. Speaking specifically to the power imbalance of the often male doctor–woman patient relationship, Mahowald rejects the "paternalistic" medical model of beneficence and do no harm, and the "maternalistic" model of patient autonomy only. Combining the two, her "parentalist" model has the doctor and patient protecting and caring for each other, and defines autonomy as a lifelong relationship between parents and children. Her relational model is based as well on concern for socioeconomic context and distributive justice. Mary B. Mahowald, "Sex-Role Stereotypes in Medicine," *Hypatia* 2, no. 2 (Summer 1987): 21–38.

21. Overall, *Ethics and Human Reproduction*, p. 6.

22. See also Valerie Hartouni, "Containing Women: Reproductive Discourse in the 1980s," in *Technoculture*, ed. Constance Penley and Andrew Ross (Minneapolis: University of Minnesota Press, 1991), pp. 27–56, especially for the prevailing view of woman as a "maternal body."

23. Donna J. Haraway, "A Cyborg Manifesto: Science, Technology, and Socialist-Feminism in the Late Twentieth Century," chapter 8 in *Simians, Cyborgs, and Women: The Reinvention of Nature* (New York: Routledge, 1991), pp. 170, 163. An earlier version of this essay was published as "Manifesto for Cyborgs: Science, Technology, and Socialist Feminism in the 1980s," *Socialist Review* 80 (1985): 65–108, and reprinted in Nicholson, *Feminism/Postmodernism*, pp. 190–233.

24. Bordo, "Feminism, Postmodernism, and Gender-Scepticism," pp. 144, 145.

25. Suzanne K. Damarin, "Technologies of the Individual: Women and Sub-jectivity in the Age of Information," in "Technology and Feminism," ed. Joan Rothschild, special issue, *Research in Technology and Philosophy: Technology and Feminism* 13 (1993): 192–93.

26. Ibid., p. 196.

27. In other words, a postmodern subjectivity that is fluid and changing and allows for difference is not incompatible with female embodiment as long as we recognize a distinction between physical self and consciousness of self derived through bodily experiences. This distinction is a dualism of a different order than are the self-other or mind-body splits characteristic of traditional reproductive ethics and practice. Recognizing this brand of dualism may be a precondition for reclaiming female bodily integrity while exploring the dimensions of a liberating and multiple female identity. I am indebted to Herta Nagl for pointing out this critical distinction to me in a conversation in Vienna in 1992. As I understand her criticism of Haraway, it is that one cannot apply a fractured postmodern subjec-tivity to the body as well as to identity. Dualism in this sense becomes a necessary concept.

28. Virginia Held, "The Meshing of Care and Justice," in "Feminist Ethics and Social Policy, Part II," special issue, *Hypatia* 10, no. 2 (Spring 1995): 132. Her article appeared in the Symposium on Care and Justice cited above.

29. Overall, *Ethics and Human Reproduction*, pp. 40–67 passim.

30. Anne Donchin, "Autonomy and Interdependence: Quandaries in Genetic Decision Making," in *Relational Autonomy: Feminist Perspectives on Autonomy, Agency, and the Social Self,* ed. Catriona Mackenzie and Natalie Stoljar (New York: Oxford University Press, 2000), p. 239.

31. Gilligan, "Hearing the Difference," pp. 122–23, 125.

32. Foucault, *History of Sexuality,* vol. 1, pp. 94–96.

33. Sawicki, *Disciplining Foucault,* pp. 81, 87. Sawicki's quotation of Foucault is from "Two Lectures," in *Power/Knowledge: Selected Interviews and Other Writ-ings, 1972–1977,* ed. Colin Gordon (New York: Pantheon, 1980). p. 82.

34. Monique Deveaux, "Shifting Paradigms: Theorizing Care and Justice in Political Theory," in "Feminist Ethics and Social Policy, Part II," special issue, *Hypatia* 10, no. 2 (Spring 1995): 117. This article is part of the Symposium on Care and Justice cited above.

35. Whitbeck, speaking to values and standards for understanding the ethical issues raised by the new reproductive technologies, states, "[i]t is unavoidable that any articulation of standards should be culturally marked. . . . Without the artic-ulation of alternative standards we are likely to adopt the assumptions of the prevalent ideology." She notes further that alternative standards must be fully stated and held open to criticism. Caroline Whitbeck, "Ethical Issues Raised by the New Reproductive Technologies," in Rodin and Collins, *Women and New Re-productive Technologies,* p. 58.

36. Rodin and Collins, introduction to *Women and New Reproductive Tech-nologies,* p. 1.

37. See Whitbeck, "Ethical Issues," pp. 58, 49–64 passim.

38. Sheryl Ruzek, "Women's Reproductive Rights: The Impact of Technology," in Rodin and Collins, *Women and New Reproductive Technologies*, p. 84. Ruzek is specifically referring to Rosalind Petchesky. See Rosalind Petchesky, "Abortion in the 1980's: Feminist Morality and Women's Health," in *Women, Health and Healing*, ed. Ellen Lewin and Virginia Oleson (New York: Tavistock, 1985), pp. 139–73.

39. Ruzek, "Women's Reproductive Rights"; and World Health Organization, "Constitution of the World Health Organization," *Chronicle of WHO* 1, no. 1 (1947).

40. See chapter 3. See also Susan Merrill Squier, *Babies in Bottles: Twentieth-Century Visions of Reproductive Technology* (New Brunswick, N.J.: Rutgers University Press, 1994).

41. Hilary Rose, "Dreaming the Future," *Hypatia* 3, no. 1 (1988): 134 and passim. This article also appears as chapter 9, "Dreaming the Future: Other Wor(l)ds," in Hilary Rose, *Love, Power and Knowledge: Towards a Feminist Transformation of the Sciences* (Bloomington: Indiana University Press, 1995), pp. 208–29.

42. Charlotte Perkins Gilman, *Herland* (1915; reprint, New York: Pantheon, 1979); Sally Miller Gearhart, *The Wanderground* (Watertown, Mass.: Persephone, 1979); Ursula K. LeGuin, *The Left Hand of Darkness* (New York: Ace, 1969); and Marge Piercy, *Woman on the Edge of Time* (New York: Fawcett Crest, 1976).

43. Shulamith Firestone, *The Dialectic of Sex: The Case for Feminist Revolution* (New York: William Morrow, 1970). See also Hilary Rose's comments on Firestone in "Dreaming the Future," p. 128. Naomi Mitchison's *Solution Three* (1975; reprint, New York: Feminist Press, 2002) projected similar goals. Mitchison, who counted several futuristic novels among her many books, was a sister of J. B. S. Haldane. She died in 1999 at the age of 101.

44. Patrocinio Schweickart, "What If . . . Science and Technology in Feminist Utopias," in *Machina Ex Dea: Feminist Perspectives on Technology*, ed. Joan Rothschild (New York: Pergamon, 1983; New York: Teachers College Press, 1992), pp. 198–211.

SELECT BIBLIOGRAPHY

Allen, Garland E. "The Eugenic Record Office at Cold Spring Harbor, 1910–1940: An Institutional History." *Osiris,* 2nd series, 2 (1986): 225–64.

———. "Genetics, Eugenics, and Class Struggle." *Genetics* 79 (1975): S29–S45.

———. "The Misuse of Biological Hierarchies: The American Eugenics Movement, 1900–1940." *History and Philosophy of the Life Sciences,* section 2 of *Pubblicazioni della Stazione Zoologica di Napoli* 5, no. 2 (1983): 105–28.

Altman, Barbara M. "Studies of Attitudes toward the Handicapped: The Need for a New Direction." *Social Problems* 28, no. 3 (February 1981): 321–37.

American Society for Reproductive Medicine. "2002 Guidelines for Gamete and Embryo Donation." *Fertility & Sterility* 77, no. 6 (June 2002): S1–S16.

Americans with Disabilities Act. Public Law No. 101-336, 1990.

Anderson, W. French. "Human Gene Therapy: Scientific and Ethical Considerations." *Journal of Medicine and Philosophy* 10, no. 3 (August 1985): 275–91.

———. "Human Gene Therapy: Why Draw a Line?" *Journal of Medicine and Philosophy* 14, no. 6 (December 1989): 681–93.

Andrews, Lori B., Jane E. Fullarton, Neil A. Holtzman, and Arno Motulsky, eds. *Assessing Genetic Risks: Implications for Health and Social Policy.* Washington, D.C.: National Academy Press, 1994.

Annas, George J. "Who's Afraid of the Human Genome?" *Hastings Center Report* 19, no. 4 (July–August 1989), 19–21.

Annas, George J., and Sherman Elias. *Gene Mapping: Using Law and Ethics as Guides.* New York: Oxford University Press, 1992.

Apple, Rima D., ed. *Women, Health and Medicine in America: A Historical Handbook.* 1990. Reprint, New Brunswick, N.J.: Rutgers University Press, 1992.

Appleyard, Bryan. *Brave New Worlds: Staying Human in the Genetic Future.* New York: Viking, 1998.

Arditti, Rita, Renate Duelli Klein, and Shelley Minden, eds. *Test-Tube Women: What Future for Motherhood?* London: Pandora, 1984.

Arney, William Ray. *Power and the Profession of Obstetrics.* Chicago: University of Chicago Press, 1982.

Asch, Adrienne. "Prenatal Diagnosis and Selective Abortion: A Challenge to Practice and Policy." *American Journal of Public Health* 89, no. 11 (November 1999): 1649–57.

———. "Why I Haven't Changed My Mind about Prenatal Diagnosis: Reflections and Refinements." In Parens and Asch, *Prenatal Testing and Disability Rights,* pp. 234–58.

Asch, Adrienne, and Michelle Fine, eds. "Moving Disability beyond 'Stigma.' " Special issue, *Journal of Social Issues* 44, no. 1 (Spring 1988).

——. "Shared Dreams: A Left Perspective on Disability Rights and Reproductive Rights." In Fine and Asch, *Women with Disabilities,* pp. 297–305.

Baker, Robert B., Arthur L. Caplan, Linda L. Emanuel, and Stephen R. Latham, eds. *The American Medical Ethics Revolution: How the AMA's Code of Ethics Has Transformed Physicians' Relationships to Patients, Professionals, and Society.* Baltimore: Johns Hopkins University Press, 1999.

Barber, Bernard. *Informed Consent in Medical Therapy and Research.* New Brunswick, N.J.: Rutgers University Press, 1980.

Baruch, Elaine Hoffman, Amadeo F. D'Adamo, Jr., and Joni Seager, eds. *Embryos, Ethics, and Women's Rights: Exploring the New Reproductive Technologies.* New York: Harrington Park, 1988.

Baskin, Yvonne. *The Gene Doctors: Medical Genetics at the Frontier.* New York: William Morrow, 1984.

Beauchamp, Tom L., and LeRoy Walters, eds. *Contemporary Issues in Bioethics.* 6th ed. Belmont, Calif.: Thomson/Wadsworth, 2003.

Becker, Carl L. *The Heavenly City of the Eighteenth-Century Philosophers.* New Haven: Yale University Press, 1932.

Becker, Howard S., ed. *The Other Side: Perspectives on Deviance.* New York: Free Press, 1967.

Beckwith, Jon. "Social and Political Uses of Genetics in the United States: Past and Present." In Lappé and Morison, *Ethical and Scientific Issues,* pp. 46–58.

Begab, Michael J. "The Major Dilemma of Mental Retardation: Shall We Prevent It?" *American Journal of Mental Deficiency* 78, no. 5 (March 1974): 519–29.

Benn, Peter A., Lillian Y. F. Hsu, Ann Carlson, and Hody L. Tannenbaum. "The Centralized Prenatal Genetics Screening Program of New York City III: The First 7,000 cases." *American Journal of Medical Genetics* 20, no. 2 (February 1985): 369–84.

Berger, Edward M., and Bernard M. Gert. "Genetic Disorders and the Ethical Status of Germ-Line Gene Therapy." *Journal of Medicine and Philosophy* 16, no. 6 (December 1991): 667–83.

Bergsma, Daniel, with Marc Lappé, Richard Roblin, and James M. Gustafson, eds. *Ethical, Social and Legal Dimensions of Screening for Human Genetic Disease.* Birth Defects Original Article Series 10, no. 6. New York: Stratton Intercontinental Medical Book Corp., 1974.

Bernal, J. D. *The World, the Flesh and the Devil: An Inquiry into the Future of the Three Enemies of the Rational Soul.* 1929. Reprint, London: Jonathan Cape, 1970.

Bernhardt, Barbara A., Gail Geller, Theresa Doksum, S. M. Larson, D. Roter, and Neil A. Holtzman. "Prenatal Genetic Testing: Content of Discussions between Obstetric Providers and Pregnant Women." *Obstetrics and Gynecology* 91, no. 5, pt. 1 (May 1998): 648–55.

Biesecker, Barbara Bowles, and Lori Hamby. "What Difference the Disability Community Arguments Should Make for the Delivery of Genetic Services." In Parens and Asch, *Prenatal Testing and Disability Rights,* pp. 340–57.

Biesecker, Barbara, Patricia A. Magyari, and Natalie W. Paul, eds. *Religious, Cultural and Ethnic Influences on the Counseling Process.* Part 2 of *Strategies in Genetic Counseling.* Birth Defects Original Article Series 23, no. 6. White Plains, N.Y.: March of Dimes Birth Defects Foundation, 1987.

Biklen, Douglas. "Framed: Print Journalism's Treatment of Disability Issues." In Gartner and Joe, *Images of the Disabled,* pp. 79–95.

Birth Defects Prevention Act of 1998. Public Law 105-68, 1998.

Blatt, Robin J. "To Choose or Refuse Prenatal Testing." *GeneWatch,* January–February 1987, pp. 3–5.

Bogdan, Janet Carlisle. "Childbirth in America, 1650 to 1990." In Apple, *Women, Health and Medicine in America,* chapter 4.

Bogdan, Robert. *Freak Show: Presenting Human Oddities for Amusement and Profit.* Chicago: University of Chicago Press, 1988.

Bogdan, Robert, and Douglas Biklen. "Handicapism." *Social Policy* 7, no. 5 (March–April 1977): 14–19.

Bogdan, Robert, and Steven J. Taylor. *Inside Out: The Social Meaning of Mental Retardation.* Toronto: University of Toronto Press, 1982.

Bondeson, William B., H. Tristram Englehardt, Jr., Stuart F. Spicker, and Daniel Winship, eds. *Abortion and the Status of the Fetus,* Dordrecht, Holland: D. Reidel, 1983.

Bordo, Susan R. "The Body and the Reproduction of Femininity: A Feminist Appropriation of Foucault." In Jaggar and Bordo, *Gender/Body/Knowledge,* pp. 13–33.

———. "Feminism, Postmodernism, and Gender-Scepticism." In Nicholson, *Feminism/Postmodernism,* pp. 133–56.

Borst, Charlotte G. "The Professionalization of Obstetrics: Childbirth Becomes a Medical Specialty." In Apple, *Women, Health and Medicine in America,* pp. 197–216.

Boyle, T. Coraghessan. *The Road to Wellville.* New York: Viking, 1993.

Browner, Carole H., and H. Mabel Preloran. "Male Partners' Role in Latinas' Amniocentesis Decisions." *Journal of Genetic Counseling* 8, no. 2 (April 1999): 85–108.

———. "*Para Sacarse la Espina* (To Get Rid of the Doubt): Mexican Immigrant Women's Amniocentesis Decisions." In Saetnan, Oudshoorn, and Kirejczyk, *Bodies of Technology,* 368–83.

Browner, Carole H., H. Mabel Preloran, and Simon J. Cox. "Ethnicity, Bioethics, and Prenatal Diagnosis: The Amniocentesis Decisions of Mexican-Origin Women and Their Partners." *American Journal of Public Health* 89, no. 11 (November 1999): 1658–66.

Browner, Carole H., Mabel Preloran, and Nancy A. Press. "The Effects of Ethnicity, Education and an Informational Video on Pregnant Women's Knowledge and Decisions about a Prenatal Diagnostic Screening Test." *Patient Education and Counseling* 27, no. 2 (March 1996): 135–46.

Buchanan, Allen E., Dan W. Brock, Norman Daniels, and Daniel Wickler. *From Chance to Choice: Genetics and Justice.* Cambridge: Cambridge University Press, 2000.

Buck v. Bell, 274 U.S. 200 (1927).

Bulger, Roger J., and Victoria P. Rostow, eds. *An Interdisciplinary Review.* Vol. 2 of *Medical Professional Liability and the Delivery of Obstetrical Care.* Washington, D.C.: National Academy of Sciences, 1989.

Burgess, Michael, and Lori d'Agincourt-Canning. "Genetic Testing for Hereditary Disease: Attending to Relational Responsibility." *Journal of Clinical Ethics* 12, no. 4 (Winter 2001): 361–72.

Burke, B. Meredith, and Aliza Kolker. "Directiveness in Prenatal Genetic Counseling." *Women & Health* 22, no. 2 (1994): 31–53.

Callahan, Daniel. "Bioethics, Our Crowd, and Ideology." Part of a symposium: "In Search of the Good Society: The Work of Daniel Callahan." *Hastings Center Report* 26, no. 6 (November–December 1996): 3–4.

———. "The Meaning and Significance of Genetic Disease: Philosophical Perspectives." In Hilton et al., *Ethical Issues in Human Genetics,* pp. 83–90.

Callahan, Joan C., ed. *Reproduction, Ethics, and the Law: Feminist Perspectives.* Bloomington: Indiana University Press, 1995.

Cameron, Paul, Donna Gnadinger Titus, John Kostin, and Marilyn Kostin. "The Life Satisfaction of Nonnormal Persons." *Journal of Consulting and Clinical Psychology* 41, no. 2 (October 1973): 207–14.

Caplan, Arthur L. *Am I My Brother's Keeper? The Ethical Frontiers of Biomedicine.* Bloomington: Indiana University Press, 1997.

———. "Genetic Counseling, Medical Genetics and Theoretical Genetics: An Historical Overview." In Capron et al., *Genetic Counseling,* pp. 21–31.

Capron, Alexander Morgan, Marc Lappé, Robert F. Murray, Jr., Tabitha M. Powledge, Sumner B. Twiss, and Daniel Bergsma, eds. *Genetic Counseling: Facts, Values and Norms.* Birth Defects Original Article Series 15, no. 2. New York: Alan R. Liss, 1979.

Carlson, Dru E., and Lawrence D. Platt. "Ultrasound Detection of Genetic Anomalies." *Journal of Reproductive Medicine* 37, no. 5 (May 1992): 419–27.

Carrel, Alexis. *Man, the Unknown.* 1935. Reprint, New York: MacFadden, 1961.

Casper, Monica J. *The Making of the Unborn Patient: A Social Anatomy of Fetal Surgery.* New Brunswick, N.J.: Rutgers University Press, 1998.

Cassell, Eric J. "The Principles of the Belmont Report Revisited: How Have Respect for Persons, Beneficence, and Justice Been Applied to Clinical Medicine?" *Hastings Center Report* 30, no. 4 (July–August 2000): 12–21.

———. "The Sorcerer's Broom: Medicine's Rampant Technology." *Hastings Center Report* 23, no. 6 (November–December 1993): 32–39.

Chadwick, Ruth F., ed. *Ethics, Reproduction and Genetic Control.* London: Croom Helm, 1987.

Chambers, Robert. *Vestiges of the Natural History of Creation.* London: George Routledge and Sons, 1890.

———. *Vestiges of the Natural History of Creation and Other Evolutionary Writings.* Edited by James A. Secord. Chicago: University of Chicago Press, 1994.

Chambers, Tod. *The Fiction of Bioethics: Cases as Literary Texts.* New York: Routledge, 1999.

Chapman, Audrey R., and Mark S. Frankel, eds. *Designing Our Descendants: The Promises and Perils of Genetic Modifications.* Baltimore: Johns Hopkins University Press, 2003.

Chase, Allan. *The Legacy of Malthus: The Social Costs of the New Scientific Racism.* New York: Alfred A. Knopf, 1977.

Chervenak, Frank A., and Asim Kurjak, eds. *Current Perspectives on the Fetus as a Patient.* New York: Parthenon, 1996.

Chitty, Lyn S. "Ultrasound Screening for Fetal Abnormalities." *Prenatal Diagnosis* 15, no. 13 (December 1995): 1241–57.

Code, Lorraine, Sheila Mullett, and Christine Overall, eds. *Feminist Perspectives: Philosophical Essays on Method and Morals.* Toronto: University of Toronto Press, 1988.

Coleman, Lerita M. "Stigma: An Enigma Demystified." In Davis, *Disability Studies Reader,* pp. 216–31.

Collins, Francis S., Ari Patrinos, Elke Jordan, Aravinda Chakravarti, Raymond Gestelend, and LeRoy Walters. "New Goals for the U.S. Human Genome Project: 1998–2003." *Science* 282, no. 5389 (October 23, 1998): 682–89.

Comte, Auguste. *Auguste Comte and Positivism: The Essential Writings.* Edited by Gertrude Lenzer. 1975. Reprint, Chicago: University of Chicago Press, 1983.

Condorcet, Jean-Antoine-Nicolas de Caritat, Marquis de. *Sketch for a Historical Picture of the Progress of the Human Mind.* Translated by June Barraclough. New York: Noonday, 1955.

"Congenital Malformations Surveillance Report: A Report from the National Birth Defects Prevention Network." *Teratology, The Journal of Abnormal Development* 56, nos. 1–2 (July–August 1997): 115–75.

Corea, Gena. *The Mother Machine: Reproductive Technologies from Artificial Insemination to Artificial Wombs.* New York: Harper & Row, 1985.

Council for Responsible Genetics. "Position Paper on Human Genome Initiative." Boston, Mass.: Council for Responsible Genetics, 1989.

Council on Ethical and Judicial Affairs, American Medical Association. "Ethical Issues Related to Prenatal Genetic Testing." *Archives of Family Medicine* 3, no. 7 (July 1994): 633–42.

Cravens, Hamilton. *The Triumph of Evolution: American Scientists and the Heredity-Environment Controversy, 1900–1941.* Baltimore: Johns Hopkins University Press, 1978.

Damarin, Suzanne K. "Technologies of the Individual: Women and Subjectivity in the Age of Information." In Rothschild, "Technology and Feminism," special issue, *Research in Technology and Philosophy* 13 (1993): 183–98.

Darling, Rosalyn Benjamin, and Jon Darling. *Children Who Are Different: Meeting the Challenge of Birth Defects in Society.* St. Louis: C. V. Mosby, 1982.

Darwin, Charles. *The Descent of Man.* London: John Murray, 1871.

Davenport, Charles Benedict. *Heredity in Relation to Eugenics.* New York: H. Holt, 1911.

Davies, Stanley. *Social Control of the Mentally Deficient.* New York: Thomas Y. Crowell, 1930.

Davis, Lennard J., ed. *The Disability Studies Reader.* New York: Routledge, 1997.

de Beauvoir, Simone. *The Second Sex.* Edited and translated by H. M. Parshley. New York: Alfred A. Knopf, 1953.

Delhanty, J. D., and J. C. Harper. "Pre-implantation Genetic Diagnosis." *Baillière's Best Practices Research: Clinical Obstetrics and Gynaecology* 14, no. 4 (August 2000): 691–708.

Dice, Lee R. "Heredity Clinics, Their Value for Public Service and for Research." *American Journal of Human Genetics* 4, no. 1 (1952): 1–13.

———. "Resources of Mental Ability: How Can the Supply of Superior Ability Be Conserved and Perhaps Increased?" *Eugenics Quarterly* 7, no. 1 (March 1960): 9–22.

DiQuinzio, Patrice, and Iris Marion Young. Introduction to "Feminist Ethics and Social Policy." Special issue, *Hypatia* 10, no. 1 (Winter 1995): 1–7.

Dobzhansky, Theodosius. *Heredity and the Nature of Man.* New York: Harcourt, Brace & World, 1964.

———. *Mankind Evolving.* New Haven: Yale University Press, 1962.

Doksum, Teresa, and Barbara A. Bernhardt. "Population-Based Carrier Screening for Cystic Fibrosis." *Clinical Obstetrics and Gynecology* 39, no. 4 (December 1996): 763–71.

Donchin, Anne. "Autonomy and Interdependence: Quandaries in Genetic Decision Making." In Mackenzie and Stoljar, *Relational Autonomy*, pp. 236–58.

Drugan, Arie, Anne Greb, Mark Paul Johnson, Eric L. Krivchenia, Wendy R. Uhlmann, Kamran S. Moghissi, and Mark I. Evans. "Determinants of Parental Decisions to Abort for Chromosome Abnormalities." *Prenatal Diagnosis* 10, no. 8 (August 1990): 483–90.

Dunn, Rex. "Eugenic Sterilization Statutes: A Constitutional Re-evaluation." *Journal of Family Law* 14, no. 2 (1975): 280–308.

Duster, Troy. *Backdoor to Eugenics.* New York: Routledge, 1990.

Easlea, Brian. *Fathering the Unthinkable: Masculinity, Scientists and the Nuclear Arms Race.* London: Pluto, 1983.

Edwards, R. G., and Jean M. Purdy, eds. *Human Conception in Vitro: Proceedings of the First Bourn Hall Meeting.* London: Academic Press, 1982.

Edwards, R. G., and Patrick Steptoe. *A Matter of Life: The Story of a Medical Breakthrough.* New York: William Morrow, 1980.

Ehrenreich, Barbara, and Deirdre English. *For Her Own Good: 150 Years of the Experts' Advice to Women*. Garden City, N.Y.: Anchor/Doubleday, 1979.

Ekirch, Arthur A., Jr. *The Idea of Progress in America, 1815–1860*. New York: Columbia University Press, 1944.

Elias, Sherman, and George J. Annas. *Reproductive Genetics and the Law*. Chicago: Year Book Medical Publishers, 1987.

ELSI Project Descriptions. NHGRI ELSI Program—1990 to the Present. Bethesda, Md.: Ethical, Legal, and Social Implications Program, Division of Extramural Research, NHGRI, NIH/DOE, 1999.

Ethics Committee, American College of Obstetricians and Gynecologists. "Sterilization of Women Who Are Mentally Handicapped." In Evans et al., *Fetal Diagnosis and Therapy*, 110–13.

Ethics Committee, American Society for Reproductive Medicine. "Preconception Gender Selection for Nonmedical Reasons." *Fertility & Sterility* 75, no. 5 (May 2001): 861–64.

———. "Sex Selection and Preimplantation Genetic Diagnosis." *Fertility & Sterility* 72, no. 4 (October 1999): 595–98.

Evans, Mark I., ed. *Reproductive Risks and Prenatal Diagnosis*. Norwalk, Conn.: Appleton and Lange, 1992.

Evans, Mark I., John C. Fletcher, Alan O. Dixler, and Joseph D. Schulman, eds. *Fetal Diagnosis and Therapy: Science, Ethics and the Law*. Philadelphia: J. B. Lippincott, 1989.

Evans, Mark I., and Mark Paul Johnson. "Prenatal Diagnosis in the '90s: A Symposium." *Journal of Reproductive Medicine* 37, no. 5 (May 1992): 387–88.

Evans, Mark I., Mark P. Johnson, and Kamran S. Moghissi, eds. *Invasive Outpatient Procedures in Reproductive Medicine*. Philadelphia: Lippincott-Raven, 1997.

Evans, Mark I., Michelle A. Sobiecki, Eric L. Krivchenia, Debra A. Duquette, Arie Drugan, Roderick F. Hume, Jr., and Mark P. Johnson. "Parental Decisions to Terminate/Continue following Abnormal Cytogenetic Prenatal Diagnosis: 'What' Is Still More Important Than 'When.'" *American Journal of Medical Genetics* 61, no. 4 (February 1996), 353–55.

Evers-Kiebooms, Gerry, Jean-Jacques Cassiman, Herman Vanden Berghe, and Gery d'Ydevalle, eds. *Genetic Risk, Risk Perception, and Decision Making*. Birth Defects Original Article Series 23, no. 2. New York: Alan R. Liss, 1987.

Evers-Kiebooms, Gerry, Jean-Pierre Fryns, and Jean-Jacques Cassiman, eds. *Psychosocial Aspects of Genetic Counseling*. Birth Defects Original Article Series 28, no. 1. New York: Wiley-Liss, 1992.

Ewigman, Bernard G., James P. Crane, Frederic D. Frigoletto, Michael L. LeFevre, Raymond P. Bain, Donald McNellis, and the RADIUS Study Group. "Effect of Prenatal Ultrasound Screening on Perinatal Outcome." *New England Journal of Medicine* 329, no. 12 (September 16, 1993): 821–27.

Ferguson, Philip M., Alan Gartner, and Dorothy K. Lipsky. "The Experience of Disability in Families: A Synthesis of Research and Parent Narratives." In Parens and Asch, *Prenatal Testing and Disability Rights*, pp. 72–94.

Fiedler, Leslie. *Freaks: Myths and Images of the Secret Self.* 1977. Reprint, New York: Anchor, 1993.

———. "Pity and Fear: Images of the Disabled in Literature and the Popular Arts." In Fiedler, *Tyranny of the Normal,* pp. 33–47. (Originally published 1982.)

———. "The Tyranny of the Normal." In Fiedler, *Tyranny of the Normal,* pp. 147–55. (Originally published 1984.)

———. *Tyranny of the Normal: Essays on Bioethics, Theology & Myth.* Boston: David R. Godine, 1996.

Figlio, Karl. "The Historiography of Scientific Medicine: An Invitation to the Human Sciences." *Comparative Studies in Society and History* 19, no. 3 (1977): 262–86.

Fine, Michelle, and Adrienne Asch, eds. *Women with Disabilities: Essays in Psychology, Culture, and Politics.* Philadelphia: Temple University Press, 1988.

Finger, Anne. "Claiming *All* of Our Bodies: Reproductive Rights and Disability." In Arditti, Klein, and Minden, *Test-Tube Women,* pp. 281–97.

Firestone, Shulamith. *The Dialectic of Sex: The Case for Feminist Revolution.* New York: William Morrow, 1970.

Fischer, Claude S., Michael Hout, Martin Sanchez Jankowski, Samuel R. Lucas, Ann Swidler, and Kim Voss. *Inequality by Design: Cracking the Bell Curve Myth.* Princeton, N.J.: Princeton University Press, 1996.

Fletcher, John C. "Ethical Issues in and beyond Prospective Clinical Trials of Human Gene Therapy." *Journal of Medicine and Philosophy* 10, no. 3 (August 1985): 293–309.

———. "What Are Society's Interests in Human Genetics and Reproductive Technologies?" *Law, Medicine and Health Care* 16, nos. 1–2 (Spring–Summer 1988): 131–37.

Fletcher, John C., and Gerd Richter. "Human Fetal Gene Therapy: Moral and Ethical Questions." *Human Gene Therapy* 7, no. 13 (August 20, 1996): 1605–14.

Fletcher, Joseph. "Ethical Aspects of Genetic Control: Designed Genetic Changes in Man." *New England Journal of Medicine* 285, no. 14 (September 30, 1971): 776–83.

———. "Ethics and Genetic Control." In Monagle and Thomasma, *Medical Ethics,* pp. 3–11.

Foucault, Michel. *Discipline and Punish: The Birth of the Prison.* Translated by Alan Sheridan. New York: Pantheon, 1977.

———. *The History of Sexuality, Volume 1: An Introduction.* Translated by Robert Hurley. New York: Vintage, 1980.

Frankel, Charles. *The Faith of Reason: The Idea of Progress in the French Enlightenment.* New York: Octagon, 1969.

Franklin, Sarah, and Helena Ragoné, eds. *Reproducing Reproduction: Kinship, Power and Technological Innovation.* Philadelphia: University of Pennsylvania Press, 1998.

Fraser, Steven, ed. *The Bell Curve Wars: Race, Intelligence, and the Future of America.* New York: Basic, 1995.

Freidson, Eliot. *Profession of Medicine: A Study of the Sociology of Applied Knowledge.* 1970. Reprint, Chicago: University of Chicago Press, 1988.

Friedmann, Theodore. "Experiment or Treatment? A Personal View." In *Gene Therapy: Fact and Fiction in Biology's New Approach to Disease.* Cold Spring Harbor, N.Y.: Cold Spring Harbor Laboratory, 1983.

——. "The Human Genome Project—Some Implications of Extensive 'Reverse Genetic' Medicine." *American Journal of Human Genetics* 46, no. 3 (March 1990): 407–14.

——. "Prenatal Diagnosis of Genetic Disease." *Scientific American* 225, no. 5 (November 1971): 34–42.

Fuchs, Fritz. "Symposium on Amnio Fluid: Foreword." *Clinical Obstetrics and Gynecology* 9, no. 2 (June 1966): 425–26.

Fuchs, Fritz, and Povl Riis. "Antenatal Sex Determination." Letter. *Nature* 177, no. 4503 (February 18, 1956): 330.

Funk, Robert. "Disability Rights: From Caste to Class in the Context of Civil Rights." In Gartner and Joe, *Images of the Disabled,* pp. 7–30.

Galton, Francis. *Hereditary Genius: An Inquiry into Its Laws and Consequences.* Rev. ed. New York: D. Appleton, 1900.

Gardner, William. "Can Human Genetic Enhancement Be Prohibited?" *Journal of Medicine and Philosophy* 20, no. 1 (February 1995): 65–84.

Gartner, Alan, and Tom Joe, eds. *Images of the Disabled, Disabling Images.* New York: Praeger, 1987.

Garver, Kenneth L., and Bettylee Garver. "The Human Genome Project and Eugenic Concerns." *American Journal of Human Genetics* 54, no. 1 (January 1994): 148–58.

Garver, Kenneth L., Nadene Henderson, and Kay A. LeChien. "New Genetic Technologies: Our Added Responsibilities." *American Journal of Human Genetics* 54, no. 1 (January 1994): 120.

Gearhart, Sally Miller. *The Wanderground.* Watertown, Mass.: Persephone, 1979.

"Genetic Grammar: 'Health,' 'Illness,' and the Human Genome Project." *Hastings Center Report,* special supplement 22, no. 4 (July–August 1992): S1–S20.

Gilligan, Carol. "Hearing the Difference: Theorizing the Connection," In "Feminist Ethics and Social Policy, Part II," special issue, *Hypatia* 10, no. 2 (Spring 1995): 120–27.

——. *In a Different Voice: Psychological Theory and Women's Development.* Cambridge, Mass.: Harvard University Press, 1982.

Gilman, Charlotte Perkins. *Herland.* 1915. Reprint, New York: Pantheon, 1979.

Glass, Bentley. "Human Heredity and Ethical Problems." *Perspectives in Biology and Medicine* 15, no. 2 (Winter 1972): 237–53.

——. *Progress or Catastrophe: The Nature of Biological Science and Its Impact on Human Society.* New York: Praeger, 1985.

Gliedman, John, and William Roth. *The Unexpected Minority: Handicapped Children in America.* New York: Harcourt Brace Jovanovich, 1980.

Goffman, Erving. *Stigma: Notes on the Management of Spoiled Identity.* Englewood Cliffs, N.J.: Prentice Hall, 1963.

Goodfield, June. *Playing God: Genetic Engineering and the Manipulation of Life.* New York: Random House, 1977.

Gould, Carol C., ed. *Beyond Domination: New Perspectives on Women and Philosophy.* Totowa, N.J.: Rowman & Allanheld, 1983.

Gould, Stephen Jay. "Curveball." *New Yorker,* November 28, 1994, pp. 139–49.

———. *Full House: The Spread of Excellence from Plato to Darwin.* New York: Harmony, 1996.

———. *The Mismeasure of Man.* New York: W. W. Norton, 1981.

Graber, Glenn C. "Basic Theories in Medical Ethics." In Monagle and Thomasma, *Medical Ethics,* pp. 462–75.

Granberg, Donald, and Beth Wellman Granberg. "Abortion Attitudes, 1965–1980: Trends and Determinants." *Family Planning Perspectives* 12, no. 5 (September–October 1980): 250–61.

Green, Harvey. *Fit for America: Health, Fitness, Sport, and American Society.* New York: Pantheon, 1986.

Greene, John C. *Darwin and the Modern World View.* Baton Rouge: Louisiana State University Press, 1961.

———. *The Death of Adam: Evolution and Its Impact on Western Thought.* Ames: Iowa State University Press, 1959.

Grimes, David A. "Technology Follies: The Uncritical Acceptance of Medical Innovation." Commentary. *Journal of the American Medical Association* 269, no. 23 (June 16, 1993): 3030–33.

Hahn, Harlan. "Civil Rights for Disabled Americans: The Foundation of a Political Agenda." In Gartner and Joe, *Images of the Disabled,* pp. 181–203.

———. "Paternalism and Public Policy." *Society* 20, no. 3 (March–April 1983): 36–46.

———. "The Politics of Physical Differences: Disability and Discrimination." In Asch and Fine, "Moving Disability beyond 'Stigma,' " special issue, *Journal of Social Issues* 44, no. 1 (Spring 1988): 39–48.

Haldane, J. B. S. *Daedalus, or Science and the Future.* New York: E. P. Dutton, 1924.

———. *Heredity and Politics.* New York: W. W. Norton, 1938.

Hall, Robert E. "Therapeutic Abortion, Sterilization, and Contraception." *American Journal of Obstetrics and Gynecology* 91 (February 15, 1965): 518–32.

Haller, John S., Jr. *Outcasts from Evolution: Scientific Attitudes of Racial Inferiority, 1859–1900.* Urbana: University of Illinois Press, 1971.

Hammons, Helen G., ed. *Heredity Counseling.* New York: Paul B. Hoeber, 1959.

Handyside, Alan H., John G. Lesko, Juan J. Tarin, Robert M. L. Winston, and Mark R. Hughes. "Birth of a Normal Girl after In Vitro Fertilization and Pre-implantation Diagnostic Testing for Cystic Fibrosis." *New England Journal of Medicine* 327, no. 13 (September 24, 1992): 905–909.

Haraway, Donna J. "A Cyborg Manifesto: Science, Technology, and Socialist-Feminism in the Late Twentieth Century." In *Simians, Cyborgs, and Women: The Reinvention of Nature*, pp. 149–81. New York: Routledge, 1991.

Harper, Joyce C. "Preimplantation Diagnosis of Inherited Disease by Embryo Biopsy: An Update of the World Figures." *Journal of Assisted Reproduction and Genetics* 13, no. 2 (February 1996): 90–95.

Harris, Maureen, ed. *Early Diagnosis of Human Genetic Defects: Scientific and Ethical Considerations.* Washington, D.C.: U.S. Government Printing Office, 1972.

Harrison, Beverly Wildung. *Making the Connections: Essays in Feminist Social Ethics.* Edited by Carol S. Robb. Boston: Beacon, 1985.

Harrison, Michael R., Mitchell S. Golbus, and Roy A. Filly. *The Unborn Patient: Prenatal Diagnosis and Treatment.* Orlando, Fla.: Grune & Stratton, 1984.

Hartouni, Valerie. "Containing Women: Reproductive Discourse in the 1980s." In *Technoculture,* ed. Constance Penley and Andrew Ross, pp. 27–56. Minneapolis: University of Minnesota Press, 1991.

Hartz, Louis. *The Liberal Tradition in America.* New York: Harcourt, Brace & World, 1955.

Heffernan, Roy J., and William A. Lynch. "What Is the Status of Therapeutic Abortion in Modern Obstetrics?" *American Journal of Obstetrics and Gynecology* 66, no. 2 (August 1953): 335–45.

Held, Virginia. "The Meshing of Care and Justice." *Hypatia* 10, no. 2 (Spring 1995): 128–32.

Herndon, C. Nash. "III. Heredity Counseling." *Eugenics Quarterly* 2, no. 2 (June 1955): 83–89.

Herrnstein, Richard J., and Charles A. Murray. *The Bell Curve: Intelligence and Class Structure in American Life.* New York: Free Press, 1994.

Hevey, David. *The Creatures Time Forgot: Photography and Disability.* New York: Routledge, 1992.

Hill, Edward C. "Your Morality or Mine? An Inquiry into the Ethics of Human Reproduction." *American Journal of Obstetrics and Gynecology* 154, no. 6 (June 1986): 1173–80.

Hillyer, Barbara. "Women and Disabilities." *NWSA Journal* 4, no. 1 (Spring 1992): 106–14.

Hilton, Bruce, Daniel Callahan, Maureen Harris, Peter Condliffe, and Burton Berkley, eds. *Ethical Issues in Human Genetics: Genetic Counseling and the Use of Genetic Knowledge.* New York: Plenum, 1973.

Hoagland, Hudson, and Ralph W. Burhoe, eds. *Evolution and Man's Progress.* New York: Columbia University Press, 1962.

Holmes, Helen B., Betty B. Hoskins, and Michael Gross, eds. *The Custom-Made Child? Women's Perspectives.* Clifton, N.J.: Humana, 1981.

Holmes, Steven A. "Sweeping U.S. Law to Help Disabled Goes into Effect." *New York Times,* January 27, 1992, pp. A1, A12.

Holtzman, Neil A. *Proceed with Caution: Predicting Genetic Risks in the Recombinant DNA Era.* Baltimore: Johns Hopkins University Press, 1989.

Holtzman, Neil A., and Michael S. Watson, eds. *Promoting Safe and Effective Genetic Testing in the United States: Final Report of the Task Force on Genetic Testing.* Bethesda, Md.: NIH-DOE Working Group on Ethical, Legal, and Social Implications of Human Genome Research, National Human Genome Research Institute, National Institutes of Health, 1997.

Horton, Richard. "Is Homosexuality Inherited?" Review of *The Sexual Brain,* by Simon LeVay, and *The Science of Desire: The Search for the Gay Gene and the Biology of Behavior,* by Dean Hamer and Peter Copeland. *New York Review of Books* 42, no. 12 (July 13, 1995): 36–41.

Howard, Ted, and Jeremy Rifkin. *Who Should Play God? The Artificial Creation of Life and What It Means for the Future of the Human Race.* New York: Dell, 1977.

Howe, Edmund G. "Implementing Feminist Perspectives in Clinical Care." *Journal of Clinical Ethics* 7, no. 1 (Spring 1996): 2–12.

———. "*The Journal of Clinical Ethics:* Genesis, Purposes, and Scope." *Journal of Clinical Ethics* 1, no. 1 (Spring 1990).

———. "The Need for Original Ethical Analyses for Women." *Journal of Clinical Ethics* 10, no. 4 (Winter 1999): 333–40.

Hubbard, Ruth, and Elijah Wald. *Exploding the Gene Myth: How Genetic Information Is Produced and Manipulated by Scientists, Physicians, Employers, Insurance Companies, Educators, and Law Enforcers.* Boston: Beacon, 1993.

Huxley, Julian. *Essays of a Humanist.* New York: Harper & Row, 1964.

———. *Evolution: The Modern Synthesis.* New York: Harper & Brothers, 1942. 3rd edition, New York: Hafner, 1974.

———. "The Evolutionary Vision." In Tax and Callender, *Issues in Evolution,* pp. 249–61.

Imber, Jonathan B. *Abortion and the Private Practice of Medicine.* New Haven: Yale University Press, 1986.

Institute of Medicine. *Professional Liability and the Delivery of Obstetrical Care.* Edited by Victoria P. Rostow and Roger J. Bulger. Washington, D.C.: National Academy Press, 1989.

Jacobs, Allan J. "Liberty, Equality, and Genetic Selection." *The Pharos* 64, no. 1 (Winter 2001): 15–20.

Jacoby, Russell, and Naomi Glauberman, eds. *The Bell Curve Debate: History, Documents, Opinions.* New York: Times Books, 1995.

Jaggar, Alison M. *Feminist Politics and Human Nature.* Totowa, N.J.: Rowman & Allanheld, 1983.

Jaggar, Alison M., and Susan R. Bordo, eds. *Gender/Body/Knowledge: Feminist Reconstructions of Being and Knowing.* New Brunswick, N.J.: Rutgers University Press, 1989.

Jennings, Herbert S. *Prometheus, or Biology and the Advancement of Man.* New York: E. P. Dutton, 1925.

Johnson, Susan R., and Thomas E. Elkins. "Ethical Issues in Prenatal Diagnosis." *Clinical Obstetrics and Gynecology* 31, no. 2 (June 1988): 408–17.

Kaback, Michael M., ed. *Genetic Issues in Pediatric and Obstetric Practice.* Chicago: Year Book Medical Publishers, 1981.

Kaiser Family Foundation. *National Survey of Physicians, Part III: Doctors' Opinions about Their Profession.* March 2002. Highlights and chart pack available on line at http://www.kff.org/kaiserpolls/20020426c-index.cfm, accessed September 20, 2004.

Kaplan, Deborah. "Prenatal Screening and Its Impact on Persons with Disabilities." *Clinical Obstetrics and Gynecology* 36, no. 3 (September 1993): 605–12.

Karp, Laurence E. "Genetic Drift toward the Perfect Child." *American Journal of Medical Genetics* 5, no. 2 (1980): 115–16.

Karson, Evelyn M., William Polvino, and W. French Anderson. "Prospects for Human Gene Therapy." *Journal of Reproductive Medicine* 37, no. 6 (June 1992): 508–14.

Keller, Evelyn Fox. *The Century of the Gene.* Cambridge, Mass.: Harvard University Press, 2000.

Kenen, Regina H. "Genetic Counseling: The Development of a New Interdisciplinary Occupational Field." *Social Science and Medicine* 18, no. 7 (1984): 541–49.

———. "A Look at Prenatal Diagnosis within the Context of Changing Parental and Reproductive Norms." In Holmes, Hoskins, and Gross, *Custom-Made Child,* pp. 67–73.

Kent-First, M. "The Critical and Expanding Role of Genetics in Assisted Reproduction." *Prenatal Diagnosis* 20, no. 7 (July 2000): 536–51.

Kessler, Seymour. "Process Issues in Genetic Counseling." In Evers-Kiebooms, Fryns, and Cassiman, *Psychosocial Aspects of Genetic Counseling,* pp. 1–10.

Kevles, Daniel J. *In the Name of Eugenics: Genetics and the Uses of Human Heredity.* Berkeley: University of California Press, 1985.

Kevles, Daniel J., and Leroy Hood, eds. *The Code of Codes: Scientific and Social Issues in the Human Genome Project.* Cambridge, Mass.: Harvard University Press, 1992.

Keymer, Eduardo, Edna Silva-Inzunza, and Waldeman E. Coutts. "Contribution to the Antenatal Determination of Sex." *American Journal of Obstetrics and Gynecology* 74, no. 5 (November 1957): 1098–1101.

Kincheloe, Joe L., Shirley R. Steinberg, and Aaron D. Gresson III, eds. *Measured Lies: The Bell Curve Examined.* New York: St. Martin's, 1996.

Kitcher, Philip. *The Lives to Come: The Genetic Revolution and Human Possibilities.* New York: Simon & Schuster, 1996.

Klass, Perri. "The Perfect Baby." *New York Times Magazine,* January 29, 1989, pp. 45–46.

Kloepfer, H. Warner. "Genetic Signposts of Preventive Medicine." *Eugenics Quarterly* 7, no. 2 (June 1960): 69–76.

Kocun, C. C., J. T. Harrigan, J. C. Canterino, S. M. Feld, and C. O. Fernandez. "Changing Trends in Patient Decisions concerning Genetic Amniocentesis." *American Journal of Obstetrics and Gynecology* 182, no. 5 (May 2000): 1018–20.

Kolata, Gina. "Cell Error Pinpointed in Down Syndrome." *New York Times,* May 28, 1991, p. C3.

———. "Scientists Brace for Changes in Path of Human Evolution." *New York Times,* March 21, 1998, pp. A1, A12.

Kolker, Aliza, and B. Meredith Burke. *Prenatal Diagnosis: A Sociological Perspective.* Westport, Conn.: Bergin & Garvey, 1994.

Kongstvedt, Peter R., ed. *Essentials of Managed Health Care.* 4th ed. Gaithersberg, Md.: Aspen, 2001.

Kroeger-Mappes, Joy. "The Ethic of Care vis-à-vis the Ethic of Rights: A Problem for Contemporary Moral Theory." *Hypatia* 9, no. 3 (Summer 1994): 108–31.

Kuliev, Anver, Laird Jackson, Ursula Froster, Bruno Brambati, Joe Leigh Simpson, Yury Verlinsky, Norman Ginsburg, Steen Smidt-Jensen, and Haim Zakut. "Chorionic Villus Sampling Safety. Report of World Health Organization/ EURO Meeting in Association with the Seventh International Conference on Early Prenatal Diagnosis of Genetic Diseases, Tel-Aviv, Israel, May 21, 1994." *American Journal of Obstetrics and Gynecology* 174, no. 3 (March 1996): 807–11.

Kuller, Jeffrey A., and Steven A. Laifer. "Contemporary Approaches to Prenatal Diagnosis." *American Family Physician* 52, no. 8 (December 1995): 2277–83.

Kumar, Krishan. *Prophecy and Progress: The Sociology of Industrial and Post-industrial Society.* Harmondsworth: Penguin, 1978.

Kuppermann, Miriam, James D. Goldberg, Robert F. Nease, Jr., and A. Eugene Washington. "Who Should Be Offered Prenatal Diagnosis? The 35-Year-Old Question." *American Journal of Public Health* 89, no. 2 (February 1999): 160–63.

Kurjak, Asim, and Frank A. Chervenak, eds. *The Fetus as a Patient: Advances in Diagnosis and Therapy.* New York: Parthenon, 1994.

Ladd, John. "Physicians and Society: Tribulations of Power and Responsibility." In *The Law-Medicine Relation: A Philosophical Exploration,* ed. S. F. Spicker, J. M. Healey, and H. T. Engelhardt, pp. 33–52. Dordrecht: Reidel, 1981.

LaPlante, Mitchell P. "How Many Americans Have a Disability?" Disabilities Statistics Abstract 5. San Francisco: Disability Statistics Rehabilitation Research and Training Center, June 1992.

Lappé, Marc. "Ethical Issues in Manipulating the Human Germ Line." *Journal of Medicine and Philosophy* 16, no. 6 (December 1991): 621–39.

Lappé, Marc, and Robert S. Morison, eds. *Ethical and Scientific Issues Posed by Human Uses of Molecular Genetics.* New York: New York Academy of Sciences, 1976.

Lasker, Judith N., and Susan Borg. *In Search of Parenthood: Coping with Infertility and High-Tech Conception.* Boston: Beacon, 1987.

Laughlin, Harry H. *Report of the Committee to Study and to Report on the Best Practical Means of Cutting off the Defective Germ-Plasm in the American Population. 1. The Scope of the Committee's Work.* Bulletin No. 10A. Cold Spring Harbor, N.Y.: Eugenics Record Office, February 1914.

Leavitt, Judith Walzer. *Brought to Bed: Childbearing in America, 1750 to 1950.* New York: Oxford University Press, 1986.

Lebacqz, Karen. "The Ghosts Are on the Wall: A Parable for Manipulating Life." In *The Manipulation of Life,* ed. Robert Esbjornson, pp. 22–41. New York: Harper & Row, 1984.

LeGuin, Ursula K. *The Left Hand of Darkness.* New York: Ace, 1969.

Lemonick, Michael D. "Smart Genes?" *Time,* September 13, 1999, pp. 54–62.

Lewontin, R. C., Steven Rose, and Leon J. Kamin. *Not in Our Genes: Biology, Ideology, and Human Nature.* New York: Pantheon, 1984.

Lipkin, Jr., Mack, and Peter T. Rowley, eds. *Genetic Responsibility: On Choosing Our Children's Genes.* New York: Plenum, 1974.

Lippman, Abby. "Prenatal Diagnosis: Reproductive Choice? Reproductive Control?" In Overall, *Future of Human Reproduction,* pp. 182–94.

——. "Prenatal Genetic Testing and Screening: Constructing Needs and Reinforcing Inequities." *American Journal of Law and Medicine* 17, nos. 1–2 (1991): 15–50.

Lippman-Hand, Abby, and F. Clarke Fraser. "Genetic Counseling: Provision and Perception of Information." *American Journal of Medical Genetics* 3, no. 2 (1979): 113–27.

Livneh, Hanoch. "On the Origins of Negative Attitudes toward People with Disabilities." *Rehabilitation Literature* 43, nos. 11–12 (November–December 1982): 338–47.

Lloyd, Genevieve. *The Man of Reason: "Male" and "Female" in Western Philosophy.* Minneapolis: University of Minnesota Press, 1985.

Longmore, Paul K. "Screening Stereotypes: Images of Disabled People in Television and Motion Pictures." In Gartner and Joe, *Images of the Disabled,* pp. 65–78.

Love, Rosaleen. " 'Alice in Eugenics-Land': Feminism and Eugenics in the Scientific Careers of Alice Lee and Ethel Elderton." *Annals of Science* 36, no. 2 (March 1979): 145–58.

Lovejoy, Arthur O. *The Great Chain of Being: A Study of the History of an Idea.* 1936. Reprint, Cambridge, Mass.: Harvard University Press, 1964.

Lublin, Nancy. *Pandora's Box: Feminism Confronts Reproductive Technology.* Lanham, Md.: Rowman & Littlefield, 1998.

Ludmerer, Kenneth M. *Genetics and American Society: A Historical Appraisal.* Baltimore: Johns Hopkins University Press, 1972.

Luker, Kristin. *Abortion and the Politics of Motherhood.* Berkeley: University of California Press, 1984.

Lutz, Jacqueline A., and Hindy J. Shaman. "The Impact of Consumerism on Managed Health Care." In Kongstvedt, *Essentials of Managed Care,* pp. 566–86.

Mackenzie, Catriona, and Natalie Stoljar, eds. *Relational Autonomy: Feminist Perspectives on Autonomy, Agency, and the Social Self.* New York: Oxford University Press, 2000.

MacKenzie, Donald. "Karl Pearson and the Professional Middle Class." *Annals of Science* 36, no. 2 (March 1979): 125–43.

Macklin, M. T. "Medical Genetics: An Essential Part of the Medical Curriculum from the Standpoint of Prevention." *Journal of the Association of American Medical Colleges* 8 (1933): 291–301.

——. "The Need of a Course in Medical Genetics in the Medical Curriculum: A Pivotal Point in the Eugenic Program." In *A Decade of Progress in Eugenics: Scientific Papers of the Third International Congress of Eugenics*, 157–58. American Museum of Natural History, New York, August 21–23, 1932. Baltimore: Williams and Wilkins, 1934.

Macpherson, C. B. *The Political Theory of Possessive Individualism: Hobbes to Locke.* Oxford: Clarendon, 1962.

Mahowald, Mary B. "Sex-Role Stereotypes in Medicine." *Hypatia* 2, no. 2 (Summer 1987): 21–38.

Makowski, E. L., K. A. Prem, and I. H. Kaiser. "Detection of Sex of Fetuses by the Incidence of Sex Chromatin Body in Nuclei of Cells in Amniotic Fluid." *Science* 123, no. 3196 (March 30, 1956): 542–43.

Mansfield, Caroline, Suellen Hopfer, and Theresa M. Marteau. "Termination Rates after Prenatal Diagnosis of Down Syndrome, Spina Bifida, Anencephaly, and Turner and Klinefelter Syndromes: A Systematic Literature Review." *Prenatal Diagnosis* 19, no. 9 (September 1999): 808–12.

Manuel, Frank E. *The Prophets of Paris.* 1962. Reprint, New York: Harper & Row, 1965.

Maranto, Gina. *Quest for Perfection: The Drive to Breed Better Human Beings.* New York: Scribner, 1996.

"Marching toward a Future without Birth Defects." *New York Times Magazine,* supplement, April 2, 1995.

Markens, Susan, Carole H. Browner, and Nancy Press. " 'Because of the Risks': How U.S. Pregnant Women Account for Refusing Prenatal Screening." *Social Science & Medicine* 49, no. 3 (August 1999): 359–69.

Marteau, Theresa, Susan Michie, Harriet Drake, and Martin Bobrow. "Public Attitudes towards the Selection of Desirable Characteristics in Children." *Journal of Medical Genetics* 32, no. 10 (October 1995): 796–98.

Mattingly, Susan S. "The Maternal-Fetal Dyad: Exploring the Two-Patient Obstetric Model." *Hastings Center Report* 22, no. 1 (January–February 1992): 13–18.

Mayr, Ernst. "Comments on Genetic Evolution." In Hoagland and Burhoe, *Evolution and Man's Progress,* pp. 50–51.

McCormick, Richard A. *How Brave a New World? Dilemmas in Bioethics.* Garden City, N.Y.: Doubleday, 1981.

McCusick, Victor A. *Human Genetics.* 2nd ed. Englewood Cliffs, N.J.: Prentice-Hall, 1969.

——. "Mapping and Sequencing the Human Genome." *New England Journal of Medicine* 320, no. 14 (April 6, 1989): 910–15.

McElheny, Victor K. *Watson and DNA: Making a Scientific Revolution.* Cambridge, Mass.: Perseus, 2003.

Meyerson, Lee. "The Social Psychology of Physical Disability: 1948 and 1988." In Asch and Fine, "Moving Disability beyond 'Stigma,'" special issue, *Journal of Social Issues* 44, no. 1 (Spring 1988): 173–88.

Midgely, Mary. *Evolution as a Religion: Strange Hopes and Stranger Fears.* London: Methuen, 1985.

Milunsky, Aubrey. *Choices, Not Chances: An Essential Guide to Your Heredity and Health.* Boston: Little, Brown, 1989.

———. *Choices Not Chances: How to Have the Healthiest Baby You Can.* New York: Simon & Schuster, 1986.

———, ed. *Genetic Disorders and the Fetus: Diagnosis, Prevention, and Treatment.* 2nd ed. New York: Plenum, 1986.

———, ed. *Genetic Disorders and the Fetus: Diagnosis, Prevention, and Treatment.* 3rd ed. Baltimore: Johns Hopkins University Press, 1992.

———, ed. *Genetic Disorders and the Fetus: Diagnosis, Prevention, and Treatment.* 4th ed. Baltimore: Johns Hopkins University Press, 1998.

———. *Heredity and Your Family's Health.* New York: Simon & Schuster, 1987.

———. *How to Have the Healthiest Baby You Can.* Baltimore: Johns Hopkins University Press, 1992.

———. *Know Your Genes.* Boston, Mass.: Houghton Mifflin, 1977.

———. *The Prevention of Genetic Disease and Mental Retardation.* Philadelphia: Saunders, 1975.

Milunsky, Aubrey, and George J. Annas, eds. *Genetics and the Law.* New York: Plenum, 1976.

Mitchison, Naomi. *Solution Three.* 1975. Reprint, New York: Feminist Press, 2002.

Monagle, John F., and David C. Thomasma, eds. *Medical Ethics: A Guide for Health Professionals.* Rockville, Md.: Aspen, 1988.

Morgan, Thomas Hunt. "Chromosomes and Heredity." *American Naturalist* 44, no. 524 (August 1910): 449–96.

Mulkay, Michael. "Changing Minds about Embryo Research." *Public Understanding of Science* 3, no. 2 (April 1994): 195–213.

———. "Embryos in the News." *Public Understanding of Science* 3, no. 1 (January 1994): 33–51.

———. "Rhetorics of Hope and Fear in the Great Embryo Debate." *Social Studies of Science* 23, no. 4 (November 1993): 721–42.

Muller, Hermann J. "The Guidance of Human Evolution." In Tax, *Evolution of Man,* pp. 423–62.

———. "Our Load of Mutations." *American Journal of Human Genetics* 2 (1950): 111–76.

———. *Out of the Night: A Biologist's View of the Future.* 1935. Reprint, New York: Garland, 1984.

Muller, Virginia L. *The Idea of Perfectibility.* Lanham, Md.: University Press of America, 1985.

Mullett, Sheila. "Shifting Perspective: A New Approach to Ethics." In Code, Mullett, and Overall, *Feminist Perspectives,* pp. 109–26.

Murphy, Edmond A., Gary A. Chase, and Alejandro Rodriguez. "Genetic Intervention: Some Social, Psychological, and Philosophical Aspects." In *Genetic Issues in Public Health and Medicine,* ed. Bernice H. Cohen, Abraham M. Lilienfeld, and P. C. Huang, pp. 358–98. Springfield, Ill.: Charles C. Thomas, 1978.

Nadler, Henry L. "Antenatal Detection of Hereditary Disorders." *Pediatrics* 42, no. 6 (December 1968): 912–18.

National Center for Human Genome Research. *Progress Report: Fiscal Years 1991 and 1992.* NIH Publication No. 93-3550. Washington, D.C.: National Institutes of Health, March 1993.

National Center on Birth Defects and Developmental Disabilities. *Birth Defects: Frequently Asked Questions.* National Center on Birth Defects and Developmental Disabilities, Centers for Disease Control, 2002.

National Conference on Race Betterment. *Proceedings of the Third Race Betterment Conference, January 2–6, 1928.* Battle Creek, Mich.: The Race Betterment Foundation, 1928.

National Human Genome Research Institute, National Institutes of Health. "Ethical, Legal and Social Implications of the Human Genome Project." Fact sheet summarizing the final report of the Ethical, Legal and Social Implications (ELSI) Program. December 19, 1996.

——. "International Human Sequencing Consortium Publishes Sequence and Analysis of the Human Genome." Washington, D.C.: National Human Genome Research Institute, National Institutes of Health, February 12, 2001.

——. *A Review and Analysis of the ELSI Research Programs at the National Institutes of Health and the Department of Energy.* ERPEG Final Report. February 10, 2000.

National Research Council. *Mapping and Sequencing the Human Genome.* Washington, D.C.: National Academy Press, 1988.

Neel, James V. "Social and Scientific Priorities in the Use of Genetic Knowledge." In Hilton et al., *Ethical Issues in Human Genetics,* pp. 353–68.

Nicholson, Linda J., ed. *Feminism/Postmodernism.* New York: Routledge, 1990.

Oakley, Ann. *The Captured Womb.* Oxford: Basil Blackwell, 1984.

Oehninger, Sergio, Suheil J. Muasher, and Herbert E. Bevan. "Current Status of Preimplantation Diagnosis." *Journal of Assisted Reproduction and Genetics* 14, no. 2 (February 1997): 72–75.

Olden, Marian S. "Present Status of Sterilization in the United States." *Eugenical News* 31, no. 1 (March 1946): 3–14.

Opitz, J. M. "The American Journal of Medical Genetics—Forward." *American Journal of Medical Genetics* 1, no. 1 (1977): 1–2.

Orenstein, David M., Glenna B. Winnie, and Harold Altman. "Cystic Fibrosis: A 2002 Update." *Journal of Pediatrics* 140, no. 2 (February 2002): 156–64.

Osborn, Frederick. "The Eugenic Hypothesis: Part I: Positive Eugenics." *Eugenical News* 36, no. 2 (June 1951): 19–21.

———. "The Eugenic Hypothesis: Part II: Negative Eugenics." *Eugenical News* 37, no. 1 (March 1952): 6–9.

———. *Preface to Eugenics.* Rev. ed. New York: Harper & Brothers, 1951.

Overall, Christine. *Ethics and Human Reproduction: A Feminist Analysis.* Boston: Allen & Unwin, 1987.

———, ed. *The Future of Human Reproduction.* Toronto: Women's Press, 1989.

Parens, Erik, and Adrienne Asch. "The Disability Rights Critique of Prenatal Genetic Testing: Reflections and Recommendations." In Parens and Asch, *Prenatal Testing and Disability Rights,* pp. 3–43.

———, eds. *Prenatal Testing and Disability Rights.* Washington, D.C.: Georgetown University Press, 2000.

Passmore, John. *The Perfectibility of Man.* New York: Charles Scribner's Sons, 1970.

Paul, Diane B. "Eugenics and the Left." In Paul, *Politics of Heredity,* pp. 11–35.

———. "From Reproductive Responsibility to Reproductive Autonomy." In *Mutating Concepts, Evolving Disciplines: Genetics, Medicine, and Society,* ed. Lisa S. Parker and Rachel A. Ankeny, pp. 87–105. Boston: Kluwer Academic Publishers, 2002.

———. " 'In the Interests of Civilization': Marxist Views of Race and Culture in the Nineteenth Century." *Journal of the History of Ideas* 42, no. 1 (January–March 1981): 115–38.

———. " 'Our Load of Mutations' Revisited." *Journal of the History of Biology* 20, no. 3 (Fall 1987): 321–35,

———. *The Politics of Heredity: Essays on Eugenics, Biomedicine, and the Nature-Nurture Debate.* Albany: State University of New York Press, 1998.

Pearson, Karl. *The Academic Aspect of the Science of National Eugenics.* London: Dulau, 1911.

———. *The Groundwork of Eugenics.* London: Dulau, 1912.

———. *The Scope and Importance to the State of the Science of National Eugenics.* 3rd ed. London: Dulau, 1911.

Pennisi, E. "Human Genome. Reaching Their Goal Early, Sequencing Labs Celebrate." *Science* 300, no. 5618 (April 18, 2003): 409.

"Perfectly Beautiful." *New York Times Magazine,* supplement, March 28, 1993.

Pergament, Eugene, and Morris Fiddler. "Prenatal Gene Therapy: Prospects and Issues." *Prenatal Diagnosis* 15, no. 13 (December 1995): 1303–11.

Petchesky, Rosalind Pollack. "Foetal Images: The Power of Visual Culture in the Politics of Reproduction." In Stanworth, *Reproductive Technologies,* pp. 57–80.

Peters, Ted. *Playing God? Genetic Determinism and Human Freedom.* New York: Routledge, 1997.

Pfeffer, Naomi. *The Stork and the Syringe.* London: Blackwell, 1994.

Physician Characteristics and Distribution in the U.S., 2001–2002 Edition. Chicago: American Medical Association, 2002.

Physician Socioeconomic Statistics, 2000–2002 Edition. Chicago: Center for Health Policy Research, American Medical Association, © 1999.

Piercy, Marge. *Woman on the Edge of Time.* New York: Fawcett Crest, 1976.

Planned Parenthood of Southeastern Pennsylvania v. Casey. 112 S.Ct. 2791 (1992).

President's Commission for the Study of Ethical Problems in Medicine and Biomedical and Behavioral Research. *Screening and Counseling for Genetic Conditions: A Report on the Ethical, Social and Legal Implications of Genetic
Screening, Counseling, and Educational Programs.* Washington, D.C.: U.S.
Government Printing Office, 1983.

Press, Nancy. "Assessing the Expressive Character of Prenatal Testing: The Choices
Made or the Choices Made Available?" In Parens and Asch, *Prenatal Testing
and Disability Rights,* pp. 214–33.

Press, Nancy, and Carole H. Browner. "Collective Silences and Collective Fictions:
How Prenatal Diagnostic Testing Became Part of Routine Prenatal Care." In
Women and Prenatal Testing: Facing the Challenges of Genetic Technology, ed.
Karen H. Rothenberg and Elizabeth J. Thomson, pp. 201–18. Columbus:
Ohio State University Press, 1994.

Press, Nancy, Carole H. Browner, Diem Tran, Christine Morton, and Barbara Le
Master. "Provisional Normalcy and 'Perfect Babies': Pregnant Women's Atti-
tudes toward Disability in the Context of Prenatal Testing." In Franklin and
Ragoné, *Reproducing Reproduction,* pp. 46–65.

"Proceedings of the Heredity Counseling Symposium Held at the New York Academy of Medicine Building. Nov. 1, 1957: Sponsored by the American Eugenics Society." *Eugenics Quarterly* 5, no. 1 (March 1958): 3–62.

Pryde, Peter G., Arie Drugan, Mark P. Johnson, Nelson B. Isada, and Mark I.
Evans. "Prenatal Diagnosis: Choices Women Make about Pursuing Testing
and Acting on Abnormal Results." *Clinical Obstetrics and Gynecology* 36, no. 3
(September 1993) 496–509.

"Public and Private Eugenics." Special issue, *GeneWatch* 12, no. 3 (June 1999).

Rabinow, Paul, ed. *The Foucault Reader.* New York: Pantheon, 1984.

Ralston, Steven J. "Reflections from the Trenches: One Doctor's Encounter with
Disability Rights Arguments." In Parens and Asch, *Prenatal Testing and Disability Rights,* pp. 334–36.

Ramsey, Paul. "Screening: An Ethicist's View." In Hilton et al., *Ethical Issues in
Human Genetics,* pp. 147–60.

Rapp, Rayna. "Chromosomes and Communication: The Discourse of Genetic
Counseling." *Medical Anthropology Quarterly,* n.s. 2, no. 2 (June 1988): 143–
57.

———. "Communicating about the New Reproductive Technologies: Cultural, Interpersonal, and Linguistic Determinants of Understanding." In Rodin and
Collins, *Women and New Reproductive Technologies,* pp. 135–52.

———. "Moral Pioneers: Women, Men and Fetuses on a Frontier of Reproductive
Technology." *Women & Health* 13, nos. 1–2 (1987): 101–16.

———. *Testing Women, Testing the Fetus: The Social Impact of Amniocentesis in
America.* New York: Routledge, 2000.

Reed, Sheldon C. "Down's Syndrome (Mongolism)." *Eugenics Quarterly* 10, no. 3 (September 1963): 139–42.

———. "A Short History of Human Genetics in the USA." *American Journal of Medical Genetics* 3, no. 3 (1979): 282–95.

Reilly, Philip. *The Surgical Solution: A History of Involuntary Sterilization in the U.S.* Baltimore: Johns Hopkins University Press, 1991.

Report of the Joint NIH/DOE Committee to Evaluate the Ethical, Legal, and Social Implications of the Human Genome Project. Bethesda, Md.: National Human Genome Research Institute, National Institutes of Health, December 19, 1996.

Resnik, David. "Debunking the Slippery Slope Argument against Human Germ-Line Gene Therapy." *Journal of Medicine and Philosophy* 19, no. 1 (February 1994): 23–40.

"Review of the Literature: Feminist Approaches to Medical Ethics." *Journal of Clinical Ethics* 5, no. 1 (Spring 1994): 65–85.

"A Revolution at 50. DNA Changed the World. Now What?" Science Times. *New York Times,* section F, February 25, 2003.

Rhoads, George G., Laird G. Jackson, Sarah E. Schlesselman, Felix F. de la Cruz, Robert J. Desnick, Mitchell S. Golbus, David H. Ledbetter, Herbert A. Lubs, Maurice J. Mahoney, Eugene Pergament, Norman A. Ginsberg, James D. Goldberg, John C. Hobbins, Lauren Lynch, Patricia H. Shiono, Ronald J. Wapner, and Julia M. Zachary. "The Safety and Efficacy of Chorionic Villus Sampling for Early Prenatal Diagnosis of Cytogenic Abnormalities." *New England Journal of Medicine* 320, no. 10 (March 9, 1989): 609–17.

Richardson, Stephen A. "Age and Sex Differences in Values toward Physical Handicaps." *Journal of Health and Social Behavior* 11, no. 3 (September 1970): 207–14.

Richardson, Stephen A., Norman Goodman, Albert H. Hastorf, and Sanford M. Dornbusch. "Cultural Uniformity in Reaction to Physical Disabilities." *American Sociological Review* 26 (1961): 241–77.

Rifkin, Jeremy. *The Biotech Century: Harnessing the Gene and Remaking the World.* New York: Jeremy P. Tarcher/Putnam, 1998.

Rifkin, Jeremy, with Nicanor Perlas. *Algeny: A New Word, a New World.* New York: Penguin, 1984.

Rigotti, Francesca. "Biology and Society in the Age of Enlightenment." *Journal of the History of Ideas* 47, no. 2 (April–June 1986): 215–33.

Riis, Povl, and Fritz Fuchs. "Antenatal Determination of Foetal Sex in Prevention of Hereditary Disease." *Lancet* 276, no. 7143 (July 23, 1960): 180–82.

Riordan, J., J. Rommens, B.-S. Kerem, N. Alon, R. Rozmahel, Z. Grzelczak, et al. "Identification of the Cystic Fibrosis Gene: Cloning and Characterization of Complementary DNA." *Science* 245, no. 4922 (September 8, 1989): 1066–73.

Robertson, John. *Children of Choice: Freedom and the New Reproductive Technologies.* Princeton, N.J.: Princeton University Press, 1994.

——. "Embryo Research." *University of Western Ontario Law Review* 24, no. 1 (June 1986): 15–37.

Robinson, Arthur, Bruce G. Bender, and Mary G. Linden. "Decisions following the Intrauterine Diagnosis of Sex Chromosome Aneuploidy." *American Journal of Medical Genetics* 34, no. 4 (December 1989): 552–54.

Robitscher, Jonas, comp. and ed. *Eugenic Sterilization.* Springfield, Ill.: Charles C. Thomas, 1973.

Rodeck, Charles H., ed. *Fetal Diagnosis of Genetic Defects.* Baillière's Clinical Obstetrics and Gynaecology: International Practice and Research 1, no. 3. London: Baillière Tindall, 1987.

Rodin, Judith, and Aila Collins, eds. *Women and New Reproductive Technologies: Medical, Psychosocial, Legal, and Ethical Dilemmas.* Hillsdale, N.J.: Lawrence Erlbaum, 1991.

Rodriguez de Alba, M., P. Palomino, C. Gonzalez-Gonzalez, I. Lorda-Sanchez, M. A. Ibanez, R. Sanz, J. M. Fernandez-Moya, C. Ayuso, J. Diaz-Recasens, and C. Ramos. "Prenatal Diagnosis on Fetal Cells from Maternal Blood: Practical Comparative Evaluation of the First and Second Trimesters." *Prenatal Diagnosis* 21, no. 3 (March 2001): 165–70.

Rose, Hilary. "Dreaming the Future." *Hypatia* 3, no. 1 (1988): 119–38.

——. *Love, Power and Knowledge: Towards a Feminist Transformation of the Sciences.* Bloomington: Indiana University Press, 1995.

Rose, Steven. "DNA and the Goal of Human Perfectibility." *Monthly Review* 38, no. 3 (July–August 1986): 48–60.

Rosenberg, Charles E. "Disease and Social Order in America: Perceptions and Expectations." *Milbank Quarterly* 64, supplement 1 (1986): 34–55.

——. *No Other Gods: On Science and American Social Thought.* Baltimore: Johns Hopkins University Press, 1976. (A revised and expanded edition was published in 1997.)

Rosenkrantz, Barbara Gutmann. "Damaged Goods: The Dilemmas of Responsibility for Risk." *Milbank Memorial Fund Quarterly/Health and Society* 57, no. 1 (Winter 1979): 1–37.

Roter, D. L., G. Geller, B. A. Bernhardt, S. M. Larson, and T. Doksum. "Effects of Obstetrician Gender on Communication and Patient Satisfaction." *Obstetrics and Gynecology* 93, no. 5, pt. 1 (May 1999): 635–41.

Roth, William. "Handicap as a Social Construct." *Society* 20, no. 3 (March–April 1983): 56–61.

Rothman, Barbara Katz. *Genetic Maps and Human Imaginations: The Limits of Science in Understanding Who We Are.* New York: W. W. Norton, 1998.

——. *The Tentative Pregnancy: Prenatal Diagnosis and the Future of Motherhood.* New York: Viking, 1986.

Rothschild, Joan. "Engineering Birth: Toward the Perfectibility of *Man?*" In *Science, Technology, and Social Progress,* ed. Steven L. Goldman, pp. 93–120. Bethlehem, Pa.: Lehigh University Press, 1989.

——. "Engineering the 'Perfect Child': Feminist Responses." In *Against Patri-*

archal Thinking: A Future without Discrimination? ed. Maja Pellikan-Engel, pp. 233–41. Amsterdam: VU University Press, 1992.

——, ed. *Machina Ex Dea: Feminist Perspectives on Technology.* New York: Pergamon, 1983. New York: Teachers College Press, 1992.

——, ed. "Technology and feminism." Special issue, *Research in Technology and Philosophy* 13 (1993).

Ruddick, William. "Can Doctors and Philosophers Work Together?" *Hastings Center Report* 11, no. 2 (April 1981): 12–17.

Ruzek, Sheryl. "Women's Reproductive Rights: The Impact of Technology." In Rodin and Collins, *Women and New Reproductive Technologies,* pp. 65–87.

Sabagh, E., and R. B. Edgerton. "Sterilized Mental Defectives Look at Eugenic Sterilization." *Eugenics Quarterly* 9, no. 4 (December 1962): 213–22.

Saetnan, Ann Rudinow, Nelly Oudshoorn, and Marta Kirejczyk, eds. *Bodies of Technology: Women's Involvement with Reproductive Medicine.* Columbus: Ohio State University Press, 2000.

Safilios-Rothschild, Constantina. *The Sociology and Social Psychology of Disability and Rehabilitation.* New York: Random House, 1970.

Safir, Marilyn, Martha T. Mednick, Dafna Israeli, and Jessie Bernard, eds. *Women's Worlds: From the New Scholarship.* New York: Praeger, 1985.

Salmon, J. W., W. White, and J. Feinglass. "The Futures of Physicians: Agency and Autonomy Reconsidered." *Theoretical Medicine* 11, no. 4 (December 1990): 261–74.

Sandelowski, Margarete, and Linda Corson Jones. " 'Healing Fictions': Stories of Choosing in the Aftermath of the Detection of Fetal Anomalies." *Social Science and Medicine* 42, no. 3 (February 1996): 353–61.

Sarason, Seymour S., and John Doris. *Psychological Problems in Mental Deficiency.* 4th ed. New York: Harper & Row, 1969.

Sawicki, Jana. *Disciplining Foucault: Feminism, Power, and the Body.* New York: Routledge, 1991.

Saxton, Marsha. "Born and Unborn: The Implications of Reproductive Technologies for People with Disabilities." In Arditti, Klein, and Minden, *Test-Tube Women,* pp. 298–312.

——. "Why Members of the Disability Community Oppose Prenatal Diagnosis and Selective Abortion." In Parens and Asch, *Prenatal Testing and Disability Rights,* pp. 147–64.

Schechtman, Kenneth B., Diana L. Gray, Jack D. Baty, and Steven M. Rothman. "Decision-Making for Termination of Pregnancies with Fetal Anomalies: Analysis of 53,000 Pregnancies." *Obstetrics and Gynecology* 99, no. 2 (February 2002): 216–22.

Schulman, Joseph D. "Prenatal Diagnosis of Rare Diseases." In *Frontiers in Rare Disease Research: Proceedings of a Symposium Held in Bethesda, MD, and Washington, DC, May 2 and 3, 1990,* pp. 111–19. Publication 1992—621-953. Washington, D.C.: U.S. Government Printing Office, 1992.

Schulman, Joseph D., Andrew Dorfmann, and Mark I. Evans. "Genetic Aspects of

In Vitro Fertilization." *Annals of the New York Academy of Sciences* 442 (1985): 466–75.

Schulman, Joseph D., and Joe Leigh Simpson, eds. *Genetic Diseases in Pregnancy: Maternal Effects and Fetal Outcome.* New York: Academic Press, 1981.

Schweickart, Patrocinio. "What If . . . Science and Technology in Feminist Utopias." In Rothschild, *Machina Ex Dea,* pp. 198–211.

Schweitzer, Morton D. "What Can the Physician Make of Medical Genetics?" *Eugenical News* 6, no. 2 (May 1941): 31–35.

Scott, Joan W. "Deconstructing Equality-versus-Difference: Or, the Uses of Poststructuralist Theory for Feminism." *Feminist Studies* 14, no. 1 (Spring 1988): 33–45.

Secord, James A. *Victorian Sensation: The Extraordinary Publication, Reception, and Secret Authorship of "Vestiges of the Natural History of Creation."* Chicago: University of Chicago Press, 2001.

Seeds, John W. "The Routine or Screening Obstetrical Ultrasound Examination." *Clinical Obstetrics and Gynecology* 39, no. 4 (December 1996): 814–30.

Shaw, Margery. "Conditional Prospective Rights of the Fetus." *Journal of Legal Medicine* 5, no. 1 (March 1984): 63–116.

———. "Presidential Address. To Be or Not To Be? That Is the Question." *American Journal of Human Genetics* 36, no. 1 (January 1984): 1–9.

Shelley, Mary. *Frankenstein, or The Modern Prometheus.* 1816. Reprint, New York: New American Library, 1965.

Shettles, Landrum B. "Nuclear Morphology of Cells in Human Amniotic Fluid in Relation to Sex of Infant." *American Journal of Obstetrics and Gynecology* 71, no. 4 (April 1956): 834–38.

Siegler, Mark. "Clinical Ethics and Clinical Medicine." *Archives of Internal Medicine* 139, no. 8 (August 1979): 914–15.

Silver, Lee M. *Remaking Eden: Cloning and Beyond in a Brave New World.* New York: Avon, 1997.

Simpson, George Gaylord. *The Meaning of Evolution: A Study of the History of Life and of Its Significance for Man.* 1949. Rev. ed., New Haven: Yale University Press, 1967.

Simpson, Joe Leigh, and Sherman Elias, eds. *Essentials of Prenatal Diagnosis.* New York: Churchill Livingstone, 1993.

Singer, Eleanor. "Public Attitudes toward Genetic Testing." *Population Research and Policy Review* 10 (1991): 235–55.

Sinsheimer, Robert L. "Genetic Engineering and Gene Therapy: Some Implications." In *Genetic Issues in Public Health and Medicine,* ed. Bernice H. Cohen, Abraham M. Lilienfeld, and P. C. Huang, pp. 439–61. Springfield, Ill.: Charles C. Thomas, 1978.

———. "The Prospect of Designed Genetic Change." *American Scientist* 57, no. 1 (Spring 1969): 134–42. Reprinted in Chadwick, *Ethics, Reproduction and Genetic Control,* pp. 136–46.

———. "Prospects for Future Scientific Developments: Ambush or Opportunity." In Hilton et al., *Ethical Issues in Human Genetics*, pp. 341–52.

Skinner v. Oklahoma, 316 U.S. 535 (1942).

Smith, George P. "Genetics, Eugenics, and Public Policy." *Southern Illinois University Law Journal*, 1985, no. 3 (Summer), pp. 435–53.

———. *The New Biology: Law, Ethics, and Biotechnology*. New York: Plenum, 1989.

Spencer, Herbert. *On Social Evolution: Selected Writings*. Edited by J. D. Y. Peel. Chicago: University of Chicago Press, 1972.

Squier, Susan Merrill. *Babies in Bottles: Twentieth-Century Visions of Reproductive Technology*. New Brunswick, N.J.: Rutgers University Press, 1994.

Stafford, Barbara Maria. *Body Criticism: Imaging the Unseen in Enlightenment Art and Medicine*. Cambridge, Mass.: MIT Press, 1991.

Stafford, Barbara M., John La Puma, and David L. Schiedermayer. "One Face of Beauty, One Picture of Health: The Hidden Aesthetic of Medical Practice." *Journal of Medicine and Philosophy* 14, no. 2 (April 1989): 213–30.

Stanworth, Michelle, ed. *Reproductive Technologies: Gender, Motherhood and Medicine*. Minneapolis: University of Minnesota Press, 1987.

Steele, C. Danae, Ronald J. Wapner, J. Bruce Smith, Mark K. Hanes, and Laird G. Jackson. "Prenatal Diagnosis Using Fetal Cells Isolated from Maternal Peripheral Blood: A Review." *Clinical Obstetrics and Gynecology* 39, no. 4 (December 1996): 801–13.

Steinbrook, Robert "In California, Voluntary Mass Prenatal Screening." *Hastings Center Report* 16, no. 5 (October 1986): 5–7.

Stephenson, Sharon R., and David D. Weaver. "Prenatal Diagnosis—A Compilation of Diagnosed Conditions." *American Journal of Obstetrics and Gynecology* 141, no. 3 (October 1981): 319–43.

Stern, Curt. *Principles of Human Genetics*. 2nd ed. San Francisco: W. H. Freeman, 1960.

Tax, Sol, ed. *The Evolution of Man*. Vol. 2 of *Evolution after Darwin: The University of Chicago Centennial*. Chicago: University of Chicago Press, 1960.

Tax, Sol, and Charles Callender, eds. *Issues in Evolution*. Vol. 3 of *Evolution after Darwin: The University of Chicago Centennial*, ed. Sol Tax. Chicago: University of Chicago Press, 1960.

Teggart, Frederick J. *The Idea of Progress: A Collection of Readings*. Rev. ed. with an introduction by George H. Hildebrand. Berkeley: University of California Press, 1949.

Testart, Jacques, and B. Sele. "Towards an Efficient Medical Eugenics: Is the Desirable Always the Feasible?" *Human Reproduction* 10, no. 12 (December 1995): 3086–90.

Thomson, Elizabeth J., and Karen Rothenberg, eds. "Reproductive Genetic Testing: Impact on Women." Supplement to *Fetal Diagnosis and Therapy* 8 (April 1993).

Tocqueville, Alexis de. *Democracy in America*, vol. 2. New York: Vintage, 1945.

"Together We Can Deliver Small Miracles." *New York Times Magazine,* supplement, April 3, 1994.

Tong, Rosemary, ed. "Feminist Approaches to Bioethics." Special section, *Journal of Clinical Ethics* 7, no. 1 (Spring 1996): 13–47; 7, no. 2 (Summer 1996): 150–76; 7, no. 3 (Fall 1996): 228–42; 7, no. 4 (Winter 1996): 315–40.

U.S. Census Bureau. "Americans with Disabilities: 1997." March 1, 2001. Available on line at http://www.census.gov/hhes/www/disable/sipp/disable97.html, accessed September 20, 2004

U.S. Congress, Office of Technology Assessment. *Artificial Insemination: Practice in the United States: Summary of a 1987 Survey.* Background Paper OTA-BP-BA-48. Washington, D.C.: U.S. Government Printing Office, 1988.

———. *Mapping Our Genes: The Genome Projects—How Big, How Fast?* Washington, D.C.: U.S. Government Printing Office, 1988.

Unger, Rhoda Kesler. "Personal Appearance and Social Control." In Safir et al., *Women's Worlds,* pp. 142–51.

Van Doren, Charles. *The Idea of Progress.* New York: Frederick A. Praeger, 1967.

Verlinsky, Yury, ed. Special issue on preimplantation diagnosis. *Journal of Assisted Reproductive Genetics* 13, no. 2 (1996).

Verp, Marion S., Allan T. Bombard, Joe Leigh Simpson, and Sherman Elias. "Parental Decision following Prenatal Diagnosis of Fetal Chromosome Abnormality." *American Journal of Medical Genetics* 29, no. 3 (March 1988): 613–22.

Vogel, Friedrich, and Arno G. Motulsky. *Human Genetics: Problems and Approaches.* 2nd ed. Heidelberg: Springer, 1986.

Wachtell, S. S., L. P. Shulman, and D. Sammons. "Fetal Cells in Maternal Blood." *Clinical Genetics* 59, no. 2 (February 2001): 74–79.

Wagar, W. Warren, ed. *The Idea of Progress since the Renaissance.* New York: John Wiley & Sons, 1969.

Walgate, Robert. "In Vitro Fertilization: French Scientist Makes a Stand." *Nature* 323, no. 6087 (October 2, 1986): 385.

Walters, LeRoy, and Tamar Joy Kahn, eds. Introduction to *Bibliography of Bioethics* 24. Washington, D.C.: Kennedy Institute of Ethics, 1998.

Wapner, Ronald J., and Laird Jackson. "Chorionic Villus Sampling." *Clinical Obstetrics and Gynecology* 31, no. 2 (June 1988): 328–44.

Watson, James D., with Andrew Berry. *DNA: The Secret of Life.* New York: Alfred A. Knopf, 2003.

Watson, James D., and Francis Crick. "Molecular Structure of Nucleic Acids: Structure for Deoxyribose Nucleic Acid." *Nature* 171, no. 4356 (April 25, 1953): 737–38.

Weaver, David D. *Catalog of Prenatally Diagnosed Conditions.* Baltimore: Johns Hopkins University Press, 1989.

———. *Catalog of Prenatally Diagnosed Conditions.* 2nd ed. Baltimore: Johns Hopkins University Press, 1992.

———. *Catalog of Prenatally Diagnosed Conditions*, 3rd ed. With the assistance of Ira K. Brandt. Baltimore: Johns Hopkins University Press, 1999.

———. "A Survey of Prenatally Diagnosed Disorders." *Clinical Obstetrics and Gynecology* 31, no. 2 (June 1988): 253–69.

Webster v. Reproductive Health Services, 109 S.Ct. 3040, 3077–3079 (1989).

Weiss, Joan O. "Genetic Counseling: A Social Worker's View." *Hospital Practice* 18, no. 3 (March 1983): 40E, 40H, 40M, 40P, 40T.

Weissman, Gerald. "Foucault and the Bag Lady." In *The Woods Hole Cantata: Essays on Science and Society*, pp. 26–39. New York: Dodd, Mead, 1985.

Wells, D. Colin. "Social Darwinism." *American Journal of Sociology* 12 (March 1907): 695–716.

Wenger, Barbara L., H. Stephen Kaye, and Mitchell LaPlante. "Disabilities among Children." Disabilities Statistics Abstract 15. San Francisco: Disability Statistics Rehabilitation Research and Training Center, September 1997.

Wertz, Dorothy C., and John C. Fletcher. "Fatal Knowledge? Prenatal Diagnosis and Sex Selection." *Hastings Center Report* 19, no. 3 (May–June 1989): 21–27.

Wertz, Dorothy C., and James R. Sorenson. "Sociologic Implications." In Evans et al., *Fetal Diagnosis and Therapy*, pp. 554–65.

Wertz, Richard W., and Dorothy C. Wertz. *Lying-In: A History of Childbirth in America*. Expanded ed. New Haven: Yale University Press, 1989.

Whitbeck, Caroline. "A Different Reality: Feminist Ontology." In C. Gould, *Beyond Domination*, pp. 64–68

———. "Ethical Issues Raised by the New Reproductive Technologies." In Rodin and Collins, *Women and New Reproductive Technologies*, pp. 49–64.

———. "Fetal Imaging and Fetal Monitoring: Finding the Ethical Issues." In Baruch, D'Adamo, and Seager, *Embryos, Ethics, and Women's Rights*, pp. 47–57.

———. "The Moral Implications of Regarding Women as People: New Perspectives on Pregnancy and Personhood." In Bondeson et al., *Abortion and the Status of the Fetus*, pp. 247–72.

Williams, A. Paul, Karin Dominick Pierre, and Eugene Vayda. "Women in Medicine: Toward a Conceptual Understanding of the Potential for Change." *Journal of the American Medical Women's Association* 48, no. 8 (July–August 1993): 115–21.

Wilson, Philip K, ed. *The Medicalization of Obstetrics: Personnel, Practice, and Instruments*. Vol. 2 of *Childbirth: Changing Ideas and Practices in Britain and America, 1600 to the Present*. Hamden, Conn.: Garland, 1996.

Young, Iris Marion. "Pregnant Embodiment: Subjectivity and Alienation." *Journal of Medicine and Philosophy* 9, no. 1 (February 1984): 45–62.

———. *Throwing Like a Girl and Other Essays in Feminist Philosophy and Social Theory*. Bloomington: Indiana University Press, 1990.

Young, Robert Maxwell. *Mind, Brain and Adaptation in the Nineteenth Century: Cerebral Localization and Its Biological Context from Gall to Ferrier*. Oxford: Clarendon, 1970.

Zaner, Richard M. *Ethics and the Clinical Encounter.* Englewood Cliffs, N.J.: Prentice Hall, 1988.

Zelizer, Viviana A. *Pricing the Priceless Child: The Changing Social Value of Children.* 1985. Reprint, Princeton, N.J.: Princeton University Press, 1994.

Zimmerman, Burke K. "Human Germ-Line Therapy: The Case for Its Development and Use." *Journal of Medicine and Philosophy* 16, no. 6 (December 1991): 593–612.

INDEX

JOAN ROTHSCHILD is professor emerita at the University of Massachusetts Lowell, and research associate at the Center for Human Environments, The Graduate Center, The City University of New York. The author and editor of numerous articles and books, Rothschild was instrumental in establishing the field known as "gender and technology" with the publication of *Machina Ex Dea: Feminist Perspectives on Technology* in 1983. *The Dream of the Perfect Child* is the culmination of almost two decades of research on this topic.